T0313973

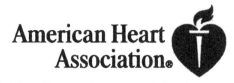

American Heart Association®

Fighting Heart Disease and Stroke

Monograph Series

INTERACTIONS OF BLOOD AND THE PULMONARY CIRCULATION

Previously published in the AHA Monograph Series:

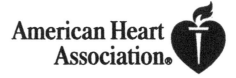

American Heart Association®

Fighting Heart Disease and Stroke

Monograph Series

INTERACTIONS OF BLOOD AND THE PULMONARY CIRCULATION

Edited by

E. Kenneth Weir, MD
Chief of Cardiology
VA Medical Center
Minneapolis;
and Professor of Medicine and Physiology
University of Minnesota
Minneapolis, Minnesota

Helen L. Reeve, PhD
Clinical Research Associate
Guidant Corporation
Minneapolis;
and Assistant Professor of Physiology
University of Minnesota
Minneapolis, Minnesota

John T. Reeves, MD
Professor Emeritus of Medicine
Pediatrics and Family Medicine
University of Colorado
Health Sciences Center
Denver, Colorado

FUTURA

Futura Publishing Company, Inc.
Armonk, NY

Copyright © 2002
Futura Publishing Company, Inc.

Published by
Futura Publishing Company
135 Bedford Road
Armonk, NY 10504
www.futuraco.com

ISBN#: 0–87993–701-7

Every effort has been made to ensure that the information in this book
is as up to date and accurate as possible at the time of publication. However, due to the constant developments in medicine, the author, the ed-
itors, and the publisher cannot accept any legal or any other responsi-
bility for any errors or omissions that may occur.

All rights reserved.

No part of this book may be translated or reproduced in any form without written permission of the publisher.

Preface

"The blood definitely permeates from the right ventricle of the heart through the artery-like vein into the lungs, thence through the vein-like artery into the left auricle, thence again into the left ventricle of the heart. I maintain, firstly, that this can happen; secondly, that it has so happened."[1] In 1628, using these words, William Harvey confirmed the prior observations of Ibn an Nafis, Michael Servetus, and Realdo Columbo that blood circulates through the lungs. To some extent he understood two of the functions of the lung circulation, other than the transfer of blood from the right to the left side of the heart. He thought that during expiration, waste products are blown outwards and "the blood is aired and purified.[1] He also concluded that "nature wished the blood to be filtered through lungs . . ."

In the subsequent period of nearly 400 years, it has been discovered that, in addition to the functions of gas exchange and filtration or sieving, the pulmonary circulation achieves the activation and, in some cases, the inactivation of chemical substances. There are also important interactions between the vascular endothelium and the erythrocytes, leukocytes, and platelets that flow repeatedly through the lungs. The contributors to this book analyze in detail the meaning of these interactions under physiological circumstances and in a variety of diseases and thrombotic states.

Unlike systemic organs, the lungs accept the entire cardiac output. As Harvey writes, they receive blood that "may be cooled, coagulated, and be figuratively worn out" and return to the systemic circulation, "mature, perfected, nutritive blood," "restored to its erstwhile state of perfection."[1] It is interesting to consider the effect of this tide in the affairs of the blood as it flows through the lungs, taking up oxygen and giving up carbon dioxide. What is the significance of the change in redox status that engulfs every cell minute by minute, as illustrated by the change in the status of hemoglobin? We are beginning to think of endothelial cells being swept from their hold and circulating briefly in the blood, perhaps being replaced by other cells, from the bone marrow. Is it possible that leukocytes (monocytes and perhaps neutrophils) not only adhere to an activated endothelium and migrate into the lungs but that some might reenter the blood and carry messages to the marrow, like a bee returning to the hive? The information in this book provides the state of the art on the interaction of the blood and the lungs in terms of adhesion molecules, inflammation, nitric oxide, oxidant stress, sickle cell disease, thrombosis, fibrinolysis, and vascular tone. As Harvey said, "the lungs and the heart contain the storehouse, source and treasury of the blood, and the laboratory in which it is brought to perfection."[1] We now understand some of the secrets of that laboratory.

E. Kenneth Weir, MD
Helen L. Reeve, PhD
John T. Reeves, MD

Reference

1. Harvey, William. *The Circulation of the Blood and Other Writings.* Translated by Kenneth J. Franklin. Introduction by Dr. Andrew Wear. Published by J. M. Dent & Sons, Ltd. London, 1990.

Contributors

William R. Auger, MD   Division of Pulmonary and Critical Care Medicine, University of California, San Diego, La Jolla, California

M. Johan Broekman, PhD   VA New York Harbor Healthcare System and Weill Medical College of Cornell University, New York, New York

Joan H.F. Drosopoulos, PhD   VA New York Harbor Healthcare System and Weill Medical College of Cornell University, New York, New York

Paul Egermayer, MA, MB, ChB   Canterbury Respiratory Research Group, Christchurch School of Medicine, Christchurch, New Zealand

Mary L. Ellsworth, PhD   Departments of Pharmacological and Physiological Science, Saint Louis University School of Medicine, Saint Louis, Missouri

Stephen H. Embury, MD   Department of Medicine, San Francisco General Hospital and the University of California, San Francisco, California

S. Bradley Forlow, PhD   Department of Biomedical Engineering, University of Virginia School of Medicine, Charlottesville, Virginia

Joe G.N. Garcia, MD   Division of Pulmonary and Critical Care Medicine, Johns Hopkins Asthma and Allergy Center, Johns Hopkins University Department of Medicine, Baltimore, Maryland

Richard B. Gayle, III, PhD   Immunex Corporation, Seattle, Washington

Elisabeth Gharehbaghi-Schnell, PhD   Department of Cardiology, and the Ludwig Boltzmann Institute for Cardiovascular Research, Vienna, Austria

Charles A. Hales, MD   Pulmonary and Critical Care Unit, Department of Medicine, Massachusetts General Hospital and Harvard Medical School, Boston, Massachusetts

Johnson Haynes Jr, MD   Pulmonary and Critical Care Division, Departments of Medicine and Physiology, University of South Alabama College of Medicine, Mobile, Alabama

Robert P. Hebbel, MD   Department of Medicine, University of Minnesota, Minneapolis, Minnesota

Cheryl A. Hillery, MD   Medical College of Wisconsin, Associate Investigator, Blood Research Institute, The Blood Center of Southeastern Wisconsin, Milwaukee, Wisconsin

May Ho, MD, MSc   Department of Microbiology and Infectious Diseases and Immunology Research Group, University of Calgary, Calgary, Alberta, Canada

Tadaatsu Imaizumi, MD   Department of Vascular Biology, Institute of Brain Sciences, Hirosaki University School of Medicine, Hirosaki, Japan

Naziba Islam, MS   VA New York Harbor Healthcare System and Weill Medical College of Cornell University, New York, New York

Keri N. Jacobs, BS   Division of Pulmonary and Critical Care Medicine, Johns Hopkins University Department of Medicine, Baltimore, Maryland

Cage Johnson, MD   Department of Medicine, University of Southern California, Keck School of Medicine, Los Angeles, California

Vijay K. Kalra, PhD   Departments of Biochemistry and Molecular Biology, University of Southern California, Keck School of Medicine, Los Angeles, California

Peter A. Lane, MD   Colorado Sickle Cell Treatment and Research Center, University of Colorado School of Medicine, Denver, Colorado

Irene M. Lang, MD   Department of Cardiology, and the Ludwig Boltzmann Institute for Cardiovascular Research, Vienna, Austria

Klaus Ley, MD   Department of Biomedical Engineering, University of Virginia School of Medicine, Charlottesville, Virginia

Andrew J. Lonigro, MD   Departments of Pharmacological and Physiological Science and Internal Medicine, Saint Louis University School of Medicine, Saint Louis, Missouri

Charles R. Maliszewski, PhD   Immunex Corporation, Seattle, Washington

Aaron J. Marcus, MD   Hematology/Medical Oncology, VA New York Harbor Healthcare System and Weill Medical College of Cornell University, New York, New York

Neil M. Matsui, PhD   Department of Pediatrics, San Francisco General Hospital and the University of California; Northern California Comprehensive Sickle Cell Center, San Francisco, California

Thomas M. McIntyre, PhD   Departments of Internal Medicine and Pathology, and the Program in Human Molecular Biology and Genetics, University of Utah School of Medicine, Salt Lake City, Utah

Boniface Obiako, MS   Pulmonary and Critical Care Division, Departments of Medicine and Physiology, University of South Alabama College of Medicine, Mobile, Alabama

Leslie V. Parise, PhD   Department of Pharmacology, Center for Thrombosis and Hemostasis, Lineberger Comprehensive Cancer Center, University of North Carolina at Chapel Hill, Chapel Hill, North Carolina

Andrew J. Peacock, MPhil, MD, FRCP   Scottish Pulmonary Vascular Unit, Western Infirmary, Glasgow, Scotland

Irina Petrache, MD   Division of Pulmonary and Critical Care Medicine, Johns Hopkins University Department of Medicine, Baltimore, Maryland

David J. Pinsky, MD   Departments of Surgery, Medicine, and Physiology and Cellular Biophysics, College of Physicians and Surgeons of Columbia University, New York, New York

Stephen M. Prescott, MD   Departments of Internal Medicine and Oncologic Sciences, The Huntsman Cancer Institute, University of Utah School of Medicine, Salt Lake City, Utah

Deborah A. Quinn, MD   Pulmonary and Critical Care Unit, Department of Medicine, Massachusetts General Hospital and Harvard Medical School, Boston, Massachusetts

Guy L. Reed, MD   Cardiovascular Biology Laboratory, Harvard School of Public Health, Boston; and Massachusetts General Hospital, Boston, Massachusetts

Helen L. Reeve, PhD   Guidant Corporation, Minneapolis; and Department of Physiology, University of Minnesota, Minneapolis, Minnesota

John T. Reeves, MD   Pediatrics and Family Medicine, University of Colorado Health Sciences Center, Denver, Colorado

C. Edward Rose, MD   Department of Medicine, Division of Pulmonary and Critical Care Medicine, University of Virginia School of Medicine, Charlottesville, Virginia

Suresh Selvaraj, PhD   Departments of Biochemistry and Molecular Biology, University of Southern California, Keck School of Medicine, Los Angeles, California

Randy S. Sprague, MD   Departments of Pharmacological and Physiological Science and Internal Medicine, Saint Louis University School of Medicine, Saint Louis, Missouri

Alan H. Stephenson, PhD   Departments of Pharmacological and Physiological Science, Saint Louis University School of Medicine, Saint Louis, Missouri

David M. Stern, MD   Departments of Surgery, Medicine, and Physiology and Cellular Biophysics, College of Physicians and Surgeons of Columbia University, New York, New York

Matthew K. Topham, MD   Department of Internal Medicine, The Huntsman Cancer Institute, University of Utah School of Medicine, Salt Lake City, Utah

G. Ian Town, MD, FRCP   Canterbury Respiratory Research Group, Christchurch School of Medicine, Christchurch, New Zealand

Stephan F. Van Eeden, MD, PhD, FRCP   University of British Columbia, Pulmonary Research Laboratory, St. Paul's Hospital, Vancouver, B.C., Canada

Wiltz W. Wagner, Jr., PhD   Departments of Physiology, Biophysics, and Pediatrics, Indiana University School of Medicine, Indianapolis, Indiana

John V. Weil, MD   Department of Cardiology, University of Colorado Health Sciences Center, Denver, Colorado

E. Kenneth Weir, MD   VA Medical Center, Minneapolis; and Departments of Medicine and Physiology, University of Minnesota, Minneapolis, Minnesota

Carolyn H. Welsh, MD   Denver Veterans Affairs Medical Center, Division of Pulmonary Sciences and Critical Care Medicine, Department of Medicine, University of Colorado Health Sciences Center, Denver, Colorado

Timothy M. Wick, PhD   School of Chemical Engineering, Georgia Institute of Technology, Atlanta, Georgia

Shi Fang Yan, MD   Departments of Surgery, Medicine, and Physiology and Cellular Biophysics, College of Physicians and Surgeons of Columbia University, New York, New York

Guy A. Zimmerman, MD   Department of Internal Medicine, and the Program in Human Molecular Biology and Genetics. University of Utah School of Medicine, Salt Lake City, Utah

Contents

xiii

SECTION III. Platelets

SECTION IV. Leukocytes

SECTION V. Thrombosis

Section I

Introduction

The Development of Concepts of the Interaction of Blood and the Pulmonary Circulation

Deborah A. Quinn, MD, and
Charles A. Hales, MD

Introduction

This book focuses on the interaction of blood with the pulmonary vessels. Discovery of receptors for neutrophils, platelets, and red cells, especially sickle cells, on the pulmonary vascular endothelium has greatly advanced our understanding of acute chest syndrome and pulmonary hypertension in patients with sickle cell anemia and of thromboembolic hypertension and acute respiratory distress syndrome.[1–6] There are other sections of this book that explain the interaction with the endothelium of sickle cells, platelets, leukocytes, and the clotting cascade in the genesis of lung injury and hypertension. This chapter will address an additional area in which the circulation interacts perhaps injuriously with the lung, which is endothelial cell stress injury as may occur when pulmonary artery pressures rise in the lung due to vasoconstriction or occlusion of part of the vascular tree. We will first present a case that highlights the complexity of the interaction.

In 1983, C.A.H. was asked to discuss a case of pulmonary hypertension for the *New England Journal of Medicine*.[7] The patient was a 40-year-old black woman with sickle cell hemoglobin C anemia. She was in excellent health and had been dancing with her husband the day before her admission to the hospital with an intracranial hemorrhage. She became febrile and hypotensive in spite of large volumes of fluid. A Swan-Ganz

From: Weir EK, Reeve HL, Reeves JT (eds). *Interactions of Blood and the Pulmonary Circulation*. Armonk, NY: Futura Publishing Company, Inc.; ©2002.

line was placed, which showed a pulmonary artery pressure of 78/40 mm Hg and a pulmonary capillary wedge pressure of 5 mm Hg. Her chest x-ray showed prominence of the main pulmonary artery with loss of definition of the small pulmonary vessels. Lung perfusion scan revealed multiple areas of decreased perfusion in the right mid-lung field posterolaterally and at the right base with no corresponding chest x-ray abnormality. A Doppler study of the legs showed no evidence of deep vein thrombosis in either leg. She underwent clipping of an aneurysm of her left ophthalmic artery and of the right anterior communicating artery. Further work-up of her pulmonary hypertension was deferred at the family's request pending any recovery of her neurological status.

Four months later she developed the abrupt onset of dyspnea and pleuritic pain over the left chest. No friction rub was heard but she now had a right ventricular heave and marked accentuation of the pulmonic component of the second heart sound. Pulmonary angiography revealed multiple small filling defects in the right lower lobe but none on the left. Most of these defects had dye surrounding them and were thus thought more likely embolic than thrombotic. Her pulmonary artery pressure had risen to 95/50 mm Hg. She died shortly thereafter and her autopsy revealed right ventricular hypertrophy and no evidence of deep venous thrombosis in the legs or pelvis. Several clots 1–3 mm in diameter were found peripherally in the lung. Microscopic exam of these clots showed recannulization and evidence of active organization with strands of fibroblasts. The most common vascular finding was subtotal occlusion of muscular arteries between 0.3 and 1 mm in diameter with concentric cellular intimal proliferation, leaving a small central lumen (Figure 1). Plexiform-like lesions were also found, although it was not possible to be certain these were not recannalizing clots. Dr. Eugene Mark, the lung pathologist, felt this pattern of concentric occlusion was most atypical for organizing pulmonary emboli, in which the fibrous cushion resulting from organization of thrombus or embolus is asymmetrical, leaving an eccentric rather than a concentric lumen.

Concentric hypertrophy of the intima of small muscular arteries seen in this case is similar to that described in other autopsy reports on pulmonary hypertension in hemoglobin S or SC disease,[8,9] although eccentric hypertrophy is perhaps more common.[10] In this case vascular occlusion by thromboembolic disease and activation of the clotting system surely played a role in the pulmonary hypertension but there was also perhaps activation of another system that caused the pathology in the small muscular vessels. Speculation about sickle cell diseases has been that the cause of the concentric intimal proliferation is due either to endothelial wall shear stress caused by the more rigid sickle cells or to the blood pressure in those vessels that are still patent, having escaped thromboembolic obliteration.[7]

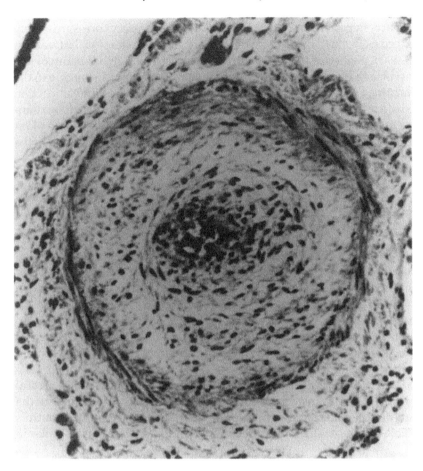

Figure 1. Small muscular pulmonary artery almost occluded by concentric cellular intimal proliferation (×256) from a patient with sickle cell disease.

There is a striking similarity in the microscopic picture of these small arteries to those seen in patients with primary pulmonary hypertension, liver disease, dietetic drug use, or cardiac left-to-right shunts.[7,11–16] There is an increase in thickness of the intima by a variable increase in the intima of endothelial cells, fibroblasts, and smooth muscle cells, and in extracellular matrix. There is an increase in smooth muscle cells and a distal extension of smooth muscle cells in the media as well, similar to what occurs in chronic hypoxic pulmonary hypertension. Rarely in hypoxic pulmonary hypertension, there is also intimal proliferation but much less commonly than in other forms of hypertension. Are these intimal changes primary to the initiating pulmonary hypertension process or are they at least in part secondary to the magnitude of the developing pulmonary hypertension? The mean pulmonary artery pressure rarely exceeds 45 mm Hg in hypoxic pulmonary hypertension but can be 50–100% higher in the other forms of hypertension. How many of the vascular changes in nonhypoxic pulmonary hypertension are due to the initiating process and how many are secondary, representing a reaction to increasing pressure and flow within the pulmonary circulation, damage to the endothelium, or activation of the clotting cascade? Several investigators have explored this phenomenon both in the normal and in the remodeling pulmonary circulation responding to another stress.

Pressure and Flow in the Hypoxic Remodeling Lung

Rabinovitch et al. did a classic study in 1979 in which they banded the left pulmonary artery of rats being exposed to chronic 10% O_2 environment.[17] This allowed them to examine the effect of a decrease in flow and pressure on hypoxic pulmonary vessel remodeling in the left lung and an increase in flow and pressure in the right. They demonstrated that in the banded pulmonary artery the pressure distal to the band increased only from 10 to 12 mm Hg during chronic hypoxia compared to the nonbanded artery which rose to a mean of 40 mm Hg. The banded pulmonary artery showed significantly less increase in medial thickness in muscular arteries and less distal extension of the media into peripheral arteries compared to the nonbanded hypoxic controls (Table 1). Loss of small precapillary and capillary vessels was similar in

Table 1

Normoxic and Hypoxic Rats (10% O_2 × 2 weeks) with Banded Left Lung

		Band + Air	Hypoxia	Band + Hypoxia
Mean PAP (nl = 18 mm Hg)		23 mm Hg	34 mm Hg	40 mm Hg
Post band left		10 mm Hg		12 mm Hg
Smooth muscle extension	(R)	+	+ +	+ + +
	(L)	+	+ +	+
Wall thickness	(R)	+	+ +	+ +
	(L)	+	+ +	+
Arterial concentration	(R)	−	--	--
	(L)	−	--	--
Neointima		0	0	0

From Rabinovitch et al., *Circ Res* 1983, with permission.

hypoxic banded and nonbanded vessels, suggesting hypoxia per se caused this remodeling. We and others have shown that endothelial cells can release growth factors such as PDGF in response to hypoxia (Figure 2) so a mechanism has been proposed that could account for direct remodeling of small vessels in response to hypoxia.[13,14] However, blood pressure or flow within the hypoxic remodeling vessels amplified the pulmonary vascular remodeling in small pulmonary arteries. In the distal pulmonary arteries in the right nonbanded lung that had a doubling of flow, there was no change in the thickness of the media compared to hypoxic nonbanded controls but there was greater distal extension of the muscle. This lung primarily had increased flow as the mean pulmonary artery pressure of 40 mm Hg was only mildly higher than the 34 mm Hg seen in the nonbanded but hypoxic rat ($P<0.05$). No intimal proliferation occurred in these rats but again their pressure elevation was modest. Systolic and diastolic pressures were not given

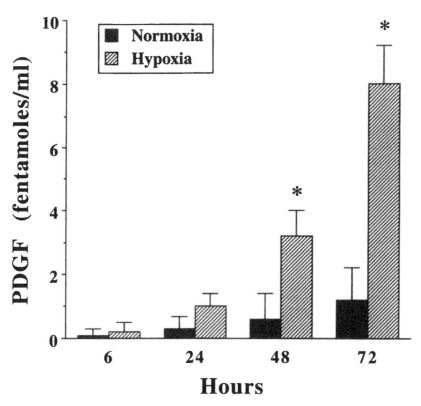

Figure 2. Platelet-derived growth factor (PDGF) released from bovine pulmonary artery endothelial cells grown in 3% O_2. * = $P<.05$ from all earlier values.

and thus an estimate of pulsatility cannot be made. Thus this study demonstrated that pulmonary artery flow and pressure are important in the vascular remodeling of the media in chronic hypoxia. There is a hint that pressure may be more important than flow in causing thickening of the media while flow has a larger role in extension of a muscular media more peripherally.

Pressure and Flow in Monocrotaline-Induced Pulmonary Vascular Remodeling

Okada et al. also have shown an important role for pulmonary artery flow and pressure in amplifying vascular remodeling following injection of monocrotaline.[18,19] Monocrotaline produces modest pulmonary hypertension in rats that is due primarily to an increase in medial thickness akin to what occurs in chronic hypoxia. They have also shown, as have many others, that performing a pneumonectomy with a resulting doubling of blood flow to the remaining lung produces only a modest rise in pulmonary artery pressure and little change in vascular remodeling, at least in the short term (Table 2). However, when the monocrotaline is given to the rats and then a pneumonectomy performed to increase flow and vascular pressure in the remaining lung, there is a dramatic increase in vascular remodeling, especially of the intima. In this model the pulmonary pressure rises to a systolic pressure of 79 with a mean pulmonary artery pressure of 47 mm Hg. Thus increased vascular pressure or flow can clearly augment pulmonary artery remodeling in monocrotaline-induced pulmonary hypertension, especially by creating intimal thickening.

Table 2

Monocrotaline (MONO) and Pneumonectomy (PNEUM)

	SHAM	PNEUM	MONO	PNEUM+MONO
Systolic PAP mm Hg	37		37	79
Mean PAP mm Hg	14	25	26	47
Wall thickness	0	?	+ +	+ +
Neointima	0	0	0	+ + +

From Tanaka et al., *JCI* 1996, with permission. ? = not reported.

Subclavian Anastamosis and
Pulmonary Hypertension

Can increased pulmonary blood flow and/or pressure produce vascular remodeling on their own? Multiple investigations have shown that pneumonectomy alone is not sufficient to induce remodeling acutely, although some species do develop medial thickening when followed for many months to years.[20,21] In this model, blood flow to the lung is doubled but resting pulmonary artery pressure is only slightly elevated initially.

Several investigators have anastomosed the subclavian artery directly to the main pulmonary artery without producing pulmonary vascular remodeling.[22 23] Ferguson et al. anastomosed the subclavian artery to the main pulmonary artery and even after a pneumonectomy were un-

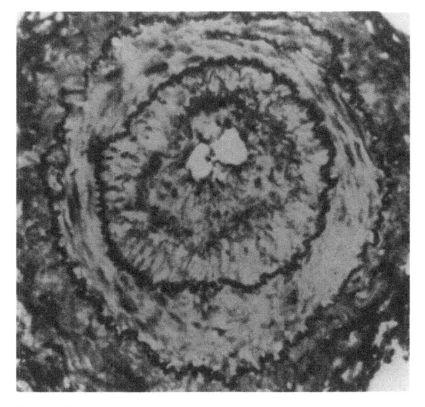

Figure 3. Photomicrograph of pulmonary arteriole from a dog with subclavian artery anastomosed to the left lower lobe pulmonary artery for 6 months (200 μ x 180). Verhoeff's and van Gieson's stains. Each of the 3 coats is greatly thickened and the lumen is nearly obliterated by the intima.

able to induce pulmonary vascular remodeling. They then tried direct anastomosis of the subclavian artery into the left upper or the left lower lobe pulmonary artery.[22] Three out of 4 animals with anastomosis to the left upper lobe died within 12 days with the lung showing pulmonary edema. The surviving animal had severe remodeling of the adventitia, media, and intima. In the dogs with anastomosis to the left lower lobe lobar artery, all survived; 7 of 21 had medial thickening and 6 of those also had moderate to severe concentric intimal thickening (Figure 3). The investigators could not reproduce this remodeling if the subclavian artery went to the main pulmonary artery before going to the lobar artery, even if other lobar arteries were excluded, making blood flow equivalent in the 2 models of lobar perfusion. They hypothesized that the lack of remodeling was because of loss of pulsatility due to buffering by the elasticity of the main pulmonary artery. They did not pursue this, however, and only reported mean pulmonary artery pressures, which were lower with an intervening main pulmonary artery. Dammon et al. also anastomosed the subclavian artery into the left upper lobe pulmonary artery, producing severe remodeling of the adventitia, media, and intima.[24] They did measure post-anastomosis cyclic pulmonary artery pressures and found them to be 18 mm Hg in the post-anastomotic lobar artery compared to 11 mm Hg in the main pulmonary artery. The 11-mm Hg control value is after ligation of the left upper lobe artery and may be slightly higher than in an animal with no intervention involving the pulmonary artery. Thus in their model, post-anastomotic pulmonary artery pressures were systemic (60–90 mm Hg) and pulse pressure was widened.

Heart Disease and Pulmonary Hypertension in Humans

Chronic mitral stenosis produces marked pulmonary hypertension with medial smooth muscle cell proliferation, smooth muscle cell distal extension, as well as intimal proliferation in both veins and arteries.[11] Of note is that 56% of these pulmonary arteries show concentric hypertrophy, which is similar to that found in most cases of advanced primary pulmonary hypertension.[11,13,15] The mitral lung thus clearly suggests that pulmonary artery pressure and not flow can induce concentric intimal thickening. Atrial septal defects, which primarily produce increased flow and not pressure in the pulmonary arteries, do produce vascular remodeling in 10–18%, which may have intimal thickening but this does not occur usually until the third or fourth decade.[25,26] Ventricular septal defects in humans produce pulmonary hypertension that is greater than in ASD, although early on this is primarily a flow insult except in very large defects. The pulmonary vessels of these patients do develop medial hypertrophy and concentric intimal thickening, often in the first decade. This flow and pressure insult, however, occurs at an early age; many investigators have found that in animal models, it predisposes to greater remodeling of the pulmonary vessels in response to several kinds of stress.[27] Interestingly, even in large ventricular septal defects of >0.5 cm/m², in which pulmonary artery pressure usually increases as well as flow, there is a bi-model distribution of pulmonary vascular resistance, with about half developing a severe increase in pulmonary vascular resistance (>12 μ/m²) with an Eisenmenger physiology, but in the rest there is only a mild increase in pulmonary vascular resistance of 3 or <3 μ/m².[28] Just as in sickle cell disease, where 10–40% of patients develop pulmonary hypertension,[29,30] there seem to be some patients who are either genetically predisposed to develop pulmonary hypertension or suffer a second environmental insult. The finding of monoclonality of endothelial cells in primary pulmonary hypertension and in anorexigenic pulmonary hypertension is intriguing and could represent such a genetic predisposition.[31] However, it leaves us looking for other predisposing factors in other nonmonoclonal pulmonary hypertensions such as right-to-left shunts and portal hypertension.

Mechanisms by Which Increased Pulmonary Artery Pressure and Flow Can Induce Pulmonary Vascular Remodeling

Waters has shown that increased shear stress caused by increased flow past lung microvascular endothelial cells grown on microbeads will increase extravascular leak.[32] In the upper lobar to subclavian anastomosis model, early pulmonary edema is a prominent part of the pathology, preceding the vascular remodeling.[22] Rabinovitch's group has demonstrated that endogenous vascular elastase plays a crucial role in the development of monocrotaline and chronic hypoxia-induced pulmonary hypertension in rats.[33,34] This enzyme's activation, however, depends on exposure to circulating serum factors. Thus stretch or shear stress on the microvascular bed could allow leakage of the serum products and initiate remodeling just as the inflammatory reaction of monocrotaline to increase permeability in the endothelium allows pulmonary vascular remodeling to occur in monocrotaline-induced pulmonary hypertension.

An alternative hypothesis is that shear stress or stretch of pulmonary endothelial cells directly activates them to produce growth factors or mediators of inflammation or to stop the production of factors that normally control smooth muscle or endothelial cell proliferation. Multiple factors have been shown to increase or decrease in systemic endothelial cells[35–38] undergoing shear stress (Table 3). Some of these are also known to occur in pulmonary artery endothelial cells, as well as several other changes[39–43] (Table 4). Certainly shear stress has the potential to contribute to pulmonary vascular remodeling in the hypertensive lung. There has been a lot of interest in ventilator-induced lung injury in which stretch of the whole lung induces release of multiple cytokines and mediators of inflammation. Increasing endothelial cell stretch also develops in the pulmonary hypertensive lung as the right ventricle struggles to maintain cardiac output by increasing ejection pressure, producing a higher mean pulmonary artery pressure but also a widened pulse pressure.

Cell stretch has been shown to cause cell hypertrophy and to alter DNA synthesis, gene expression, and protein production. The effect of stretch has been studied both in cultured cells and in isolated pulmonary arteries. Stretch of lung epithelial cells,[44] airway smooth muscle cells,[45] and pulmonary artery smooth muscle cells[46] increases DNA synthesis. In pulmonary fibroblasts exposed to cyclic stretch, mRNA expression of calcyclin, a calcium-binding protein associated with cell proliferation, is upregulated.[47] Mechanical strain of vascular smooth muscle cells induces release of fibroblast growth factor II.[48] In cardiomyocytes, cell stretch causes autocrine release of angiotensin II, a growth factor for cardiac tissue.[49] Constant stretch of whole pulmonary arteries for 4 days caused hypertrophy and hyperplasia of pulmonary artery smooth muscle cells and fibroblasts.[50] Little is understood about how cells sense external load and transduce these signals to regulate gene expression and cell function.

A group of intracellular messengers that is activated by mechanical cell stretch and fluid shear stress is the mitogen-activated protein kinases (MAPKs).[51–53] The MAPKs include the growth factor-responsive MAPKs, extracellular signal-regulated kinases, ERK 1/2, and the stress-responsive MAPKs, stress-activated protein kinase (SAPK, also known as Jun kinase), and p38.[54] These protein kinases act as signal transduction path-

---

Table 3

Shear Stress Systemic Endothelial Cells

↑ Intracellular Ca^{++}
↑ ERK 1/2
↑ Activating protein 1
↑ PDGF
↑ TGF-β
↓ Endothelin
↑ eNos

Table 4

Shear Stress Pulmonary Artery Endothelial Cells

↑ ACE Activity
↓ ACE chronically (18 hours)
↑ EDRF
↑ NOS synthase
↑ K channel
↑ Intracellular Ca
↑ PGI$_2$

ways which, when activated, result in changes in gene expression. The postulated effects of the stress-responsive MAPKs include induction of c-Jun, adhesion molecules, IL-1β, and TNF-α. In rats, blocking SAPK activation inhibited pressure overload-induced cardiac hypertrophy.[55] Platelet-derived growth factor and epidermal growth factor stimulate growth through activation of ERK 1/2.[56] Thus stretch activates pathways that can promote cell proliferation.

The patterns of stretch activation of MAPKs appear to depend on the cell type. Stretch-induced MAPK activation has been found in cardiomyocytes,[53] cardiac fibroblasts,[51] and vascular smooth muscle cells.[52] In cardiomyocytes and vascular smooth muscle cells, ERK 1/2, p38, and SAPK are activated by cell stretch. In A549 cells and type II-like alveolar epithelial cells, we found cyclic stretch resulted in activation of SAPK, but not p38 or ERK 1/2. This suggests that stretch-induced activation of the MAPKs is cell-specific. Likewise, the processes that are regulated by these kinases may differ. In A549 cells, we have found that stretch-induced IL-8 production is dependent on SAPK activation. In neutrophils[57] and vascular endothelial cells,[58] release of IL-8 is dependent on p38 activation.

We have studied the effects of cyclic stretch on human type II-like alveolar epithelial cells, or A549 cells,[59,60] and on pulmonary endothelial cells.[61] We used a cell stretch device that produces uniform biaxial strain.[62] Strain is a measure of cell stretch, expressed as the percent of the change in cell length to the resting cell length. By adjusting the cams, we can make the silastic membrane with the cells growing on its surface provide a 5% strain or a 15% strain, thus mimicking low stretch as might normally occur in the normal lung vessels or high stretch as might occur in the hypertensive lung. We exposed A549 cells and bovine and human endothelial cells to cyclic stretch at 20 cycles/minute at 5% and 15% strain for 2 hours. We found that 15% cyclic stretch induced SAPK activation, IL-8 protein production, and IL-8 mRNA expression more than did 5% stretch. We do not know the upstream kinase pathway in endothelial cells, but in A549 cells, inhibition of SAPK activity by transfection with the dominant negative mutant to SEK, the kinase upstream activator of SAPK, blocks IL-8 mRNA expression and attenuates IL-8 protein expression. Whether the SAPK pathway is also the activator of IL-8 production in endothelial cells will await further study. Nevertheless, SAPK is clearly activated in cyclically stretched endothelial cells and more so with greater stretch.

SAPK activation has been associated with apoptosis in some but not most systems and has also been implicated in cardiac cell hypertrophy.[63] We do not know what the significance of SAPK activation is in remodeling lung vessels, but it could potentially modulate or augment multiple aspects of vascular remodeling, especially as the disease progresses, producing greater cell stretch. Gupta et al. have shown that vascular endothelial growth factor (VEGF) protects static endothelial cells against noxious insults such as serum starvation by downregulating SAPK activation and upregulating MAPK in human microdermal endothelial cells.[64] It is intriguing in view of Voelkel et al.'s demonstration that blockade of the VEGF receptor promotes uncontrolled endothelial cell proliferation. Perhaps endothelial cells undergoing greater cyclic stretch, as occurs in advancing pulmonary hypertension, would increase their SAPK activity and resist VEGF's protective effect, allowing endothelial cell proliferation.

Conclusion

In conclusion, there seems to be good evidence that moderate pulmonary artery pressure and flow can magnify pulmonary vascular remodeling, at least in animals. More severe pulmonary artery pressures in humans and animals can produce not only medial but also intimal thickening. Of note is that in humans and in animals, these changes, especially of the intima, are quite variable, likely reflecting the need for a second insult or a genetic predisposition to induce the injury. Cyclic stretch of pulmonary artery endothelial cells activates SAPK and this potentially can modulate or augment pulmonary vascular remodeling, especially as it becomes advanced. Cyclic stretch adds a new variable to be accounted for in in vitro studies of pulmonary hypertension.

References

1. Hebbel RP. Clinical implications of basic research: Blockade of adhesion of sickle cells to endothelium by monoclonal antibodies. *N Engl J Med* 2000;342(25):1910–1912.

2. Hebbel RP. Prospectives series: Cell adhesion in vascular biology. Adhesive interactions of sickle erythrocytes with endothelium. *J Clin Invest* 1997;99(11):2561–2564.
3. Van Schravendijk M, Handunnetti SM, Barnwell JW, et al. Normal human erythrocytes express DC36, an adhesion molecule of monocytes, platelets, and endothelial cells. *Blood* 1992;80(8):2105–2114.
4. Chaouat A, Weitenblum E, Higenbottom T. The role of thrombosis in severe pulmonary hypertension. *Eur Respir J* 1996; 9(2):356–363.
5. Brittain HA, Eckman JR, Wick TM. Sickle erythrocyte adherence to large vessel and microvascular endothelium under physiologic flow is qualitatively different. *J Lab Clin Med* 1992;120:538–545.
6. Walzog B, Gaehtgens P. Adhesion molecules: The path to a new understanding of acute inflammation. *News Physiol Sci* 2000;15:107–113.
7. Hales CA, Mark EJ. Case 52: Pulmonary hypertension associated with abnormal hemoglobin: Case records of the Massachusetts General Hospital. *N Engl J Med* 1983; 309(26):1627–1636.
8. Yater WM, Hansmann GH. Sickle-cell anemia: a new cause of cor pulmonale: Report of two cases with numerous disseminated occlusions of the small pulmonary arteries. *Am J Med Sci* 1936;191:474–484.
9. Song J. *Pathology of Sickle Cell Disease.* Springfield, Ill: Charles C. Thomas; 1971.
10. Spencer H. *Pathology of the Lung.* Oxford, NY: Pergamon Press; 1984:598.
11. Chazova I, Loyd JE, Zhdanov VS, et al. Pulmonary artery adventitial changes and venous involvement in primary pulmonary hypertension. *Am J Pathol* 1995;146(2):389–397.
12. Palevsky HI, Schloo BL, Pietra GG, et al. Primary pulmonary hypertension: Vascular structure, morphometry, and responsiveness to vasodilator agents. *Circulation* 1989;80(5):1207–1221.
13. Pietra GG, Edwards WD, Kay JM, et al. Histopathology of primary pulmonary hypertension: A quality and quantitative study of pulmonary blood vessels from 58 patients in the National Heart, Lung, and Blood Institute, Primary Pulmonary Hypertension Registry. *Circulation* 1989;80(5):1198–1206.
14. Lebrec D, Capron JP, Dhumeaux D, et al. Pulmonary hypertension complicating portal hypertension. *Am Rev Respir Dis* 1979;120(4):849–856.
15. Chazova I, Robbins I, Loyd J, et al. Venous and arterial changes in pulmonary veno-occlusive disease, mitral stenosis and fibrosing mediastinitis. *Eur Respir J* 2000;15(1):116–122.
16. Wagenvoort CA. Open lung biopsies in congenital heart disease for evaluation of pulmonary vascular disease: Predictive value with regard to corrective operability. *Histopathology* 1985;9(4):417–436.
17. Rabinovitch M, Konstam MA, Gamble WJ, et al. Changes in pulmonary blood flow affect vascular response to chronic hypoxia in rats. *Circ Res* 1983;(52):432–441.
18. Tanaka Y, Schuster DP, Davis EC, et al. The role of vascular injury and hemodynamics in rat pulmonary artery remodeling. *J Clin Invest* 1996;98(2):434–442.
19. Okada K, Tanaka Y, Bernstein M, et al. Pulmonary hemodynamics modify the rat pulmonary artery response to injury: A neointimal model of pulmonary hypertension. *Am J Pathol* 1997;151(4):1019–1025.
20. Rudolph AM, et al. Effects of pneumonectomy on pulmonary circulation in adult and young animals. *Circ Res* 1961;9:856–861.
21. Davies P, et al. Structured changes in the canine lung and pulmonary arteries after pneumonectomy. *J Applied Physiol* 1982;53:859–864.

22. Ferguson DJ, Varco RL. The relation of blood pressure and flow to the development and regression of experimentally induced pulmonary arteriosclerosis. *Circ Res* 1955;3:152–158.
23. Rendas A, Lennox S, Reid L. Aorta-pulmonary shunts in growing pigs: Functional and structural assessment of the changes in the pulmonary circulation. *J Thorac Cardio Surg* 1979;77(1):109–118.
24. Dammon JF, Baker JP, Muller WH. Pulmonary vascular changes induced by experimentally produced pulmonary arterial hypertension. *Surg Gynecol Obstet* 1959;105:16–26.
25. Besterman E. Atrial septal defect with pulmonary hypertension. *Br Heart J* 961;23:587–598.
26. John-Sutton M, Tajik A, McGoon D. Atrial septal defect in patients age 60 or older: Operative and long-term postoperative follow-up. *Circulation* 1981;64:402–409.
27. Stenmark K, et al. Severe pulmonary hypertension and arterial adventitial changes in newborn calves at 4300M. *Am J Physiol* 1987;62:821–830.
28. Gheen KM, Reeves JT. Effect of size of ventricular septal defect and age on pulmonary hemodynamics at sea level. *Am J Cardiol* 1995;75:66–70.
29. Moser KM, Luchsinger PC, Katz S. Pulmonary and cardiac function in sickle cell lung disease: Preliminary report. *Dis Chest* 1960; 37:637–648.
30. Haupt HM, Moore GW, Bauer TW, et al. The lung in sickle cell disease. *Chest* 1982;81(3):332–337.
31. Lee SD, Shroyer KR, Markham NE, et al. Monoclonal endothelial cell proliferation is present in primary not secondary pulmonary hypertension. *J Clin Invest* 1998;101(5):927–934.
32. Waters CM. Flow-induced modulation of the permeability of endothelial cells cultured on microcarrier beads. *J Cell Physiol* 1996;168(2):403–411.
33. Cowan KN, Heilbut A, Humpl T, et al. Complete reversal of fatal pulmonary hypertension in rats by serine elastase inhibitor. *Nat Med* 2000;6(6):698–702.
34. Cowan KN, Jones PL, Rabinovitch M. Elastase and matrix metalloproteinase inhibitors induce regression and tenascin-C antisense prevents progression of vascular disease. *J Clin Invest* 2000;105(1):21–34.
35. Mo M, Eskin SG, Schilling WP. Flow-induced changes in Ca^{2+} signaling of vascular endothelial cells: Effect of shear stress and ATP. *Am J Physiol* 1991;260(5 pt 2):H1698–1707.
36. Buga GM, Gold ME, Fukuto JM, et al. Shear stress-induced release of nitric oxide from endothelial cells grown on beads. *Hypertension* 1991;17(2):187–193.
37. Akimoto S, Mitsumata M, Sasaguri T, Yoshida Y. Laminar shear stress inhibits vascular endothelial cell proliferation by inducing cyclin-dependent kinase inhibitor p21[Sdi1/Cip1/Waf1]. *Circ Res* 2000;86:185–190.
38. Ishida T, Takahashi M, Corson MA, et al. Fluid shear stress-mediated signal transduction: How do endothelial cells transduce mechanical force into biological responses? *Ann NY Acad Sci* 12–24.
39. Schilling WP, Mo M, Eskin SG. Effect of shear stress on cytosolic Ca^{2+} of calf pulmonary artery endothelial cells. *Exp Cell Res* 1992;198(1):31–35.
40. Alevriadou BR, Eskin SG, McIntire LV, et al. Effect of shear stress on 86Rb+ efflux from calf pulmonary artery endothelial cells. *Ann Biomed Eng* 1993;21(1):1–7.
41. Hakim TS. Flow-induced release of EDRF in the pulmonary vasculature: Site of release and action. *Am J Physiol* 1994;267(1 pt 2):H363–369.
42. Rieder MJ, Carmona R, Krieger JE, et al. Suppression of angiotensin-

converting enzyme expression and activity by shear stress. *Circ Res* 1997;80 (3):312–319.

43. VanGrondelle A, Worthen GS, Ellis D, et al. Altering hydrodynamic variables influences PG12 production in isolated lungs and endothelial cells. *J Appl Physiol* 1984;57(2):388–395.

44. Liu M, Xu J, Tanswell A, Post M. Stretch-induced growth-promoting activities stimulate fetal rat lung epithelial cell proliferation. *Exp Lung Res* 1993;19:505–517.

45. Smith PG, Moreno R, Ikebe M. Strain increases airway smooth muscle contractile and cytoskeletal proteins in vitro. *Am J Physiol* 1997;157:615–624.

46. Kulik TJ, Alvarado SP. Effects of stretch on growth and collagen synthesis in cultured rat and lamb pulmonary artery smooth muscle cells. *J Cell Physiol* 1993;157:615–624.

47. Breen EC, Fu Z, Normand H. Calcyclin gene expression is increased by mechanical strain in fibroblasts and lung. *Cell Mol Biol* 1999;21:746–752.

48. Cheng GC, Briggs WH, Gerson DS, et al. Mechanical strain tightly controls fibroblast growth factor-2 release from cultured human vascular smooth muscle cells. *Circ Res* 1997;80:28–36.

49. Sadoshima J, Xu Y, Slayter HS, et al. Autocrine release of angiotensin II mediates stretch-induced hypertrophy of cardiac myocytes in vitro. *Cell* 1993;75:977–984.

50. Kolpakov V, Rekhter M, Gordon D, et al. Effect of mechanical forces on growth and matrix protein synthesis in the in vitro pulmonary artery. *Circ Res* 1995;77:823–831.

51. MacKenna DA, Dolfi F, Voufri K, et al. Extracellular signal-regulated kinase and c-Jun NH$_2$-terminal kinase activation by mechanical stretch is integrin-dependent and matrix-specific in rat cardiac fibroblasts. *J Clin Invest* 1998;101:301–310.

52. Li C, Hu Y, Mayr M, et al. Cyclic strain stress-induced mitogen-activated protein kinase (MAPK) phosphatase 1 expression in vascular smooth muscle cells is regulated by Ras/Rac-MAPK pathways. *J Biol Chem* 1999;274: 25273–25280.

53. Seko Y, Seko N, Takahashi K, et al. Pulsatile stretch activates mitogen-activated protein kinase (MAPK) family members and focal adhesion kinase (pl25^{FAK}) in cultured rat cardiac myocytes. *Biochem Biophys Res Comm* 199;259:8–14.

54. Force T, Polombo CM, Avruch JA, et al. Stress-activated protein kinases in cardiovascular diseases. *Circ Res* 1996;78:947–953.

55. Choukroun G, Hajjar R, Fry S, et al. Regulation of cardiac hypertrophy in vivo by the stress-activated protein kinases/c-Jun NH$_2$-terminal kinases. *J Clin Invest* 1999;104:391–398.

56. Cooper JA, Bowen-Pope F, Raines R, et al. Similar effects of platelet-derived growth factor and epidermal growth factor on the phosphorylation of tyrosine in cellular proteins. *Cell* 1982;31:263–273.

57. Shapiro L, Dinarello, CA. Osmotic regulation of cytokine synthesis in vitro. *Proc Natl Acad Sci USA* 1995;92:12230–12234.

58. Hashimoto K, Matsumoto Y, Gon Y, et al. Mitogen-activated protein kinase regulates IL-8 expression in human pulmonary vascular endothelial cells. *Eur Respir J* 1999;13:1357–1364.

59. Quinn DA, Choukroun G, Tager A, et al. Stress-activated protein kinase regulation of stretch-induced IL-8 production in an in vitro model of ventilator-induced lung injury. *Circulation* 1998;98:1–64.

60. Makkinje A, Quinn DA, Chen A, et al. Gene 33/Mig-6: A transcriptionally inducible adapter protein that binds GTP-Cdc42 and activates SAPK/JNK. *J Biol Chem* 2000;23:17838–17847.

61. Matyal R, Hales CA, Quinn DA. Stretch-induced IL-8 production in human pulmonary artery endothelial cells. *Am J Crit Care Med* 2000;161: A417.

62. Schaffer JL, Rizen M, L'Italien GJ, et al. Device for the application of a dynamic biaxially uniform and isotropic strain to a flexible cell culture membrane. *J Orthop Res* 1994;12:709–719.

63. Tibbles LA, Woodgett JR. The stress-activated protein kinase pathways. Review article. *CMLS* 1999;55:1230–1254.

64. Gupta, K, Kshirsagar S, Li W, et al. VEGF prevents apoptosis of human microvascular endothelial cells via opposing effects on MAPK/ERK and SAPK/JNK signaling. *Exp Cell Res* 1999;247:495–504.

Section II

Erythrocytes

Chapter 2

The Endothelium in Sickle Cell Disease

Robert P. Hebbel, MD

Introduction

The vascular wall endothelium contributes in many ways to vascular physiology and disease pathobiology.[1] The endothelial cell comprises the interface between tissue and blood, thereby providing a physical barrier and an ideal biocompatible surface. It displays a host of adhesion molecules for blood cells and proteins. It contributes separately to the physiology of hemostasis and inflammation and links them by residing at their interface. It helps control the delicate balance between procoagulant and anticoagulant properties of blood and vessel wall. It controls vascular tone by elaborating several vasoconstricting and vasodilating substances. Most importantly, the endothelial cell is highly responsive to a great variety of biological stimulants. Examples of agents that cause the endothelial cell to modify its complement of surface molecules include histamine, thrombin, interleukins, hypoxia, endotoxin, oxidants, tissue necrosis factor, and growth factors.

Each of these physiological functions of the vascular endothelial cell can be implicated, at least theoretically, in the vascular pathobiology of sickle cell disease. This chapter will emphasize 3 aspects of the endothelial biology of this disease that are intimately related: adhesion biology, endothelial activation, and reperfusion injury physiology as a possible activating factor.

Supported by the National Institutes of Health (HL30160, HL55552).

From: Weir EK, Reeve HL, Reeves JT (eds). *Interactions of Blood and the Pulmonary Circulation*. Armonk, NY: Futura Publishing Company, Inc.; ©2002.

Adhesion Biology: Red Blood Cells

Sickle red blood cells (RBC), even when oxygenated, are abnormally adherent to endothelial cells. This has been shown under a variety of experimental conditions in vitro,[2,3] as well as in sickle transgenic mice in vivo.[4] In aggregate, the many investigations of RBC/endothelial interaction argue that this abnormal adhesion event comprises a trigger of vaso-occlusion in sickle cell disease. Specifically, data support the concept that vaso-occlusion is a 2-step event, with RBC adhesion com-

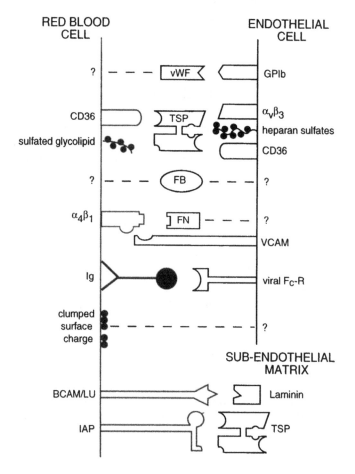

Figure 1. Mechanisms of RBC adhesion to endothelial cells. Mechanisms supported by the literature are shown for interaction of red cells (left) with endothelial cells (right). Ig = immunoglobulin; BCAM/LU = basal cell adhesion molecule, Lutheran; IAP = integrin-associated peptide; GP= glycoprotein; VCAM = vascular cell adhesion molecule; TSP = thrombospondin; FB = fibrinogen; FN = fibronectin; vWF = von Willebrand factor.

prising an initiating phase that is followed by a propagation phase caused by upstream log-jamming with poorly deformable and sickling RBC.[5-7] Therefore, there is considerable interest in the mechanisms that underlie RBC interaction with endothelium.

Not surprisingly, diverse mechanisms are reported to underlie the abnormal adhesion of sickle RBC to endothelium. Many, but not all, involve identified adhesion receptors and/or adhesogenic plasma proteins (Figure 1). The author favors thrombospondin as the likely major adhesogen involved, but this is arguable and other candidates are possible. Reasonably strong data also support roles for von Willebrand factor and for endothelial VCAM. All known RBC adhesion mechanisms were initially identified in vitro, but few have been specifically documented in vivo. One recent study of human sickle RBC infused into the rat showed that blood flow was markedly improved by antibodies that block $\alpha_V\beta_3$,[8] one of the endothelial receptors for thrombospondin. Whether this particular observation can be directly extrapolated to humans, however, is debatable.[9] Other chapters in this book add new information on RBC adhesion mechanisms and perhaps shed light on some of the extant controversies.

Contemplation of antiadhesive therapies for sickle cell disease raises a fundamental question: what is the most important RBC adhesion mechanism in vivo? The author's opinion is that there is likely no single answer to this question. Rather, it seems entirely plausible that the relevant adhesion mechanism might differ from patient to patient, from organ to organ, or even from time to time in the individual patient. Furthermore, it seems probable that multiple adhesion mechanisms would be involved at any one time. Therefore, it seems most likely that effective therapeutics based on this phenomenon will have to provide a general antiadhesive approach (a "vascular lubricant"), rather than one highly specific to a particular mechanism.

Adhesion Biology: White Blood Cells

The adhesion biology of sickle cell disease almost certainly also involves white blood cells (WBC). The nature of WBC interaction with endothelium is well known.[1,10] For granulocytes, this involves the initial rolling of WBC on endothelium, if the latter is sufficiently activated to express selectins, and this can be followed by firm adhesion if endothelium is activated to express CAMs (cell adhesion molecules) and granulocytes are activated to express integrin CD11b/CD18. Monocyte adhesion involves VCAM on activated endothelium.

Several observations suggest that WBC may be important in sickle cell disease. There is a positive relationship between leukocytosis and mortality.[11] A strong predictor of a beneficial clinical response to therapy with hydroxyurea is the consequent lowering of the white count.[12] For all the elegant studies on RBC stiffness and stickiness as impediments to optimal microvascular blood flow, it may be noted that the white cell is larger, stiffer, and stickier than red cells. It is easy to imagine that abnormal enhancement of WBC/endothelial cell interaction would lead to delayed flow and, therefore, sickling and vaso-occlusion. Supporting the likelihood that this is actually relevant to sickle vascular pathobiology, published studies have demonstrated that both granulocytes and monocytes are elevated in number[13] and abnormally activated[14–16] in sickle patients (Figure 2).

It will be argued below that the endothelium is in a chronically activated state in patients with sickle cell disease. Thus, the well-known paradigm of inflammation, with its activating and injuring consequences for the endothelium, is likely to be relevant to the vascular pathobiology of

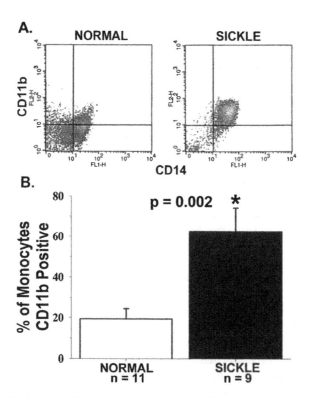

Figure 2. Monocyte activation in sickle patients. The top panels show typical flow cytometry analysis of normal and sickle monocytes for the monocyte marker CD14 (horizontal) and the activation marker CD11b (vertical). The group data comparing 11 normal patients with 9 sickle patients are shown at the bottom. Reproduced with permission from *Blood*.[16]

sickle cell disease. Conversely, potential therapeutic opportunities may be found in interruption of WBC/endothelial interaction or, alternatively, in the cell-activating events that are proximate to WBC adhesion.

Reperfusion Injury Physiology

We have hypothesized that reperfusion injury physiology is a fundamental, endothelial-activating aspect of sickle cell disease vascular pathobiology.[17,18] The reperfusion injury paradigm has been validated in a variety of vascular occlusive states[19-21] and seems likely to be relevant to sickle vaso-occlusion as well. The basic concept of reperfusion injury is that damage from a vascular occlusion occurs not only from the obstruction itself but also, and possibly mostly, to the events that accompany resolution of an occlusion. Among the biochemical changes that occur due to the low oxygen tension during occlusion are catabolism of ATP to hypoxanthine and conversion of xanthine dehydrogenase (XD) to xanthine oxidase (XO). In the presence of oxygen, XO generates superoxide when it catalyzes the conversion of xanthine or hypoxanthine to uric acid. Therefore, restitution of oxygen supply is accompanied by generation of superoxide and, ultimately, the highly damaging hydroxyl radical. Other mechanisms can also contribute to the oxygen radical generation that typifies all models of reperfusion injury (e.g., oxidants derived from activated inflammatory cells or mitochondrial metabolism). This proximate radical generation has several consequences, including peroxidation of membrane lipids and activation of nuclear factor -κB (NF-κB). The latter is also activated by elabo-

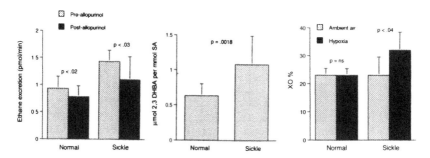

Figure 3. Biochemical footprints of reperfusion injury in the sickle mouse. At ambient air, sickle mice show greater excretion of ethane in expired gas, a marker of total body lipid peroxidation (left panel) and greater hydroxylation of salicylate, a marker of hydroxyl radical formation (middle). After a period of hypoxia, sickle animals show exaggerated increase in ethane formation (left) and conversion of XD to XO (right panel). Reproduced with permission from *Blood.*[17]

ration of cytokines during this process. The transcription factor NF-κB promotes expression of various proinflammatory molecules such as

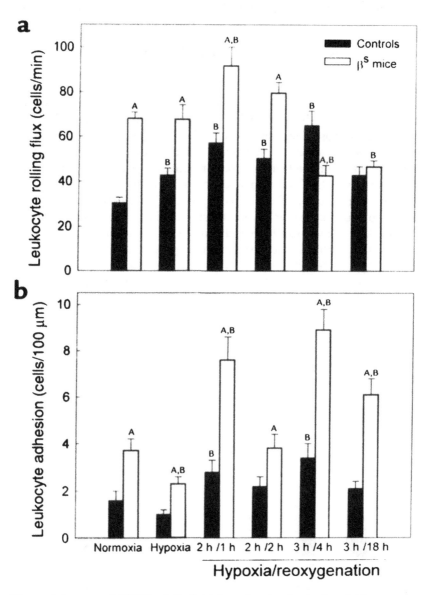

Figure 4. Increased WBC/endothelial interaction in vivo in the sickle mouse. Compared to the normal mouse (dark bars), the sickle mouse (light bars) shows exaggerated leukocyte rolling flux (top) and endothelial adhesion (bottom). Evident under baseline, ambient air conditions, this is further increased in response to hypoxia/reoxygenation. Reproduced with permission from the *Journal of Clinical Investigation*.[18]

WBC adhesion molecules. Therefore, its activation promotes neutrophil recruitment and a generalized endothelial activation state.[22] Thus, reperfusion injury states are characterized by a vigorous inflammatory response.[23,24] This could be a proximate stimulus for endothelial activation in sickle cell disease, which of course is characterized by vaso-occlusive events.

Therefore, we recently examined sickle transgenic mice for evidence of reperfusion injury physiology. In one study, we tested for biochemical footprints of reperfusion injury.[17] In sickle mice at ambient air, we observed elevated levels of ethane in expired gas (an indicator of body peroxidation) and an exaggerated conversion of salicylate to its hydroxylation products in plasma (evidence for hydroxyl radical generation) (Figure 3). Additionally, in sickle mice exposed to transient hypoxia (50 minutes of breathing 11% oxygen) followed by restoration of ambient air conditions, we observed an abnormal degree of conversion of XD to XO (Figure 3), an exaggerated increase in ethane excretion, and notable NF-κB activation in liver and kidney. In the second study, we compared the interaction of WBC with endothelium in sickle versus

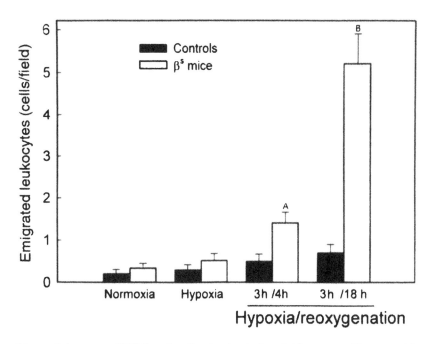

Figure 5. Increased WBC emigration in vivo in the sickle mouse. Compared to normal mouse (dark bars), the sickle mouse (light bars) shows greatly exaggerated emigration of WBC from vessel space into tissue in response to hypoxia/reoxygenation. Reproduced with permission from the *Journal of Clinical Investigation*.[18]

normal mice in vivo, using the vascular bed of the exposed cremaster muscle for observation.[18] Here, we observed sickle mice to have a greatly exaggerated inflammatory response to hypoxia/reoxygenation, as evidenced by increased WBC/endothelial interaction (both WBC rolling flux and WBC adhesion) (Figure 4) and increased WBC emigration across the endothelium into tissue (Figure 5). This was accompanied by slowed RBC transit time, as well as endothelial oxidant generation, as detected by a fluorescent oxidant detector. The mechanism of WBC/endothelial interaction in this model was observed to involve endothelial P-selectin.

Together, these studies directly demonstrate the propensity of the sickle mice to exhibit a proinflammatory phenotype. This suggests that sickle humans may also exhibit reperfusion injury physiology and are, thereby, prone to develop an inflammatory vessel wall phenotype.

Endothelial Activation Biology

Several prior observations are consistent with our view that sickle cell disease is a state of inflammation. Sickle patients have elevated levels of both acute phase reactants, such as C-reactive protein and fibrinogen, and endothelial stimulants such as IL-1, TNF, endotoxin, thrombin, hypoxia, and oxidants.[25] They also exhibit increased plasma levels of soluble adhesion molecules, a change that typically accompanies inflammation. As noted already, sickle patients have increased numbers of activated WBCs.

As a way to analyze the status of the endothelium in the living patient, we developed methods that allow assessment of circulating endothelial cells (CEC) as a surrogate for evaluation of vessel wall endothelium.[26] Briefly, from a peripheral blood sample, we make a preparation of cells enriched for CEC by using an antiendothelial antibody and immunomagnetic beads. Then, by applying standard methods of immunohistochemistry or immunofluorescence microscopy, we can assess the phenotype of the blood cells that are identified as being endothelial by virtue of being positive for endothelial antigen P1H12.

There is a wealth of evidence that the coagulation system is abnormally activated in sickle cell disease.[25] Since tissue factor is the trigger of coagulation, we are interested in the hypothesis that tissue factor on endothelium might be involved. Therefore we examined tissue factor on CEC.[27] Using an assay for expression of tissue factor antigen, we found that CEC from sickle patients are always abnormally positive (Figure 6). Interestingly, the sickle samples obtained on the first day of acute painful crisis tended to have higher degrees of activation, at least in some patients. We similarly examined sickle CEC for expression of rel-

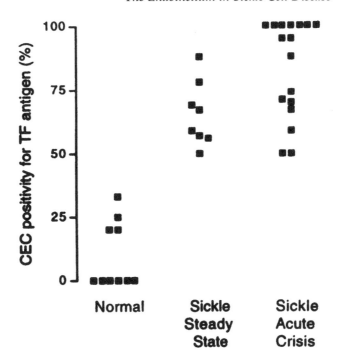

Figure 6. Abnormal expression of tissue factor (TF) on circulating endothelial cells (CEC). CEC from sickle patients show abnormal expression of TF antigen, both in steady state (middle) and at onset of acute vaso-occlusive crisis (right). Reproduced with permission from the *Journal of Clinical Investigation.*[27]

evant adhesion molecules.[26] Sickle CEC abnormally expressed ICAM-1, VCAM-1, P-selectin, and E-selectin. All 4 of these are of interest in that they promote white cell interaction with endothelium, and VCAM-1 additionally is an adhesogen for sickle RBC.

Thus, our data suggest that the endothelium in sickle patients has an abnormally proadhesive and procoagulant, i.e., an abnormally proinflammatory, phenotype. The truth of this conclusion, of course, rests on the degree to which the phenotype of CEC actually indicates the phenotype of vessel wall endothelial cells. For example, the number of tissue factor-positive CEC is probably trivial, but if vessel wall endothelium is similarly tissue factor-positive, this could be very important. We expect the phenotype of CEC to be the same, since CEC and vessel wall endothelial cells are both exposed to the same milieu of biological modifiers. Moreover, we know that phenotype of CEC is the same if they are alive or dead, indicating that they acquired their phenotype before they died. Nevertheless, the correspondence with vessel wall phenotypes remains a central issue in interpretation of CEC phenotype.

Therefore, we have examined sickle transgenic mice in an attempt to test for correspondence between phenotypes.[28] We find that CEC in sickle mice do tend to be activated, having strong positive expression of VCAM-1, ICAM-1, and E-selectin. Correspondingly, vessel endothelium in tissues also tends to be activated in these mice (Figure 7). However, the expression pattern is heterogeneous and highly complex. For example, degree of expression depends on which antigen is viewed, on vessel size, and on specific organ. Nonetheless, we can say, in the most general sense, that the activated phenotype of CEC in sickle mice does correspond to tissue endothelium phenotype. This heterogeneity of endothelial activation pattern, if it extends to the human situation, is very important and indicates that there is no such thing as "the endothelium." Rather, each organ must be considered individually to have its own pattern of endothelial activation and surface molecule expression. This, of course, has enormous implications for understanding the pathogenesis of the disease.

To further test if CEC phenotype parallels that of tissue endothelium, we treated sickle mice with a powerful inhibitor of NF-κB activation, the nuclear transcription factor that is a preeminent regulator of expression of various proinflammatory adhesion molecules (e.g., ICAM, VCAM, E-selectin) as well as a contributor to tissue factor expression. We chose to use sulfasalazine because it is reported to be a powerful inhibitor of en-

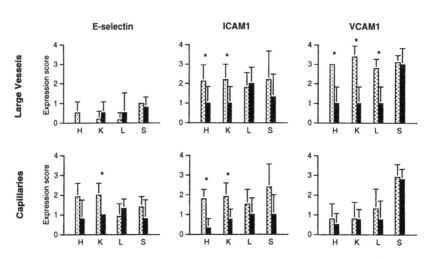

Figure 7. Tissue endothelial activation in the sickle mouse. Tissues were examined in the sickle mouse that was untreated (hatched bars) or treated with 10 days of sulfasalazine (solid bars). Endothelial expression was measured using a 0–5 scale and is shown for large vessel endothelial cells (top row) and capillary endothelial cells (bottom row). Data are illustrated for E-selectin, ICAM-1, and VCAM-1. H = heart; K = kidney; L = liver; S = spleen. Reproduced with permission from *Blood*.[28]

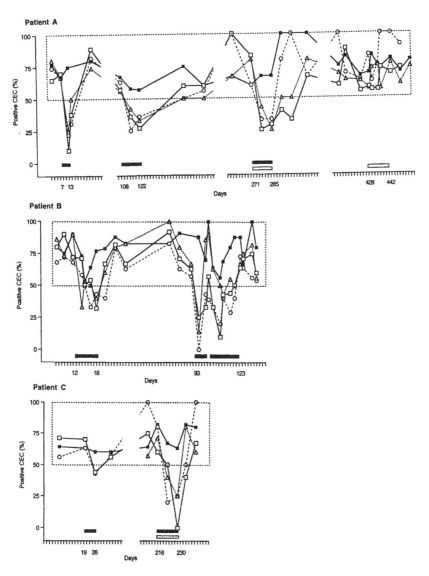

Figure 8. Sulfasalazine trial in sickle humans. Three humans with sickle cell disease were evaluated: patient A has HbSS, patient B has HbSβ^thal, and patient C has HbSC disease. Percent positivity of circulating endothelial cells (CEC) is shown on the vertical axis. In the absence of this therapeutic intervention, sickle samples are virtually always 50% or greater positive, indicated by the hatched box. During sulfasalazine treatment, indicated by solid black bars at bottom, CEC expression of ICAM-1 (open triangles), VCAM-1 (open squares), and E-selectin (open circles) diminished significantly. Tissue factor (solid squares) did not respond, even when salsalate was added, indicated by white bar at bottom. Reproduced with permission from *Blood*.[2]

dothelial cell NF-κB in vitro. This was given to sickle mice for 10 days intraperitoneally and resulted in downregulation of CEC activation. In parallel, tissues also showed some beneficial change (Figure 7). Again, the response to therapy was every bit as heterogeneous as expression profile in the starting tissues; but in a general sense CEC phenotype and tissue endothelial phenotype showed parallel downregulation.

Thus encouraged, we performed the same study on 3 human volunteers with sickle cell disease (1 each with HbSS, HbSC, and HbSβ[thal]).[28] They were given sulfasalazine for 1- or 2-week periods. As shown in Figure 8, when on drug, their degree of CEC activation dropped below the 50% level (at or above which CEC virtually always are in sickle patients, absent this therapeutic manipulation), and promptly returned to baseline values when drug was stopped. ICAM, VCAM, and E-selectin all showed this response, but tissue factor did not. In 2 of the trials we added salsalate in an attempt to recruit tissue factor responsiveness, but this failed. Insofar as CEC phenotype reflects that of vessel wall endothelium, this result suggests that this strategy of endothelial transcription factor inhibition could be useful in sickle cell disease. We would expect diminished endothelial activation to have beneficial effects on the vascular pathobiology of this disease.

These data lead us to hope that we are at the threshold of an era where status of endothelium in the patient does not have to go undiagnosed, and the contribution of the endothelium to human disease can be addressed therapeutically.

References

1. Cines DB, Pollak ES, Buck CA, et al. Endothelial cells in physiology and in the pathophysiology of vascular disorders. *Blood* 1998;91:3547–3561.
2. Hebbel RP, Mohandas N. Sickle cell adherence. In Embury SH, Hebbel RP, Mohandas N, et al., eds: *Sickle Cell Disease: Basic Principles and Clinical Practice.* New York: Raven Press; 1994:217–230.
3. Hebbel RP. Adhesion interactions of sickle erythrocytes with endothelium. *J Clin Invest* 1997;99:2561–2564.
4. Kaul DK, Fabry ME, Costantini F, et al. In vivo demonstration of red cell-endothelial interaction, sickling and altered microvascular response to oxygen in the sickle transgenic mouse. *J Clin Invest* 1995;96:2845–2853.
5. Kaul DK, Fabry ME, Nagel RL. Microvascular sites and characteristics of sickle cell adhesion to vascular endothelium in shear flow conditions: Pathophysiological implications. *Proc Natl Acad Sci USA* 1989;86:3356–3360.
6. Fabry ME, Rajanayagam V, Fine E, et al. Modeling sickle cell vasoocclusion in the rat leg: Quantification of trapped sickle cells and correlation with 31P metabolic and 1H magnetic resonance imaging changes. *Proc Natl Acad Sci USA* 1989;86:3808–3812.
7. Fabry ME, Fine E, Rajanayagam V, et al. Demonstration of endothelial adhesion of sickle cells in vivo: A distinct role for deformable sickle cell discocytes. *Blood* 1992;79:1602–1611.

8. Kaul DK, Tsai HM, Liu XD, et al. Monoclonal antibodies to $\alpha_V\beta_3$ (7E3 and LM609) inhibit sickle red blood cell-endothelium interactions induced by platelet-activating factor. *Blood* 2000;95:368–374.

9. Hebbel RP. Blockade of adhesion of sickle cells to endothelium by monoclonal antibodies. *N Engl J Med* 2000;342:1910–1912.

10. Carlos TM, Harlan JM. Leukocyte-endothelial adhesion molecules. *Blood* 1994;84:2068–2101.

11. Platt OS, Brambilla DJ, Rosse WF, et al. Mortality in sickle cell disease: Life expectancy and risk factors for early death. *N Engl J Med* 1994;330:1639–1644.

12. Charache S. Mechanism of action of hydroxyurea in the management of sickle cell anemia in adults. *Semin Hematol* 1997;34:15–21.

13. Steinberg MH, Mohandas N. Laboratory values. In Embury SH, Hebbel RP, Mohandas N, et al., eds: *Sickle Cell Disease: Basic Principles and Clinical Practice*. New York: Raven Press; 1994:469–484.

14. Hofstra TC, Kalra VK, Meiselman HJ, et al. Sickle erythrocytes adhere to polymorphonuclear neutrophils and activate the neutrophil respiratory burst. *Blood* 1996;87:4440–4447.

15. Fadlon E, Vordermeier S, Pearson TC, et al. Blood polymorphonuclear leukocytes from the majority of sickle cell patients in the crisis phase of the disease show enhanced adhesion to vascular endothelium and increased expression of CD64. *Blood* 1998;91:266–274.

16. Belcher JD, Marker PH, Weber JP, et al. Monocytes from sickle cell anemia patients activate vascular endothelium: Upregulation of NF-κB, tissue factor, E-selectin, ICAM-1, VCAM-1, and neutrophil adhesion. *Blood* 2000;96:2451–2459.

17. Osarogiagbon UR, Choong S, Belcher JD, et al. Reperfusion injury pathophysiology in sickle transgenic mice. *Blood* 2000;96:314–320.

18. Kaul DK, Hebbel RP. Hypoxia/reoxygenation causes inflammatory response in transgenic sickle mice but not in normal mice. *J Clin Invest* 2000;106:411–420.

19. McCord JM. Oxygen-derived free radicals in post-ischemic tissue injury. *N Engl J Med* 1985;312:159–163.

20. Zimmerman BJ, Granger DN. Mechanisms of reperfusion injury. *Am J Med Sci* 1994;307:284–289.

21. Freeman BA, Crapo JD. Biology of disease: Free radicals and tissue injury. *Lab Invest* 1982;47:412–426.

22. Grisham MB, Granger DN, Lefer DJ. Modulation of leukocyte-endothelial interactions by reactive metabolites of oxygen and nitrogen: Relevance to ischemic heart disease. *Free Radic Biol Med* 1998;25:404–433.

23. Gute DC, Ishida T, Yarimizu K, et al. Inflammatory responses to ischemia and reperfusion in skeletal muscle. *Mol Cell Biochem* 1998;179:169–187.

24. Granger DN, Korthuis RJ. Physiologic mechanisms of postischemic tissue injury. *Ann Rev Physiol* 1998;1995:311–332.

25. Francis RB, Jr., Hebbel RP. Hemostasis. In Embury SH, Hebbel RP, Mohandas N, et al., eds: *Sickle Cell Disease: Basic Principles and Clinical Practice*. New York: Raven Press; 1994:299–310.

26. Solovey A, Lin Y, Browne P, et al. Circulating activated endothelial cells in sickle cell anemia. *N Engl J Med* 1997;337:1584–1590.

27. Solovey A, Gui L, Key NS, et al. Tissue factor expression by endothelial cells in sickle cell anemia. *J Clin Invest* 1998;101:1899–1904.

28. Solovey AA, Solovey AN, Harkness J, et al. Modulation of endothelial cell activation in sickle cell disease: A pilot study. *Blood* 2001;97:1937–1941.

Chapter 3

Thrombin, Endothelial Gap Formation, and Erythrocyte Adhesion

Stephen H. Embury, MD, and Neil M. Matsui, PhD

Introduction

Sickle cell disease is a painful, disabling disorder of red blood cells that affects tens of thousands of Americans and millions worldwide.[1] Much of the morbidity and disability of sickle cell disease is caused by occlusion of blood flow in small blood vessels, the occurrence of which has been understood according to the following accepted interpretation. The sickle cell gene (β^S) is the result of a GAG $\rightarrow$ GTG mutation of the sixth codon of the β-globin gene. This allele directs the production of mutant β-globin (β^S-globin) having Glu $\rightarrow$ Val as the sixth amino acid. The sickle cell hemoglobin (HbS) tetramer is comprised of $\alpha_2\beta S_2$. Individuals with simple heterozygosity for β^S have approximately 60% normal hemoglobin (HbA) and 40% HbS within their erythrocytes, and those with homozygosity have virtually all HbS. Due to the profound insolubility of deoxygenated HbS, the release of oxygen from erythrocytes of individuals with homozygous sickle cell anemia results in polymerization of HbS, rigidification and sickling of red cells, and occlusion of the microvasculature. This is the traditional version of vaso-occlusion.[2,3]

Despite the widespread acceptance of this principle, there are several important aspects of sickle cell disease that are not defined by explications of polymerization.[4] One example is the assumption that rou-

From: Weir EK, Reeve HL, Reeves JT (eds). *Interactions of Blood and the Pulmonary Circulation*. Armonk, NY: Futura Publishing Company, Inc.; ©2002.

tine vaso-occlusive pain crises are the result of hypoxia-induced sick-ling of erythrocytes. This supposition ignores the fact that the average erythrocyte gives up its oxygen at least once a minute, a process that indicates sickling occurs as an ongoing constant process rather than as a sudden cataclysmic event. Moreover, the occurrence of vaso-occlusive pain crisis correlates little with accepted determinants of polymerization and cannot be predicted using polymerization formulas. Certainly, these formulas do not explain why only 5% of patients account for 30% of pain crises among patients with sickle cell disease.[5,6] While polymerization is undeniably necessary for sickle cell disease, its determinants are insufficient to define the occurrence of acute pain. In this regard, the role of polymerization in vaso-occlusion is understood best in the context of its interaction with other vaso-occlusive processes, such as coagulation, platelet activation, vascular regulation, and cytoadhesive interactions.[4,7–10]

The adherence of sickle cells to vascular endothelium is singularly important to vaso-occlusion. The initial discoveries by Hoover and by Hebbel and their colleagues that sickle cells are abnormally adherent[11,12] and by Hebbel et al. that clinical severity correlates with interpatient differences in sickle cell adhesivity[13] kindled a burst of scientific inquiry into sickle cell adhesion.[14] Justification for these studies derived from the seminal discovery by Kaul and associates that vaso-occlusion occurs ex vivo as a 2-step process, initiated by the adherence of sticky sickle cells to the endothelium and completed by the log-jamming of rigid, polymerization-prone cells.[15] The potential initiatory role of sickle cell adherence suggests that the key to comprehending the occurrence of vaso-occlusion depends on a better understanding of adhesion.

Several adhesive molecules of sickle cells are employed in adherence to resting endothelium.[16] These include CD36, integrin $\alpha_4\beta_1$, immunoglobulin, sulfated glycolipid, basal cell adhesion molecule/ Lutheran protein, band 3, and integrin-associated protein.[9,14,17–21] The soluble ligands of sickle cell adherence include high molecular weight von Willebrand factor (vWF), thrombospondin (TSP), fibrinogen, and fibronectin.[14] Unperturbed vascular endothelium utilizes GpIb, CD36, and integrins $\alpha_4\beta_1$ and $\alpha_v\beta_3$ of endothelial cells, fibronectin of the glycocalyx, and TSP, vWF, fibronectin, and laminin of the matrix.[9,14,16,17,20,22,23] This list of adhesion molecules indicates the complexity of steady-state sickle cell adhesion.

These interdependent mechanisms define a delicate equipoise between circulatory sufficiency and insufficiency. Amplification of the overall adhesiveness of this system has the potential to promote vascular occlusion. In this way the basic parameters of the system, the adhesive contributions of sickle cells, soluble ligands, and vascular endothelium, are potential triggers of vaso-occlusion. Among these, the comparatively immutable adhesivity of sickle red cells has seemed to indicate that this component of the adhesion complex is necessary but not sufficient to explain the seemingly random occurrences of painful vaso-occlusion. However, recently 2 mechanisms have been described by which temporal alterations in the adhesivity of sickle cells may contribute to vaso-occlusion. Kumar et al. found that phorbol esters enhance sickle cell adhesivity through integrin $\alpha_4\beta_1$.[24] Brittain and associates in the Parise lab discovered that the combination of shear stress and exposure to TSP transduce a G-protein, tyrosine kinase pathway that increases the integrin-associated protein-mediated adherence of sickle cells to immobilized TSP or vitronectin.[21,25] Nevertheless, sporadic pain crises are more likely related to temporal fluctuations in nonerythroid adhesive determinants. Plasma concentrations of high molecular weight vWF, TSP, fibrinogen, and fibronectin vary as acute phase reactants,[26,27] but there is no evidence that fluctuations in the level of these soluble ligands influence adherence or vaso-occlusion. More compellingly, the exquisite adhesive responses of endothelial cells to activation suggest endothelial perturbation as a potential trigger of vaso-occlusion.[14,28–30]

In fact, there is evidence that in sickle cell disease at least a fraction of endothelial cells are activated. Nadeau and associates used quantitative RT-PCR to determine that ICAM-1 and VCAM-1 mRNA levels are increased 2- to 7-fold in kidney biopsy samples from adult sickle cell patients compared to nonsickle controls.[31] Duits et al. found plasma levels of VCAM-1 to be increased in sickle cell patients in steady state and to increase further during painful vaso-occlusion.[32] Solovey and associates in the Hebbel lab reported that circulating endothelial cells are increased in number, have activated phenotypes (i.e., express ICAM-1, VCAM-1, E-selectin, and P-selectin), produce tissue factor, and increase further in number during pain crisis.[33,34] These accounts suggest the potential importance of activated endothelial cell adhesivity in sickle cell adherence and vaso-occlusion. However, they do not address the stimuli responsible for the endothelial perturbations observed. Several biological modifiers of endothelial cell adhesivity are operative in sickle cell disease, including thrombin, histamine, TNF-α, interferon-γ, IL-1β, erythropoietin, vascular endothelial growth factor (VEGF), hypoxia, reperfusion, reactive oxygen species, viruses, and sickle cells per se,[19,30,35–47] and certain of these specifically increase endothelial adhesion of sickle cells.[9,14] There is recent evidence of reperfusion injury following experimental hypoxia in a mouse sickle cell model, which was manifest by the generation of peroxide and hydroxyl and by oxygen radical-dependent adhesion of polymorphonuclear leukocytes to endothelial P-selectin.[48,49] These findings support the relevance of the finding by Setty and Stuart that VCAM-1 and $\alpha_4\beta_1$ are induced by hypoxia.[18] Hebbel and colleagues described the expression of Fc-like receptors by cells infected with herpesviruses.[19]

Shiu et al. determined that the exposure of cultured endothelium to sickle cells induced the expression of ICAM-1 and VCAM-1 by the endothelial cells.[47] Kaul and associates found that activation of endothelial cells with platelet activating factor (PAF) induced the expression of $\alpha_V\beta_3$ integrin, which in turn mediated sickle cell adherence.[50]

The Role of Thrombin in the Adhesogenic Response

The emerging recognition of sickle cell disease as a chronic inflammatory process extends the list of disease effectors to include cytokines and other mediators of inflammation.[51–55] In this regard, thrombin has dual proinflammatory and anti-inflammatory activities[56,57] and is an agonist of endothelial cells.[58] Moreover, there is considerable evidence for increased thrombin generation and activity in sickle cell disease.[7,59,60] Direct documentation includes increased levels of the activation fragment $1+2$,[7,61] fibrinopeptide A,[62] D-dimers,[62,63] thrombin-antithrombin III complexes,[62] and fragment E.[64] Indirect evidence includes increased factor VIII turnover,[62] reduced levels of contact factors,[65] factor V, antithrombin III, proteins C and S,[64,66–69] and increased activation of platelets. Platelet activation is evidenced by the presence of activation antigens on circulating platelets,[70] elevated plasma β-thromboglobulin,[67] decreased platelet content and increased plasma levels of thrombospondin,[71] and increased thromboxane generation.[72,73]

There is much evidence to support increased thrombin generation and activity in sickle cell disease, but the sources of thrombin have not been identified. It seems probable that its generation is a result of tissue factor production by endothelial cells and monocytes as part of the inflammation of sickle cell disease[62,74–78] and of the exposure of phosphatidylserine (PS) on the outer membrane leaflet of deoxygenated sickle cells and irreversibly sickled cells.[79–81] The relative contributions of these sources is unknown.

The unusual enzyme action of thrombin on endothelial cells[82–84] is the result of its proteolytic cleavage of an exodomain of a G-protein-coupled protease-activated receptor (PAR) to generate a new N-terminus, which then functions as a tethered ligand for its own PAR. Exposure of this cryptic ligand that is carried by its own receptor results in its intramolecular binding to the PAR and transduction of a signal into the cell. As an endothelial cell agonist, thrombin has the capacity to influence the pathophysiology of sickle cell vaso-occlusion.[82,84] Thrombin disrupts the integrity of endothelial monolayers by inducing endothelial cell expression of platelet-activating factor, P-selectin, and intercellular adhesion molecule-1 (ICAM-1), which facilitate adherence of polymorphonuclear leukocytes,[85,86] which in turn deliver reactive oxygen species (ROS) and proteases, leading to interendothelial cell gap formation and barrier dysfunction.[87–89] This sequence may be enhanced in sickle cell disease by the commonly elevated leukocyte counts and activation of polymorphonuclear leukocytes by sickle red cells.[90,91] Another mechanism by which thrombin disrupts endothelial monolayer integrity is the induction of endothelial cell contraction.[83,84,92–96] The integrity of endothelial cell monolayers is the result of a dynamic equilibrium between basal levels of centripetal cell tension and cell-tethering forces provided by cell-cell cadherin anchors and cell-matrix integrin moorings.[97] Thrombin shifts this equilibrium by transducing actin contraction, retraction of endothelial cells, and interendothelial cell gap formation.[83,89,98] Such endothelial cell contraction is essential to inflammation,[89] and we posited that this process may also facilitate sickle cell adherence and vaso-occlusion.

The coexistence of activated endothelial adhesivity and intercellular gap formation is critical to several normal and pathological inflammatory processes, all of which are associated with increased vascular permeability, adherence of white blood cells to the endothelium, and transendothelial migration of leukocytes.[99–103] These include wound healing, coronary and cerebral vascular diseases, ischemia-reperfusion, inflammatory reactions remote from areas of reperfusion, sepsis-thrombosis interactions, chronic venous insufficiency, cholesterol lowering, radiation injury, diabetic vasculopathy, glomerulonephritis, hyperoxic lung injury, and complications of alcoholism.[57,104–119] Whether such processes involve stimulation, activation, or injury of endothelial cells is not easily distinguished,[120] but each involves increased vascular permeability, endothelial cell adhesivity,[121] and active retraction of endothelial cells.[89,97,122] Although controversy exists regarding the exact routes of vascular permeability,[123–126] the process necessarily exposes circulating blood cells to cryptic endothelial cell adhesion molecules and matrix proteins. Some of the latter, such as TSP, vWF, laminin, and fibronectin, have adhesivity for sickle cells.[14,17,23,127–131] We have studied the molecules involved in thrombin-activated sickle cell adherence and evaluated whether interendothelial gap formation is involved in the process.

Endothelial Adhesivity for Sickle Cells Is Enhanced by Thrombin and Associated With Interendothelial Cell Gap Formation In Vitro

We began our studies of thrombin as an endothelial cell agonist by assessing the effects of increasing concentrations of thrombin (0.01 to 0.5 U/mL for 5 minutes) on the adhesivity of human umbilical vein monolayers for sickle cells using a static gravity adherence, dip rinse assay that employs microscopic visualization of adherent cells. Adherence increased in a dose-dependent manner, peaking at 0.1 U/mL (Figure 1). This curve for sickle cell adherence is similar to that for thrombin-induced gap formation in endothelial monolayers.[93] Based on these data, we chose 0.1 U/mL for 5 minutes as our working conditions of thrombin exposure to obtain maximal adhesogenic effect.

We next compared the adherence of sickle and nonsickle red blood cells to thrombin-treated monolayers (Figure 2). The mean number of nonsickle cells adherent to unstimulated endothelial cells was $2.2/mm^2$ (n=9) and of sickle cells was $6.3/mm^2$ (n=9). The greater adherence of sickle cells has been observed by others.[10] Thrombin treatment caused a significant increase in adherence of both erythrocyte populations. Mean values of adherence increased from 2.2 to 5.8 nonsickle cells per mm^2 and from 6.3 to 12.4 sickle cells per mm^2. Thus, thrombin influences endothelial cell adhesivity for both nonsickle and sickle red cells, but has a greater effect on the latter.

In our microscopic visualization of adherence, it appeared that the erythrocytes adhered mainly to the edges of endothelial cells where the cells were separated from their neighbors, and seldom to areas of the monolayer where the endothelial cells remained tightly adherent. This

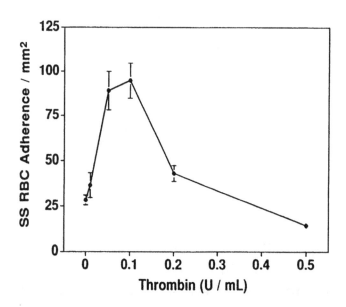

Figure 1. Dose response curve for thrombin-induced adherence. Each point represents the mean number from 4 static assays of sickle cell (SS RBC) adherent to 1 mm^2 of human umbilical cord endothelial cells (HUVEC) treated with thrombin concentrations ranging from 0 to 0.5 NIH U/mL.

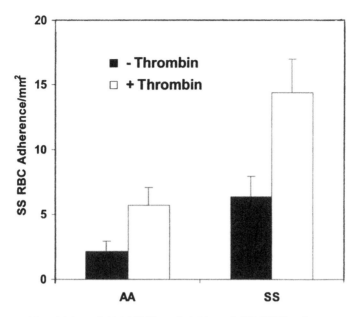

Figure 2. Nonsickle cell (AA RBC) and sickle cell (SS RBC) adherence to human umbilical cord endothelial cells (HUVEC) that had been treated with thrombin or with control buffer. The mean ± SEM number adherent RBC/mm² human umbilical cord endothelial cells (HUVEC) treated with 0.1 NIH U/mL for 5 minutes is shown (n=9).

distribution existed in both unperturbed and thrombin-treated monolayers, in which it appeared that the gap areas were substantially greater. To quantify this relationship, in 3 experiments we determined the site of adherence of adherent sickle cells. Table 1 demonstrates that the distribution of adherent sickle cells to unperturbed monolayers was 65% to endothelial cell edges, 22% to the luminal surface, and 12% in the gaps with no contact to an endothelial cell. To thrombin-treated monolayers, the distribution was 66% to the edges, 21% to the luminal surface, and 13% in the gaps. The same distribution pattern after thrombin treatment, taken together with a 2-fold overall increase in adherence, indicates equal increases at all 3 sites: cell edges, luminal surfaces, and bared matrix.

We used computerized morphometry and a test of monolayer permeability to Evans blue albumin to confirm the effects of thrombin on endothelial cell contraction and gap formation that was apparent during the adherence assays. Photographs of the same microscopic field taken at 0, 2, 5, 10, 20, and 40 minutes after a 5-minute exposure to 0.1 U/mL thrombin revealed a swift and obvious contraction of endothelial cells and gap formation (Figure 3 A–F). In contrast, a 5-minute exposure to medium alone resulted in neither contraction nor gap formation, as

Table 1

Distribution of Adherent Red Blood Cells (RBC) to Endothelial
Cell (EC) Monolayers Before and After Thrombin Treatment

	No Thrombin		With Thrombin	
Sickle Cell Location	# RBC	%	# RBC	%
EC edges	143	65	204	66
EC luminal surface	49	22	65	21
Within gaps	27	12	39	13
Total	219	100	308	100

Locations of an arbitrary number of adherent sickle cells (RBC) on endothelial cell (EC)
monolayers in 3 separate experiments were tabulated. These distributions reflect locations only, not quantitative differences in overall adherence. RBC adhered primarily to
the sides of EC that were pulled apart, and the distribution did not change after thrombin treatment.

demonstrated by photographs taken before and 40 minutes after a 5-
minute exposure to medium alone (Figure 3 G, H). Quantification of the
relative areas of gaps and cells in scans of these photomicrographs using computerized morphometry with the Melanie gel analysis system
(BioRad) demonstrated a prompt 14-fold increase in the area of the gaps
(Table 2). Using this method to assess the influence of different thrombin concentrations on gap formation revealed that a degree of gap formation matching that observed with 0.1 U/mL thrombin was induced
by 0.2 and 0.5 U/mL thrombin, concentrations at which adherence was
substantially diminished (Figure 1). Thrombin also induced a prompt
increase in permeability of monolayers to Evans blue albumin. Figure 4
shows that the same thrombin conditions resulted in a 3-fold increase in
permeability within 5 minutes, which persisted at approximately that
level throughout the 40-minute period of measurement. No change was
induced by medium alone. These data confirm that, in addition to its effect on endothelial adhesivity for sickle and nonsickle erythrocytes,
thrombin induced intercellular gap formation.

This apparent association of adherence and gap formation was
tested further by determining whether nonspecific mechanisms of gap
formation also increased erythrocyte adherence. We treated monolayers briefly with a low concentration of edetic acid (EDTA) to disrupt
cell-matrix and cell-cell interactions or with an antilaminin polyclonal
antibody to disrupt cell-matrix tethers. After a 10-second exposure to
0.5 mM EDTA that caused the cells to round up slightly, the EDTA was
washed away and the adherence assay was performed in the presence
of divalent cations. This treatment increased the mean adherence of

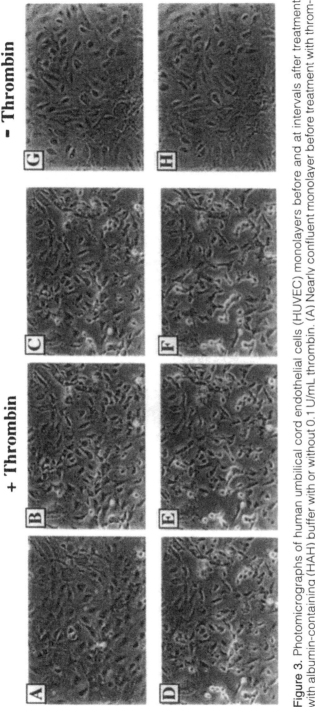

Figure 3. Photomicrographs of human umbilical cord endothelial cells (HUVEC) monolayers before and at intervals after treatment with albumin-containing (HAH) buffer with or without 0.1 U/mL thrombin. (A) Nearly confluent monolayer before treatment with thrombin. (B–F) The same microscope field 2 minutes (B), 5 minutes (C), 10 minutes (D), 20 minutes (E), and 40 minutes (F) after a 5-minute exposure to thrombin. (G) Nearly confluent monolayer before treatment with HAH buffer. (H) The same microscope field as in (G) 40 minutes after a 5-minute exposure to HAH alone. The monolayer treated with thrombin (panels B–F) demonstrates a progressive and pronounced ICGF, compared to the pretreatment monolayer (A). The monolayer exposed to HAH alone demonstrated no detectable ICGF after 40 minutes (G and H). Morphometric quantification of gap formation is tabulated in Table 2.

Table 2

Morphometric Studies of Thrombin-Induced ICGF

	PT[a]	Time after 5 min treatment w/ 0.1 U/mL thrombin in buffer					
		5 sec	2 in	5 min	10 min	20 min	40 min
Total area	7638	7545	7584	7638	7578	7612	7621
Cell area	7286	3647	3248	2669	2487	2342	2291
Gaps[b]	352	3898	4336	4969	5091	5270	5330
% Gaps[c]	4.6%	51.7%	57.2%	65.1%	67.2%	69.2%	69.9%
Fold gap Inc[d]	None	10	11	13	14	14	14

	PT[a]	Time after 5 min treatment w/ thrombin-free buffer
		40 min
Total area	7603	7603
Cell area	7514	7531
Gaps[b]	89	72
% Gaps[c]	1.2%	0.9%
Fold gap Inc[d]	None	0

[a]PT, prior to treatment.
[b]Gaps = Total Area − Cell Area.
[c]% Gaps = Gaps ÷ Total Area.
[d]Fold Gap Increase = [% Gaps (at time point) − % Gaps (at PT)] ÷ % Gaps (at PT).

sickle cells from 5.1 to 15.5 /mm² (Figure 5). Exposure of the monolayer to antilaminin antibody before testing adherence also increased the mean adherence of sickle cells (Figure 5). These results corroborate the association between gap formation and sickle cell adherence.

We tested this association also by pretreating the monolayers with agents that prevent gap formation prior to exposing the cells to agents that we had found to induce both adhesivity and gap formation. We used bromo-cAMP to prevent the gap formation induced by thrombin or EDTA. Bromo-cAMP is a cAMP analog that protects endothelial cell barrier function by inhibiting cell contraction.[132] EDTA was used as a positive control for gap formation. Cellular actions of these agents are revealed in the immunofluorescence photomicrographs of rhodamine-labeled actin filaments, which define the endothelial cytoskeleton and monolayer integrity (Figure 6). Untreated cells were closely adjacent and had no intercellular gaps and peripheral bands of actin stress fibers (Figure 6 A). Thrombin-exposed cells had intercellular gaps, reorganized stress fibers, and a few actin fibers apparently across the gaps

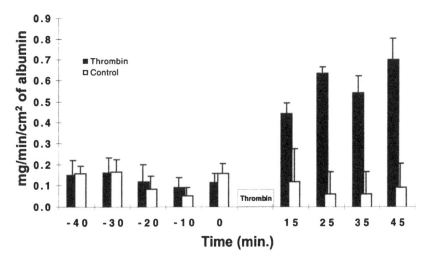

Figure 4. Evans blue albumin (EBA) permeability of HUVEC monolayers. The diffusion of Evans blue albumin (EBA) from the luminal buffer in the transwell to the abluminal buffer in the lower well is shown as mg albumin/minute/cm2 monolayer from 60 minutes before until 40 minutes after exposure to 0.1 U/mL thrombin in albumin-containing buffer (black bars) or to albumin-containing buffer alone (shaded bars). Samples were taken at several time points prior to and after treatment; the zero time point is equivalent to the start of the 5-minute treatment. Thrombin exposure resulted in a rapid increase in monolayer permeability to EBA, which was sustained for the duration of these measurements.

(Figure 6 B). Cells exposed to EDTA also had intercellular gaps, but had less well-defined actin fibers than the thrombin-treated cells, and were connected by fine processes (Figure 6 C). The combination of bromo-cAMP plus the phosphodiesterase inhibitor IBMX induced no changes in intercellular gaps or actin fibers (Figure 6 D), prevented thrombin-induced changes in actin stress fibers and ICGF (compare Figure 6 E and 6 B), but did not prohibit the gap formation caused by EDTA (compare Figure 6 F and 6 C).

Having found an effect of bromo-cAMP on gap formation, we tested its effect on adherence. The effects of bromo-cAMP pretreatment on thrombin- and EDTA-induced sickle cell adherence shown in Figure 7 are presented as a percent of control adherence. As with thrombin-induced gap formation, bromo-cAMP reduced mean thrombin-enhanced sickle cell adherence (from 243% to 122% of baseline). As with EDTA-induced gap formation, bromo-cAMP had no significant effect on EDTA-induced adherence. The similarities in adherence to cells treated with buffer alone, bromo-cAMP pretreated cells treated with buffer alone, or to bromo-

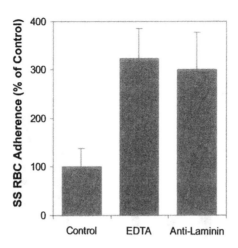

Figure 5. Effect of nonspecific mechanisms of intercellular gap formation (ICGF) on sickle cell (SS RBC) adherence. Human umbilical cord endothelial cells (HUVEC) were treated briefly with a low concentration of EDTA to remove the divalent cations necessary for cell-matrix and cell-cell interactions or with an antilaminin polyclonal antibody to disrupt EC-matrix tethers. After a brief exposure to 0.5 mM EDTA or antilaminin antibody, the cells were seen to separate slightly under visual microscopic monitoring. At that point the adherence assay was performed as usual in the presence of divalent cations.

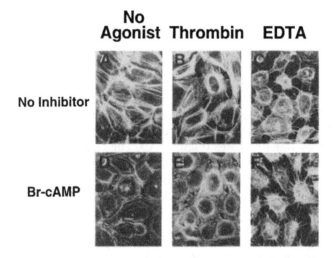

Figure 6. Immunofluorescence microscopy (IF) shows the effect of thrombin and EDTA, and inhibitors of EC contraction on actin and intercellular gap formation (ICGF). Actin was stained with rhodamine-labeled phalloidin. The camera shutter speed was set automatically so the intensities are not relative. These representative photos show that thrombin-induced but not EDTA-induced intercellular gap formation (ICGF) was blocked by the inhibitor, bromo-cAMP. Human umbilical cord endothelial cells (HUVEC) in the photos were: (A) untreated; (B) thrombin-stimulated; (C) EDTA-treated; (D) incubated with bromo-cAMP before treating with control buffer; (E) incubated with bromo-cAMP before treating with thrombin; (F) incubated with bromo-cAMP before treating with EDTA.

cAMP pretreated cells treated with thrombin are mirrored by the effects of bromo-cAMP on gap formation (Figure 6 D–F). Bromo-cAMP inhibited adherence and gap formation induced by thrombin but neither effect of EDTA.

These results demonstrate that thrombin treatment of endothelial cells increases their adhesivity for sickle cells in vitro and that there is a linkage between thrombin-induced adherence and gap formation.[36] Others have reported that endothelial cell gap formation was associated with increased adherence of phosphatidylserine-expressing nonsickle erythrocytes.[133] Our data supporting the linkage of adherence and gap formation demonstrate the existence of additional mechanisms of thrombin-enhanced adhesivity, since inhibition of actin contraction and cell retraction with bromo-cAMP only partially blocked thrombin-enhanced adhesivity (Figure 7) and the use of high thrombin concentrations revealed a dissociation between effects on gap formation and adhesivity.[36] Clearly mechanisms exist that are independent of gap formation.

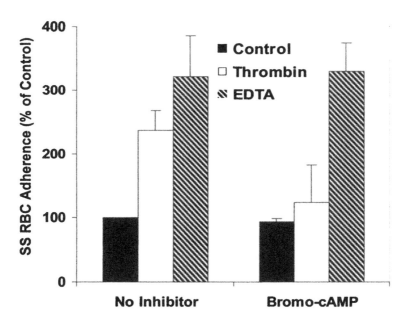

Figure 7. Effect of inhibition of cell contraction by bromo-cAMP and glutaraldehyde on sickle cell (SS RBC) adherence. Treatment of human umbilical cord endothelial cells (HUVEC) with bromo-cAMP prevented thrombin-induced but not EDTA-induced adherence. Results are presented as a percent of control adherence.

Thrombin-Enhanced Sickle Cell Adhesion Is Partly to β_1 and β_3 Integrins and Fibronectin

The association we have shown of increased adherence and gap formation led us to explore endothelial adhesion molecules and matrix proteins as possible mediators of the thrombin-induced adhesogenic response. We used our static adherence assay to assess whether adherence of sickle cells to thrombin-treated endothelial cells involved fibronectin or laminin. We found that polyclonal antibody to fibronectin partially blocked sickle cell adherence to both untreated and thrombin-treated endothelial cell monolayers but that polyclonal antilaminin antibody did not (data not shown). These results show that the adherence of sickle cells to thrombin-treated endothelial monolayers is partly to matrix fibronectin.

To determine whether the static adherence of sickle erythrocytes to thrombin-treated endothelial cells was to specific integrins, we used AIIB2 and SZ-21 mAb to block the contributions of β_1 and β_3 integrins, respectively. Despite the known source-dependent variability in endothelial cell responses[18,36,93] and sickle cell adhesivity,[13] we observed a similar and partial inhibition of thrombin-enhanced adherence by anti-β_1 mAb or anti-β_3 mAb (data not shown).

To determine whether this integrin-mediated adhesion is the result of quantitatively increased integrin on the endothelial cell surface, we used flow cytometry to quantify the expression of the β_1 and β_3 integrin subunits before and after thrombin treatment. We mobilized endothelial cells using protease-free cell dissociation solution (Sigma) and labeled endothelial cell suspensions with either AIIB2 or P5D2 against β_1 or with AP3 against β_3. Thrombin exposure resulted in no significant increase in β_1 or β_3 integrin on the surface of suspended endothelial cells (data not shown). Taken together with the mAb-blocking data, these flow cytometry studies suggest that thrombin-enhanced adhesivity is not due to quantitatively increased expression, but rather to cellular changes that redistribute cytoadhesive molecules from the abluminal cell surface to endothelial cell surfaces where they can bind sickle cells.[131]

Others have reported that these integrins are distributed on both the luminal and abluminal surface of resting endothelial cells,[134,135] but the treatment of cells with lactoperoxidase beads for iodination of membrane proteins and the solubilization of cell membranes with acetone prior to immunofluorescence microscopy, respectively, lend uncertainty to the conclusions. For instance, when we exposed resting cultured endothelial cells to lactoperoxidase beads prior to immunofluorescence microscopy, the cells retracted and rounded up as if they had been activated. Moreover, the β_1 integrin on the cell surface identified using the anti-β_1 mAb P5D2 in immunofluorescence microscopy redistributed from the ablu-

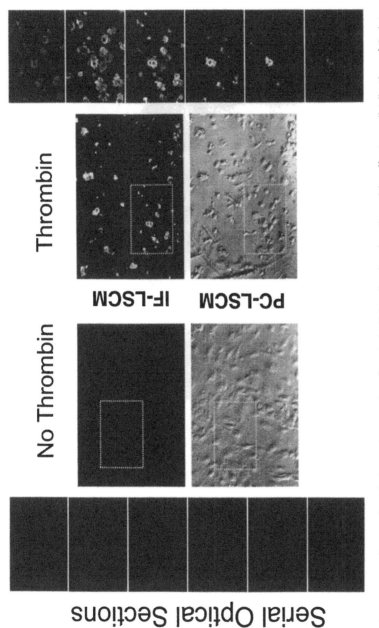

Figure 8. Laser scanning confocal photomicrographs of endothelial cells showing thrombin effect on distribution of β_1 integrin. Endothelial cells were treated with thrombin or medium alone, labeled with anti-β_1 mAb, and observed under a phase-contrast (PC) or fluorescent (IF) filter of a laser scanning confocal microscope (LSCM). Dashed boxes indicate portions of microscope fields that were used for optical sectioning. The serial optical sections represent 3-μm steps from the bottom of the cell.

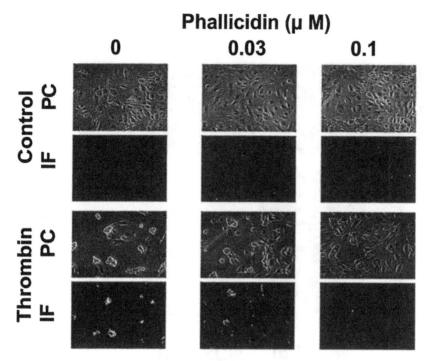

Figure 9. Laser scanning confocal photomicrographs of endothelial cells showing the inhibition by phallicidin of thrombin-induced redistribution of β_1 integrin.
Endothelial cells were pretreated with phallicidin then treated with thrombin or
medium alone. Cells were fixed, stained with anti-integrin β_1 antibody, and observed under a phase-contrast (PC) or fluorescent (IF) LSCM.

minal surface of the cells, where it had been confined in resting cells, to
the edges and luminal surface of the cells (data not shown). When we
acetone-fixed endothelial cells prior to immunofluorescence microscopy,
the permeabilized membranes of untreated cells allowed labeling of both
luminal and abluminal aspects with the anti-β_1 mAb P5D2 or the anti-β_3
mAb AP3 (data not shown).

However, a different distribution was observed using a more precise method for defining the membrane location of integrins: laser scanning confocal microscopy (LSCM). After treating endothelial monolayers with thrombin or thrombin-free buffer for 5 minutes at 37°C, the cells
were fixed with 2% paraformaldehyde (which does not permeabilize
cell membranes), stained with AIIB2 anti-β_1 mAb or AP3 anti-β_3 mAb,
reacted with biotinylated goat antimouse polyvalent immunoglobulins
secondary antibody, and then treated with FITC-conjugated avidin.
Thrombin-treated cells were found by phase contrast-LSCM (PC-
LSCM) to be retracted while untreated endothelial cells were comparatively flat (Figure 8; PC-LSCM). Immunofluorescence-LSCM (IF-LSCM)

revealed that β_1 expression is strong on the thrombin-treated cells and not detected on control-treated cells (Figure 8; IF-LSCM). Using IF-LSCM to obtain serial optical sections revealed that the retracted thrombin-treated cells express β_1 on the abluminal surface, edges, and luminal surface of the cells, but not in the interior of the cells (Figure 8, right).

0 min

1 min

2 min

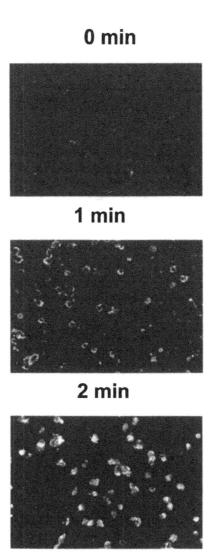

Figure 10. Laser scanning confocal photomicrographs of endothelial cells showing time course of thrombin effect on distribution of β_1 integrin. Endothelial cells were treated with thrombin for 0, 1, or 2 minutes then immediately fixed and stained. Whole cell fluorescence was observed using laser scanning confocal microscopy.

Serial sections of untreated cells showed no β_1 signal (Figure 8, left).[131] Similar results were observed for integrin β_3 expression on thrombin-treated endothelial cells (data not shown).

To further test the association between endothelial cell contraction and the availability of β_1 integrins, we pretreated cells with phallicidin, an inhibitor of actin-mediated cell contraction,[122] before thrombin exposure. Phallicidin concentrations ≤ 0.1 μM did not cause cytotoxicity, as measured by trypan blue dye exclusion, but, as shown in Figure 9 did protect against thrombin-induced endothelial cell contraction (phase contrast, PC) and against β_1 integrin expression (immunofluorescence, IF). These data further document a correlation between cell contraction and β_1 expression.[131]

We predicted that if β_1 integrins were being redistributed from the basal surface to the luminal surface, they should first appear at the edges of the contracting cell before they diffuse to the luminal membrane surface. When thrombin-treated cells are imaged using IF-LSCM, after 0 minutes minimal β_1 expression is seen (Figure 10), after 1 minute most of the cell edges express β_1, and after 2 minutes redistribution is complete on most cells, with integrin β_1 seen over the entire luminal surface.[131]

These results indicate that fibronectin and the β_1 and β_3 integrins provide a portion of the thrombin-induced adhesogenic response, and others have posited that matrix thrombospondin also contributes to this process.[135] Our data indicate that the integrins are liberated from their abluminal matrix tethers to redistribute over the cell membrane by means of an actin-dependent mechanism. Since in our studies the adhesivity attributable to β_1 or β_3 integrins or to gap formation does not account for all of thrombin-enhanced adhesivity, we conclude that other mechanisms also must participate in this adhesogenic response.

Thrombin-Enhanced Sickle Cell Adhesion Is Partly to P-selectin

The rapidity of thrombin-induced endothelial adhesogenic response is similar to the rate of P-selectin relocation from storage in Weibel-Palade bodies to the plasma membrane.[136–138] Accordingly, we tested for the participation of P-selectin in the thrombin-induced adhesogenic response we had been studying.[138a] Despite the temporal consistency of our findings with the participation of P-selectin, this C-type selectin and its counter-receptors and ligands are known to provide specificity to adhesive interactions among endothelial cells, platelets, and leukocytes,[139–144] but not erythrocytes.[145] P-selectin ligands on the opposing cells derive specificity from their component fucose, sialic acid, and sulfate recognition determinants and from the particular transferases employed in their generation.[139–144,146]

To assess whether P-selectin on thrombin-treated endothelial cells was active in the adhesogenic response, we compared the effects of P-selectin blocking and nonblocking mAb on the static adherence of nonsickle and sickle red cells to thrombin-treated and untreated HU-VEC monolayers. The data shown in Figure 11 A are consistent with the known greater adherence of sickle cells to resting endothelial cells compared to nonsickle erythrocytes and the enhanced adherence of both by thrombin-treatment of the endothelium. Figure 11 A also shows that blocking endothelial monolayers with mAb 9E1 reduced the adherence of nonsickle red cells by 21% to untreated endothelium and 51% to thrombin-treated endothelium and of sickle cells by 30% to un-treated endothelium and 76% to thrombin-treated endothelium. We also compared the effects of paired blocking and nonblocking P-se-lectin mAb 9E1 and AC1.2. Treatment of the monolayer with AC1.2 failed to reduce significantly the adherence of either nonsickle or sickle cells from that observed without mAb. Treatment with 9E1 signifi-cantly reduced adherence by 48% for nonsickle cells and 58% for sickle cells from the levels of adherence observed with AC1.2. Taken together, these data provide evidence for the novel adherence of normal and, to a greater extent, sickle erythrocytes to endothelial cell P-selectin. [138a] The incomplete inhibition afforded by P-selectin mAb indicates that P-selectin independent pathways also contribute to thrombin-en-hanced adherence. Further evidence for the involvement of other path-ways was derived from a concentration curve experiment, in which we found that the adherence of nonsickle and sickle cells was reduced, re-spectively, 64% and 70% by a 1:2000 dilution of the mAb, 72% and 84% by a 1:200 dilution, and 66% and 83% by a 1:20 dilution (Figure 11 B). The failure of a 1:20 titer to abrogate adherence totally further supports the involvement of other adhesion pathways.[138a]

Because sialyl Lewis X antigen (sLeX) is a recognition determinant for selectins that selectively inhibits their adhesivity,[139–141,143,144,146] we compared the inhibitory effects of adding sLeX tetrasaccharide or sLac (3'-sialyl-lactose, a structurally related saccharide that does not bind to P-selectin) to the static adherence assay. We compared the static ad-herence of red cells to endothelial cells in the absence of saccharide and the presence of sLac or sLeX. The level of adherence to untreated or to thrombin-treated endothelial cells was not reduced significantly by the addition of sLac for either nonsickle or sickle cells (Figure 12). The in-hibitory effect of sLeX on adherence was not significant with untreated endothelial cells but was significant with thrombin-treated cells. Al-though not significant, the adherence to untreated endothelial cells was reduced by sLeX 48% for nonsickle and 37% for sickle cells, compared

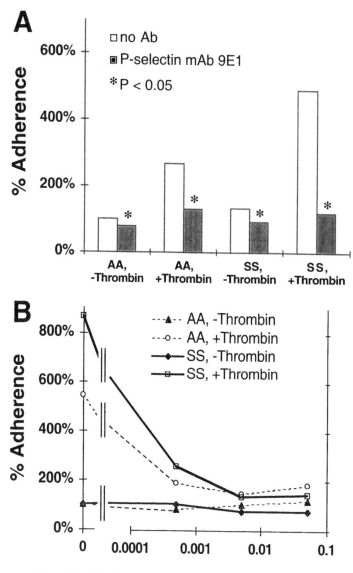

Figure 11. Effect of P-selectin antibodies on the adherence of nonsickle (AA) and sickle (SS) erythrocytes (RBC) to HUVEC treated with (+) or without (−) thrombin. The data shown are the static adherence of red blood cells (RBC) to HUVEC that were treated with thrombin or medium alone and then exposed to medium with or without blocking P-selectin antibody 9E1. 100% adherence is the mean number of AA RBC/field adherent to untreated HUVEC. A, the reduction of erythrocyte adherence to untreated or thrombin-treated HUVEC in the presence or absence of mAb 9E1. The data are mean % adherence from 12 replicate experiments. Significant inhibition of adherence due to mAb 9E1 with $P<0.05$ was denoted by an asterisk (*). B, titration of adhesion inhibition by mAb 9E1. The data from this experiment are mean % adherence plotted vs. the dilution of mAb 9E1.

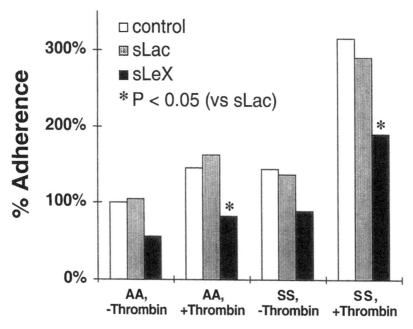

Figure 12. Effect of sLeX tetrasaccharide on the adherence of nonsickle (AA) and sickle (SS) erythrocytes to HUVEC treated with (+) or without (−) thrombin. The data shown are the static adherence of red blood cells (RBC) to HUVEC that were treated with thrombin or medium alone. 100% adherence is the mean number of AA RBC/field adherent to untreated HUVEC. There is a reduction of erythrocyte adherence to untreated or thrombin-treated HUVEC in the presence of sLeX tetrasaccharide. The data are mean % adherence from 4 replicate experiments. Significant inhibition of adherence due to sLeX with $P<0.05$ was denoted by an asterisk (*).

to adherence levels with sLac present. Adherence to thrombin-treated monolayers was reduced significantly by sLeX 49% for nonsickle and 36% for sickle cells, compared to levels with sLac present. These findings are consistent with the adhesion of nonsickle and sickle erythrocytes to P-selectin on activated endothelial cells.[138a] The incomplete inhibition observed with sLeX is not surprising since the inhibitory potency of this saccharide for P-selectin, while specific, is not strong.[143] The lack of sLac effect confirms the specificity of sLeX for P-selectin in the static adhesion assay. To confirm that the P-selectin mAb 9E1 and sLeX affect the same molecular interaction,[143] we compared these inhibitors singly and in combination. Adherence to thrombin-treated endothelial cells was inhibited to similar levels by mAb 9E1, sLeX, and their combination for nonsickle cells (17–22%) and for sickle cells (43–47%). The lack of additive effect confirms that in our system, sLeX and P-selectin participate in the same molecular interaction. Since the combination of inhibitors failed to completely abrogate adherence, these data provide further evidence for a P-selectin independent adhesion pathway to thrombin-treated endothelial cells. We also performed a flow cytometry study of nonsickle and sickle red cells using P-selectin mAb AC1.2 and 9E1 to confirm that the P-selectin blocking by sLeX was on endothelial rather than red cells. We detected no signal indicative of the presence of P-selectin on either type of erythrocyte (data not shown), which is consistent with the reported absence of P-selectin from erythroid cells.[147]

The results from our studies on thrombin-activated endothelial cells reflect the participation of adhesion molecules besides P-selectin, as with leukocyte-endothelial interactions. Selectin interactions initiate and are required for leukocyte adherence. To confirm the role of P-selectin in sickle cell adhesion, we used a rotatory adherence assay[148] to test the nonstatic adhesion of erythrocytes to a recombinant P-selectin-Ig chimera[149] immobilized on plastic microtiter wells. The data in Figure 13 compare the adherence of red cells to P-selectin, BSA, or nonbinding Siglec-6 or mutated Siglec-7 chimeras that share the Ig-Fc domain with the P-selectin construct.[149,150] The adherence of nonsickle cells to P-selectin is a significant 46% greater than to BSA and a nearly significant 41% greater than to Siglec-6 or mutated Siglec-7, and of sickle cells to P-selectin is 72% greater than to BSA and 74% greater than to Siglec-6 or mutated Siglec-7. 5 mM EDTA reduced the adherence to P-selectin by 35% for nonsickle cells and 32% for sickle cells. These differences provide further evidence that normal and, to a larger measure, sickle erythrocytes adhere to P-selectin.[138a] The significant reduction of binding caused by chelating calcium with EDTA confirms the specificity of P-selectin binding. It has been established that P-selectin has 2 binding components: one that is EDTA sensitive and one that is relatively EDTA insensitive (requiring 20 mM).[151] The second component, which is inhibited by the polycarboxylic acid nature of EDTA rather than its calcium-chelating capacity, may represent the second anion binding site of P-selectin. Our finding of nontotal inhibition of erythrocyte adherence to thrombin-activated endothelial cells using blocking P-selectin mAb, sLeX, or 5 mM EDTA indicates the presence of P-selectin independent mechanisms. Other possible mechanisms include the use of the second binding site of endothelial P-selectin[151] and the adhesion of endothelial P-selectin to sulfatide in erythrocyte membranes.[152–155] A sulfated lipid purified from sickle cell membranes that binds TSP and laminin and is resistant to sialidase treatment[23] may comprise at least a portion of the sialidase-resistant component that we identified.

The above findings indicate the presence of a P-selectin ligand on normal erythrocytes, which is enhanced markedly on sickle cells. The only published description of P-selectin binding activity by mature erythrocytes is that of malarial parasitized cells, which appears to have

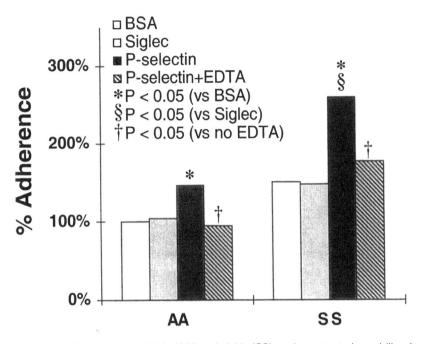

Figure 13. Adhesion of nonsickle (AA) and sickle (SS) erythrocytes to immobilized siglec-6, P-selectin, or P-selectin in the presence of EDTA. The data shown are the nonstatic adherence (in the rotatory adhesion assay) of untreated or sialidase-treated red blood cells (RBC) to immobilized BSA, Siglec-Ig chimera, P-selectin-Ig chimera, or P-selectin-Ig chimera in the presence of 5-mM EDTA. 100% adherence is the mean number of untreated AA RBC/field in a well in which BSA was immobilized. The data are mean % adherence for 4 nonsickle and 6 sickle red cell samples. Significant differences in adherence with $P<0.05$ was determined to be significant. We use symbols to designate significant adhesion compared to adhesion to BSA (*), significant adhesion compared to adhesion to Siglec (§), and significant inhibition of adhesion to P-selectin due to EDTA (†).

been malarial in origin.[156,157] Ligand activity for P-selectin is conveyed by sialylated, fucosylated, sulfated recognition determinants of membrane glycoproteins and glycolipids.[141,144] We found no flow cytometry signal using the mAb 2PH1, which is specific for P-selectin glycoprotein ligand-1 (PSGL-1), and KPL1, which is specific for tyrosine sulfated PSGL-1, which indicates that the erythrocyte binding determinant is distinct from previously known P-selectin ligands (data not shown).[146] However, we did detect a signal from a fraction of sickle cells using the sLeX mAb HECA-452,[141] the intensity of which varied among patients and over time (data not shown).

To assess the role of membrane sialic acid as a P-selectin binding determinant we treated red cells with sialidase before assaying their static adherence to endothelial cell monolayers.[148] Sialidase treatment reduced

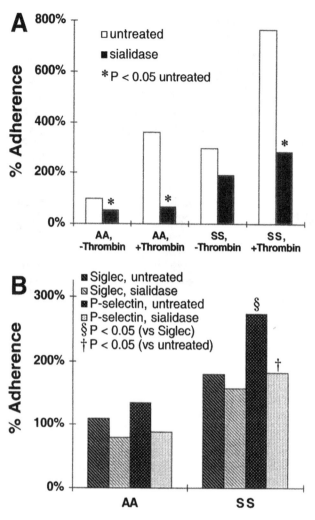

Figure 14. Effect of sialidase treatment of nonsickle (AA) and sickle (SS) erythrocytes on their adherence to HUVEC treated with (+) or without (−) thrombin and to immobilized siglec-6 or P-selectin. The data shown are the adherence of red blood cells (RBC) that had or had not been treated with sialidase either to HUVEC which had been treated with thrombin or medium alone or to immobilized BSA, Ig-Ig chimera, or P-selectin-Ig chimera. 100% adherence is the mean number of untreated AA RBC/field adherent to untreated HUVEC. (A) the reduction of static erythrocyte adherence to untreated or thrombin-treated HUVEC due to treatment of the red cells with sialidase. The data are mean % adherence from 4 replicate experiments. Significant inhibition due to sialidase with P<0.05 was denoted by an asterisk (*). (B) the reduction of nonstatic erythrocyte adherence to immobilized Siglec-6 or P-selectin due to treatment of the red cells with sialidase. The data are mean % adherence for 3 nonsickle and 5 sickle red cell samples. We use symbols to designate significant adhesion (P<0.05) compared to adhesion to Siglec-6 (§) and significant inhibition of adhesion to P-selectin due to sialidase (†).

adherence to untreated monolayers by 47% for nonsickle cells and by 36% for sickle cells and to thrombin-treated monolayers by 81% for nonsickle and 63% for sickle cells (Figure 14 A). To confirm the importance of sialic acid to the erythrocyte P-selectin ligand, we also treated red cells with sialidase before assaying their nonstatic adherence to P-selectin or to control Siglec-6. The results (Figure 14 B) demonstrate that sialidase had no significant effect on the adherence of nonsickle cells to Siglec-6 or to P-selectin. Sialidase also had no significant effect on the adherence of sickle cells to Siglec-6 ($P=0.089$) but caused a significant 33% reduction in their adherence to P-selectin ($P=0.004$). The finding that sialidase causes a statistically significant reduction in the adherence of sickle cells to P-selectin is consistent with the sialidase effects on sickle cell binding to thrombin-treated HUVEC described above. These results further support the partial characterization of a sickle cell P-selectin ligand, which employs sialic acid as a recognition determinant.[138a] Thus, this novel erythrocyte P-selectin ligand has sialic acid as a recognition determinant. To verify the canonical requirement for sialic acid of P-selectin binding,[143,148] we compared the singular and combined effects of treating red cells with sialidase and endothelial cells with mAb 9E1. Adherence to thrombin-treated endothelial cells was inhibited similarly by sialidase, mAb 9E1, and their combination for nonsickle (17–24%) and for sickle cells (29–38%). The lack of additive effect supports the participation of sialic acid and P-selectin in the same molecular interaction and confirms that red cell adhesion to P-selectin requires sialidase as a recognition determinant. The possibility of a sialidase-sensitive pathway not involving P-selectin exists.

Summary and Conclusions

The importance of vascular contributions to sickle cell pathophysiology is now widely accepted. Besides the abnormal adhesivity of sickle red cells, conditions and agonists that elicit endothelial cell adhesogenic responses also promote vaso-occlusion. We and others have shown that thrombin enhances the adhesivity of the vascular endothelium, and work from our laboratory has demonstrated the novel adhesion of sickle cells to P-selectin on activated endothelial cells. Comparisons of the molecular mechanisms of sickle cell adhesion with those of leukocyte adhesion may disclose the importance of P-selectin to sickle cell vaso-occlusion. Transient adhesion and rolling of leukocytes are facilitated by the rapid on-off kinetics of selectins, and firm adhesion is mediated by higher affinity receptors. For leukocyte adherence, the action of selectins is essential. Now P-selectin has joined integrins and members of the immunoglobulin superfamily as a molecule of sickle cell adherence. Whether it is required for sickle cell adhesion remains to be determined.

Opportunities for therapy based on inhibiting cell activation via PAR,[58,158] preventing activation of NF-κB,[159] and inhibiting upregulated integrins[16,50,160] have been described. The recognition of P-selectin as a participant in sickle cell adhesion and vaso-occlusion now presents an opportunity to explore therapeutic approaches involving inhibition of P-selectin. Such approaches include anti-P-selectin antibodies, P-selectin-Ig chimeras, inhibitory peptides derived from P-selectin sequences, glycan components of known P-selectin ligands, and pharmacomimetic agents of endogenous ligands such as sLeX mimics, and heparin.[23,151,161–163] The report that heparin therapy may be efficacious prophylactically[164] suggests that heparin therapy be validated promptly since there is much clinical experience with the use of heparin.

References

1. Embury SH, Hebbel RP, Mohandas N, Steinberg MH. *Sickle Cell Anemia: Basic Principles and Clinical Practice.* New York: Raven Press; 1994:1–902.
2. Eaton WA, Hofrichter J. Sickle cell hemoglobin polymerization. *Adv Prot Chem* 1990;40:63–279.
3. Dean J, Schechter AN. Sickle cell anemia: Molecular and cellular basis of therapeutic approaches. *N Engl J Med* 1978;299:752–870.
4. Embury SH, Hebbel RP, Mohandas N, Steinberg MH. Pathogenesis of vasoocclusion. In Embury SH, Hebbel RP, Mohandas N, et al., eds: *Sickle Cell Disease: Basic Principles and Clinical Practice.* New York: Raven Press; 1994:311–326.
5. Ferrone FA, Cho MR, Bishop MF. Can a successful mechanism for HbS gelation predict sickle cell crisis? In Beuzard Y, Charache S, Galacteros F, eds: *Approaches to the Therapy of Sickle Cell Anemia.* Paris: Les Editions Inserm; 1985:53–66.
6. Platt OS, Thorington BD, Brambilla DJ, et al. The Cooperative Study of Sickle Cell Disease. Pain in sickle cell disease: Rates and risk factors. *N Engl J Med* 1991;325:11–16.
7. Francis RB, Johnson CS. Vascular occlusion in sickle cell disease: Current concepts, unanswered questions. *Blood* 1991;77:1405–1414.
8. Faller DV. Vascular modulation. In Embury SH, Hebbel RP, Mohandas N, et al., eds: *Sickle Cell Disease: Basic Principles and Clinical Practice.* New York: Raven Press; 1994:235–246.
9. Wick TM, Eckman JR. Molecular basis of sickle cell-endothelial cell interactions. *Curr Opin Hematol* 1996;3:118–124.
10. Hebbel RP, Mohandas N. Sickle cell adherence. In Embury SH, Hebbel RP, Mohandas N, et al., eds: *Sickle Cell Disease: Basic Principles and Clinical Practice.* New York: Raven Press; 1994:217–230.
11. Hoover R, Rubin R, Wise G, Warren R. Adhesion of normal sickle erythrocytes to endothelial monolayer cultures. *Blood* 1979;54:872–876.
12. Hebbel RP, Yamada O, Moldow CF, et al. Abnormal adherence of sickle erythrocytes to cultured vascular endothelium: Possible mechanism for microvascular occlusion in sickle cell disease. *J Clin Invest* 1980;65:154–160.

13. Hebbel RP, Boogaerts MAB, Eaton JW, et al. Erythrocyte adherence to endothelium in sickle cell anemia. *N Engl J Med* 1980;302:992–995.
14. Hebbel RP. Adhesive interactions of sickle erythrocytes with endothelium. *J Clin Invest* 1997;99:2561–2564.
15. Kaul DK, Fabry ME, Nagel RL. Microvascular sites and characteristics of sickle cell adhesion to vascular endothelium in shear flow conditions: Pathophysiological implications. *Proc Natl Acad Sci USA* 1989;86:3356–3360.
16. Harlan JM. Introduction: Anti-adhesion therapy in sickle cell disease. *Blood* 2000;95:365–367.
17. Udani M, Zen Q, Cottman M, Leonard N, et al. Basal cell adhesion molecule/Lutheran protein: The receptor critical for sickle cell adhesion to laminin. *J Clin Invest* 1998;101:2550–2558.
18. Setty BN, Stuart MJ. Vascular cell adhesion molecule-1 is involved in mediating hypoxia-induced sickle red blood cell adherence to endothelium: Potential role in sickle cell disease. *Blood* 1996;88:2311–2320.
19. Hebbel RP, Visser MR, Goodman JL, Jacob HS, et al. Potentiated adherence of sickle erythrocytes to endothelium infected by virus. *J Clin Invest* 1987;80:1503–1506.
20. Thevenin BJM, Crandall I, Ballas SK, Sherman IW, et al. Band 3 peptides block the adherence of sickle cells to endothelial cells in vitro. *Blood* 1997;90:4172–4179.
21. Brittain JE, Mlinar KJ, Anderson CS, et al. Activation of sickle red blood cell adhesion via integrin-associated protein/CD47-induced signal transduction. *J Clin Invest* 2001;107:1555–1562.
22. Kaul DK. Flow properties and endothelial adhesion of sickle erythrocytes in an *ex vivo* microvascular preparation. In Ohnishi ST, Ohnishi T, eds: *Membrane Abnormalities in Sickle Cell Disease and in Other Red Blood Cell Disorders: CRC Series in Membrane-Linked Diseases*. Boca Raton: CRC Press; 1994:217–240.
23. Hillery CA, Du MC, Montgomery RR, Scott JP. Increased adhesion of erythrocytes to components of the extracellular matrix: Isolation and characterization of a red blood cell lipid that binds thrombospondin and laminin. *Blood* 1996;87:4879–4886.
24. Kumar A, Eckman JR, Swerlick RA, Wick TM. Phorbol ester stimulation increases sickle erythrocyte adherence to endothelium: A novel pathway involving alpha 4 beta 1 integrin receptors on sickle reticulocytes and fibronectin. *Blood* 1996;88:4348–4358.
25. Brittain JE, Mlinar KJ, Anderson CS, et al. Integrin-associated protein is an adhesion receptor on sickle red blood cells for immobilized thrombospondin. *Blood* 2001;97:2159–2164.
26. Gabay C, Kushner I. Acute-phase proteins and other systemic responses to inflammation. *N Engl J Med* 1999;340:448–454.
27. Stuart J, Stone PC, Akinola NO, et al. Monitoring the acute phase response to vaso-occlusive crisis in sickle cell disease. *J Clin Pathol* 1994;47:166–169.
28. Ginsberg MH, Ruggeri ZV, Varki AP. Perspectives series: Cell adhesion in vascular biology. *J Clin Invest* 1997;100(Suppl):S1–S105.
29. Moore CM, Ehlayel M, Leiva LE, Sorensen RU. New concepts in the immunology of sickle cell disease. *Ann Allergy Asthma Immunol* 1996;76:385–400.
30. Cines DB, Pollak ES, Buck CA, Loscalzo J, et al. Endothelial cells in phys-

iology and in the pathophysiology of vascular disorders. *Blood* 1998;91: 3527–3561.

31. Nadeau K, Gee B, Jennette JC, et al. Increased inflammatory and endothelial cell factors in tissues from humans and mice with sickle cell disease. *Blood* 1997;90 (Suppl 1):125A (abstract).
32. Duits AJ, Pieters RC, Saleh AW, et al. Enhanced levels of soluble VCAM-1 in sickle cell patients and their specific increment during vasoocclusive crisis. *Clin Immunol Immunopathol* 1996;81:96–98.
33. Solovey A, Lin Y, Browne P, et al. Circulating activated endothelial cells in sickle cell anemia. *N Engl J Med* 1997;337:1584–1589.
34. Solovey A, Gui L, Key NS, Hebbel RP. Tissue factor expression by endothelial cells in sickle cell anemia. *J Clin Invest* 1998;101:1899–1904.
35. Zimmerman GA, McIntyre TM, Prescott SM. Thrombin stimulates the adherence of neutrophils to human endothelial cells in vitro. *J Clin Invest* 1985;76:2235–2246.
36. Manodori AB, Matsui NM, Chen JY, Embury SH. Enhanced adherence of sickle erythrocytes to thrombin-treated endothelial cells involves interendothelial cell gap formation. *Blood* 1998;92:3445–3454.
37. Natarajan M, Udden MM, McIntire LV. Adhesion of sickle red blood cells and damage to interleukin-1β stimulated endothelial cells under flow in vitro. *Blood* 1996;87:4845–4852.
38. Vordermeier S, Singh S, Biggerstaff J, et al. Red blood cells from patients with sickle cell disease exhibit an increased adherence to cultured endothelium pretreated with tumour necrosis factor (TNF). *Br J Haematol* 1992;81:591–597.
39. Tannenbaum SH, Gralnick HR. Gamma-interferon modulates von Willebrand factor release by cultured human endothelial cells. *Blood* 1990;75: 2177–2184.
40. Asako H, Kurose I, Wolf R, et al. Role of H1 receptors and P-selectin in histamine-induced leukocyte rolling and adhesion in postcapillary venules. *J Clin Invest* 1994;93:1508–1515.
41. Defilippi P, Truffa G, Stefanuto G, et al. Tumor necrosis factor α and interferon γ modulate the expression of the vitronectin receptor (integrin β₃) in human endothelial cells. *J Biol Chem* 1991;266:7638–7645.
42. Ribatti D, Presta M, Vacca A, et al. Human erythropoietin induces a proangiogenic phenotype in cultured endothelial cells and stimulates neovascularization in vivo. *Blood* 1999;93:2627–2636.
43. Carlini RG, Reyes AA, Rothstein M. Recombinant human erythropoietin stimulates angiogenesis in vitro. *Kidney Int* 1995;47:740–745.
44. Patel KD, Zimmerman GA, Prescott SM, et al. Oxygen radicals induce human endothelial cells to express GMP-140 and bind neutrophils. *J Cell Biol* 1991;112:749–759.
45. Rank BH, Carlsson J, Hebbel RP. Abnormal redox status of membrane-protein thiols in sickle erythrocytes. *J Clin Invest* 1985;75:1531–1537.
46. Smolinski PA, Offerman MK, Eckman JR, Wick TM: Double-stranded RNA induces sickle erythrocyte adherence to endothelium: A potential role for viral infection in vaso-occlusive pain episodes in sickle cell anemia. *Blood* 1995;85:2945–2950.
47. Shiu YT, Udden MM, McIntire LV. Perfusion with sickle erythrocytes upregulates ICAM-1 and VCAM-1 gene expression in cultured human endothelial cells. *Blood* 2000;95:3232–3241.

48. Osarogiagbon UR, Choong S, Belcher JD, et al. Reperfusion injury pathophysiology in sickle transgenic mice. *Blood* 2000;96:314–320.
49. Kaul DK, Hebbel RP. Hypoxia/reoxygenation causes inflammatory response in transgenic sickle mice but not in normal mice. *J Clin Invest* 2000;106:411–420.
50. Kaul DK, Tsai HM, Liu XD, et al. Monoclonal antibodies to $\alpha_V\beta_3$ (7E3 and LM609) inhibit sickle red blood cell-endothelium interactions induced by platelet-activating factor. *Blood* 2000;95:368–374.
51. Makis AC, Hatzimichael EC, Bourantas KL. The role of cytokines in sickle cell disease. *Ann Hematol* 2000;79:407–413.
52. Bourantas KL, Dalekos GN, Makis A, et al. Acute phase proteins and interleukins in steady state sickle cell disease. *Eur J Haematol* 1998;61:49–54.
53. Taylor SC, Shacks SJ, Qu Z. In vivo production of type 1 cytokines in healthy sickle cell disease patients. *J Natl Med Assoc* 1999;91:619–624.
54. Wun T. The role of inflammation and leukocytes in the pathogenesis of sickle cell disease. *Ann Hematol* 2001;5:403–412.
55. Chui DH, Dover GJ. Sickle cell disease: No longer a single gene disorder. *Curr Opin Pediatr* 2001;13:22–27.
56. Esmon CT. Inflammation and thrombosis: The impact of inflammation on the protein C anticoagulant pathway. *Haematologica (Pavia)* 1995;80(Suppl 2):49–56.
57. Esmon CT. Introduction: Are natural anticoagulants candidates for modulating the inflammatory response to endotoxin? *Blood* 2000;95:1113–1116.
58. Coughlin SR. Thrombin signaling and protease-activated receptors. *Nature* 2000;407:258–264.
59. Francis RB. Platelets, coagulation, and fibrinolysis in sickle cell disease: Their possible role in vascular occlusion. *Blood Coagul Fibrinol* 1991;2:341–353.
60. Francis RB Jr, Hebbel RP. Hemostasis. In Embury SH, Hebbel RP, Mohandas N, et al., eds: *Sickle Cell Disease: Basic Principles and Clinical Practice*. New York: Raven Press; 1994:299–310.
61. Wolters HJ, ten Cate H, Thomas LLM, et al. Low-intensity oral anticoagulation in sickle-cell disease reverses the prothrombotic state: Promises for treatment? *Br J Haematol* 1995;90:715–717.
62. Kurantsin-Mills J, Ofosu FA, Safa TK, et al. Plasma factor VII and thrombin-antithrombin III levels indicate increased tissue factor activity in sickle cell patients. *Br J Haematol* 1992;81:539–544.
63. Francis RB. Elevated fibrin D-dimer fragment in sickle cell anemia: Evidence for activation of coagulation during the steady state as well as in painful crisis. *Haemostasis* 1989;19:105–111.
64. Leslie J, Langler D, Serjeant GR, et al. Coagulation changes during the steady state in homozygous sickle-cell disease in Jamaica. *Br J Haematol* 1975;30:159–166.
65. Gordon EM, Klein BL, Berman BW, et al. Reduction of contact factors in sickle cell disease. *J Pediatr* 1985;106:427–430.
66. Famodu AA. Coagulation changes in homozygous sickle cell disease in Nigeria [letter]. *J Clin Pathol* 1987;40:1487.
67. Green D, Scott JP. Is sickle cell crisis a thrombotic event? *Am J Hematol* 1986;23:317–321.
68. Francis RB Jr. Protein S deficiency in sickle cell anemia. *J Lab Clin Med* 1988;111:571–576.
69. Karayalcin G, Chung D, Pinto P, Lanzkowsky P. Plasma antithrombin III

levels in children with homozygous sickle cell disease (SCD). *Pediatr Res* 1984;18:242A (abstract).

70. Sugihara K, Sugihara T, Mohandas N, Hebbel RP. Thrombospondin mediates adherence of CD 36+ sickle reticulocytes to endothelial cells. *Blood* 1992;80:2634–2642.

71. Browne PV, Mosher DF, Steinberg MH, Hebbel RP. Disturbance of plasma and platelet thrombospondin levels in sickle cell disease. *Am J Hematol* 1996;51:296–301.

72. Foulon I, Bachir D, Galacteros F, Maclouf J. Increased in vivo production of thromboxane in patients with sickle cell disease is accompanied by an impairment of platelet functions to the thromboxane A2 agonist U46619. *Arterioscler Thromb* 1993;13:421–426.

73. Ibe BO, Kurantsin-Mills J, Raj JU, Lessin LS. Plasma and urinary leukotrienes in sickle cell disease: Possible role in the inflammatory process [see comments]. *Eur J Clin Invest* 1994;24:57–64.

74. Key NS, Slungaard A, Dandelet L, et al. Whole blood tissue factor procoagulant activity is elevated in patients with sickle cell disease. *Blood* 1998;91:4216–4223.

75. Collins PW, Noble KE, Reittie JR, et al. Induction of tissue factor expression in human monocyte/endothelium cocultures. *Br J Haematol* 1995;91: 963–970.

76. Lewis JC, Jones NL, Hermanns MI, et al. Tissue factor expression during coculture of endothelial cells and monocytes. *Exp Mol Pathol* 1995;62: 207–218.

77. Lo SK, Cheung A, Zheng Q, Silverstein RL. Induction of tissue factor on monocytes by adhesion to endothelial cells. *J Immunol* 1995;154:4768–4777.

78. Key NS, Slungaard A, Dandelet L, et al. Whole blood tissue factor procoagulant activity is elevated in patients with sickle cell disease. *Blood* 1998;91:4216–4223.

79. Chiu DD, Lubin B, Shohet SB. Erythrocyte membrane lipid reorganization during the sickling process. *Br J Haematol* 1979;41:223–234.

80. Chiu D, Lubin B, Roelofsen B, van Deenen LLM. Sickled erythrocytes accelerate clotting in vitro: An effect of abnormal membrane lipid assymetry. *Blood* 1981;58:398–401.

81. Lubin B, Chiu D, Bastacky J, et al. Abnormalities in membrane phospholipid organization in sickled erythrocytes. *J Clin Invest* 1981;67:1643.

82. Shuman MA. Thrombin-cellular interactions. *Ann NY Acad Sci* 1986;485: 228–239.

83. Garcia JG, Pavalko FM, Patterson CE. Vascular endothelial cell activation and permeability responses to thrombin. *Blood Coagul Fibrinol* 1995;6: 609–626.

84. Garcia JGN. Molecular mechanisms of thrombin-induced human and bovine endothelial cell activation. *J Lab Clin Med* 1992;120:513–519.

85. Carveth HJ, Shaddy RE, Whatley RE, et al. Regulation of platelet-activating factor (PAF) synthesis and PAF-mediated neutrophil adhesion to endothelial cells activated by thrombin. *Semin Thrombos Hemostas* 1992;18:126–134.

86. Sugama Y, Tiruppathi C, Janakidevi K, et al. Thrombin-induced expression of endothelial P-selectin and intercellular adhesion molecule-1: A mechanism for stabilizing neutrophil adhesion. *J Cell Biol* 1992;119:935–944.

87. Granger DN, Korthuis RJ. Physiologic mechanisms of postischemic tissue injury. *Ann Rev Physiol* 1995;57:311–332.

88. Harlan JM, Killen PD, Harker LA, et al. Neutrophil-mediated endothelial injury in vitro mechanisms of cell detachment. *J Clin Invest* 1981;68:1394–1403.

89. Lum H, Malik AB. Regulation of vascular endothelial barrier function. *Am J Physiol* 1994;267:L223–L241.
90. West MS, Wethers D, Smith J, Steinberg M. The Cooperative Study of Sickle Cell Disease. Laboratory profile of sickle cell disease: A cross-sectional analysis. *J Clin Epidemiol* 1992;45:893–909.
91. Hofstra TC, Kalra VK, Meiselman HJ, Coates TD. Sickle erythrocytes adhere to polymorphonuclear neutrophils and activate the neutrophil respiratory burst. *Blood* 1996;87:4440–4447.
92. Lum H, Aschner JL, Phillips PG, et al. Time course of thrombin-induced increase in endothelial permeability: Relationship to $Ca^{2+}i$ and inositol polyphosphates. *Am J Physiol Lung Cell Mol Physiol* 1992;263:L219–L225.
93. Laposata M, Dovnarsky DK, Shin HS. Thrombin-induced gap formation in confluent endothelial cell monolayers in vitro. *Blood* 1983;62:549–556.
94. Patterson CE, Rhoades RA, Garcia JG. Evans blue dye as a marker of albumin clearance in cultured endothelial monolayer and isolated lung. *J Appl Physiol* 1992;72:865–873.
95. Stasek JE Jr, Garcia JG. The role of protein kinase C in alpha-thrombin-mediated endothelial cell activation. *Semin Thromb Hemostas* 1992;18:117–125.
96. Verin AD, Patterson CE, Day MA, Garcia JG. Regulation of endothelial cell gap formation and barrier function by myosin-associated phosphatase activities. *Am J Physiol* 1995;269:L99–108.
97. Garcia JG, Schaphorst KL. Regulation of endothelial cell gap formation and paracellular permeability. *J Invest Med* 1995;43:117–126.
98. Goeckeler ZM, Wyslomerski RB. Myosin light chain kinase-regulated endothelial cell contraction: The relationship between isometric tension, actin polymerization, and myosin phosphorylation. *J Cell Biol* 1995;130:613–627.
99. Albelda SM, Smith CW, Ward PA. Adhesion molecules and inflammatory injury. *FASEB J* 1994;8:504–512.
100. Cotran RS, Mayadas-Norton T. Endothelial adhesion molecules in health and disease. *Pathol Biol (Paris)* 1998;46:164–170.
101. Celi A, Lorenzet R, Furie B, Furie BC. Platelet-leukocyte-endothelial cell interaction on the blood vessel wall. *Semin Hematol* 1997;34:327–335.
102. Winn R, Vedder N, Ramamoorthy C, et al. Endothelial and leukocyte adhesion molecules in inflammation and disease. *Blood Coagul Fibrinolysis* 1998;9(Suppl 2):S17–S23.
103. Pober JS. Immunobiology of human vascular endothelium. *Immunol Res* 1999;19:225–232.
104. Subramanian M, Saffaripour S, Van De Water L, et al. Role of endothelial selectins in wound repair. *Am J Pathol* 1997;150:1701–1709.
105. Jordan JE, Zhao ZQ, Vinten-Johansen J. The role of neutrophils in myocardial ischemia-reperfusion injury. *Cardiovasc Res* 1999;43:860–878.
106. Granger DN. Ischemia-reperfusion: Mechanisms of microvascular dysfunction and the influence of risk factors for cardiovascular disease. *Microcirculation* 1999;6:167–178.
107. del Zoppo G, Ginis I, Hallenbeck JM, et al. Inflammation and stroke: Putative role for cytokines, adhesion molecules and iNOS in brain response to ischemia. *Brain Pathol* 2000;10:95–112.
108. Barone FC, Feuerstein GZ. Inflammatory mediators and stroke: New opportunities for novel therapeutics. *J Cereb Blood Flow Metab* 1999;19:819–834.
109. Granger DN, Kvietys PR, Perry MA. Leukocyte-endothelial cell adhesion induced by ischemia and reperfusion. *Can J Physiol Pharmacol* 1993;71:67–75.
110. Sobral do Rosario H, Saldanha C, Martins S. Increased leukocyte-en-

dothelial interaction in the mesenteric microcirculation following remote ischemia-reperfusion. *Microvasc Res* 1999;57:199–202.

111. Esmon CT, Fukudome K, Mather T, et al. Inflammation, sepsis, and coagulation. *Haematologica* 1999;84:254–259.

112. Smith PD: Neutrophil activation and mediators of inflammation in chronic venous insufficiency. *J Vasc Res* 1999;36(Suppl 1):24–36.

113. Vogel RA. Cholesterol lowering and endothelial function. *Am J Med* 1999;107:479–487.

114. Quarmby S, Kumar P, Kumar S. Radiation-induced normal tissue injury: Role of adhesion molecules in leukocyte-endothelial cell interactions. *Int J Cancer* 1999;82:385–395.

115. Salas A, Panes J, Elizalde JI, et al. Mechanisms responsible for enhanced inflammatory response to ischemia-reperfusion in diabetes. *Am J Physiol* 1998;275:H1773–H1781.

116. Cosentino F, Luscher TF. Endothelial dysfunction in diabetes mellitus. *J Cardiovasc Pharmacol* 1998;32(Suppl 3):S54–S61.

117. Rosenkranz AR, Mendrick DL, Cotran RS, et al. P-selectin deficiency exacerbates experimental glomerulonephritis: A protective role for endothelial P-selectin in inflammation. *J Clin Invest* 1999;103:649–659.

118. Piedboeuf B, Gamache M, Frenette J, et al. Increased endothelial cell expression of platelet-endothelial cell adhesion molecule-1 during hyperoxic lung injury. *Am J Respir Cell Mol Biol* 1998;19:543–553.

119. Takaishi M, Kurose I, Higuchi H, et al. Ethanol-induced leukocyte adherence and albumin leakage in rat mesenteric venules: Role of CD18/intercellular adhesion molecule-1. *Alcohol Clin Exp Res* 1996;20:347A–349A.

120. Blann AD, Taberner DA. A reliable marker of endothelial cell dysfunction: Does it exist? *Br J Haematol* 1995;90:244–248.

121. Kvietys PR, Granger DN. Endothelial cell monolayers as a tool for studying microvascular pathophysiology. *Am J Physiol* 1997;273:G1189–G1199.

122. Phillips PG, Lum H, Malik AB, Tsan M-F. Phallicidin prevents thrombin-induced increases in endothelial permeability to albumin. *Am J Physiol* 1989;257:C562–C567.

123. Curry FE, Adamson RH. Transendothelial pathways in venular microvessels exposed to agents which increase permeability: The gaps in our knowledge [editorial]. *Microcirculation* 1999;6:3–5.

124. Mcdonald DM, Thurston G, Baluk P. Endothelial gaps as sites for plasma leakage in inflammation. *Microcirculation* 1999;6:7–22.

125. Feng D, Nagy JA, Pyne K, et al. Pathways of macromolecular extravasation across microvascular endothelium in response to VPF/VEGF and other vasoactive mediators. *Microcirculation* 1999;6:23–44.

126. Michel CC, Neal CR. Openings through endothelial cells associated with increased microvascular permeability. *Microcirculation* 1999;6:45–54.

127. Joneckis CC, Shock DD, Cunningham ML, et al. Glycoprotein IV-independent adhesion of sickle red blood cells to immobilized thrombospondin under flow conditions. *Blood* 1996;87:4862–4870.

128. Hillery CA, Scott JP, Du MC. The carboxy-terminal cell-binding domain of thrombospondin is essential for sickle red blood cell adhesion. *Blood* 1999;94:302–309.

129. Lee SP, Cunningham ML, Hines PC, et al. Sickle cell adhesion to laminin: Potential role for the alpha5 chain. *Blood* 1998;92:2951–2958.

130. Kasschau MR, Barabino GA, Bridges KR, et al. Adhesion of sickle neutrophils and erythrocytes to fibronectin. *Blood* 1996;87:771–780.

131. Matsui NM, Chen JY, Sanan DA, et al. Thrombin-enhanced sickle cell adherence correlates with exposure of matrix fibronectin and endothelial integrins and with membrane redistribution of integrins. Submitted for publication 2001.
132. Garcia JG, Davis HW, Patterson CE. Regulation of endothelial cell gap formation and barrier dysfunction: Role of myosin light chain phosphorylation. *J Cell Physiol* 1995;163:510–522.
133. Manodori AB, Barabino GA, Lubin BH, Kuypers FA. Adherence of phosphatidylserine-exposing erythrocytes to endothelial matrix thrombospondin. *Blood* 2000;95:1293–1300.
134. Conforti G, Dominguez-Jimenez C, Zanetti A, et al. Human endothelial cells express integrin receptors on the luminal aspect of their membrane. *Blood* 1992;80:437–446.
135. Manodori AB. Sickle erythrocytes adhere to fibronectin-thrombospondin-integrin complexes exposed by thrombin-induced endothelial cell contraction. *Microvasc Res* 2001;61:263–274.
136. Stenberg PE, McEver RP, Shuman MA, et al. A platelet alpha-granule membrane protein (GMP-140) is expressed on the plasma membrane after activation. *J Cell Biol* 1985;101:880–886.
137. McEver RP, Beckstead JH, Moore KL, et al. GMP-140 a platelet a-granule membrane protein is also synthesized by vascular endothelial cells is localized in Weibel-Palade bodies. *J Clin Invest* 1989;84:92–99.
138. Barkalow FJ, Goodman MJ, Gerritsen ME, Mayadas TN. Brain endothelium lacks one of two pathways of P-selectin-mediated neutrophil adhesion. *Blood* 1996;88:4585–4593.
138a. Matsui NM, Borsig L, Rosen SD, et al. P-selectin mediates the adhesion of sickle erythrocytes to the endothelium. *Blood* 2001;98:1955–1962.
139. Rosen SD, Bertozzi CR. The selectins and their ligands. *Curr Opin Cell Biol* 1994;6:663–673.
140. Furie B, Furie BC. The molecular basis of platelet and endothelial cell interaction with neutrophils and monocytes: Role of P-selectin and the P-selectin ligand, PSGL-1. *Thromb Haemost* 1995;74:224–227.
141. Kansas GS. Selectins and their ligands: Current concepts and controversies. *Blood* 1996;88:3259–3287.
142. Rosen SD, Bertozzi CR. Two selectins converge on sulphate: Leukocyte adhesion. *Curr Biol* 1996;6:261–264.
143. Varki A. Selectin ligands: Will the real ones please stand up? *J Clin Invest* 1997;99:158–162.
144. Varki A, Cummings R, Esko J, et al. *Essentials of Glycobiology.* Cold Spring Harbor: Cold Spring Harbor Laboratory Press; 1999:1–653.
145. Telen MJ. Red blood cell surface adhesion molecules: Their possible roles in normal human physiology and disease. *Semin Hematol* 2000;37:130–142.
146. Wagers AJ, Stoolman LM, Kannagi R, et al. Expression of leukocyte fucosyltransferases regulates binding to E- selectin: Relationship to previously implicated carbohydrate epitopes. *J Immunol* 1997;159:1917–1929.
147. Beckstead JH, Stenberg PE, McEver RP, et al. Immunohistochemical localization of membrane α-granule proteins in human megakaryocytes: Application to plastic-embedded bone marrow biopsy specimens. *Blood* 1986;67:285–293.
148. Rosen SD, Singer MS, Yednock TA, Stoolman LM. Involvement of sialic acid on endothelial cells in organ-specific lymphocyte recirculation. *Science* 1985;228:1005–1007.

149. Patel N, Brinkman-Van der Linden EC, Altmann SW, et al. OB-BP1/ Siglec-6. a leptin- and sialic acid-binding protein of the immunoglobulin superfamily [erratum]. *J Biol Chem* 1999;274:22729–22738.
150. Angata T, Varki A. Siglec-7: A sialic acid-binding lectin of the immuno-globulin superfamily. *Glycobiology* 2000;10:431–438.
151. Koenig A, Norgard-Sumnicht K, Linhardt R, Varki A. Differential inter-actions of heparin and heparan sulfate glycosaminoglycans with the se-lectins: Implications for the use of unfractionated and low molecular weight heparins as therapeutic agents. *J Clin Invest* 1998;101:877–889.
152. Roberts DD, Ginsburg V. Sulfated glycolipids and cell adhesion. *Arch Biochem Biophys* 1988;267:405–415.
153. Aruffo A, Kolanus W, Walz G, et al. CD62/P-selection recognition of myeloid and tumor cell sulfatides. *Cell* 1991;67:35–44.
154. Serra MV, Mannu F, Matera A, et al. Enhanced IgG- and complement-independent phagocytosis of sulfatide-enriched human erythrocytes by human monocytes. *FEBS Lett* 1992;311:67–70.
155. Needham LK, Schnaar RL. The HNK-1 reactive sulfoglucuronyl glycol-ipids are ligands for L-selectin and P-selectin but not E-selectin. *Proc Natl Acad Sci USA* 1993;90:1359–1363.
156. Ho M, Schollaardt T, Niu X, et al. Characterization of *Plasmodium falciparum*-infected erythrocyte and P-selectin interaction under flow con-ditions. *Blood* 1998;91:4803–4809.
157. Yipp BG, Anand S, Schollaardt T, et al. Synergism of multiple adhesion molecules in mediating cytoadherence of *Plasmodium falciparum*-infected erythrocytes to microvascular endothelial cells under flow. *Blood* 2000;96: 2292–2298.
158. Bernatowicz MS, Klimas CE, Hartl KS, et al. Development of potent thrombin receptor antagonist peptides. *J Med Chem* 1996;39:4879–4887.
159. Solovey AA, Solovey AN, Harkness J, Hebbel RP. Modulation of endo-thelial cell activation in sickle cell disease: A pilot study. *Blood* 2001;97: 1937–1941.
160. Hebbel RP. Clinical implications of basic research: Blockade of adhesion of sickle cells to endothelium by monoclonal antibodies. *N Engl J Med* 2000;342:1910–1912.
161. Lowe JB, Ward PA. Therapeutic inhibition of carbohydrate-protein inter-actions in vivo. *J Clin Invest* 1997;99:822–826.
162. Nelson RM, Cecconi O, Roberts WG, et al. Heparin oligosaccharides bind L- and P-selectin and inhibit acute inflammation. *Blood* 1993;82:3253–3258.
163. Gupta K, Gupta P, Solovey A, Hebbel RP. Mechanism of interaction of thrombospondin with human endothelium and inhibition of sickle eryth-rocyte adhesion to human endothelial cells by heparin. *Biochim Biophys Acta* 1999;1453:63–73.
164. Chaplin H Jr, Monroe MC, Malecek AC, et al. Preliminary trial of minidose heparin prophylaxis for painful sickle cell crises. *East Afr Med J* 1989;66: 574–584.

Chapter 4

Adhesion of Sickle Erythrocytes to Extracellular Matrix

Cheryl A. Hillery, MD

Pathogenesis of Vaso-Occlusion

Sickle cell disease is caused by a single amino acid substitution within the beta chain of hemoglobin (hemoglobin βGlu6Val) that results in hemolytic anemia. The major clinical manifestation of sickle cell disease is vaso-occlusion that results in tissue ischemia and infarction and can involve any organ. The pathogenesis of this vascular obstruction is complex and likely involves multiple sequential pathological steps related to the many primary and secondary effects of sickle hemoglobin on the erythrocyte membrane, vascular endothelium, and circulating platelets, leukocytes, and coagulant proteins.[1-3] The enhanced adhesion of sickle erythrocytes to the endothelial cells and the subendothelial matrix likely plays a significant role in the pathogenesis of vascular occlusion in sickle cell disease.

Figure 1 shows a hypothetical scenario for the evolution of vaso-occlusion in sickle cell disease based on multiple observations in patients with sickle cell disease as well as in vitro characterization. The increased adhesion of sickle erythrocytes to vascular endothelium in vitro has been described using both static adhesion assays[4] and endothelialized flow chambers.[5,6] These observations have been confirmed using live animal models either by infusing human sickle red cells into rats[7,8] or by studying transgenic sickle cell mouse models.[9,10] Sickle erythrocyte adhesion to endothelial cells can adversely affect the morphological characteristics and synthetic function of endothelial cells.

This work was in part supported by Public Health Services grant K08-HL02858 and American Heart Association Grant-in-Aid 0050467N.

From: Weir EK, Reeve HL, Reeves JT (eds). *Interactions of Blood and the Pulmonary Circulation*. Armonk, NY: Futura Publishing Company, Inc.; ©2002.

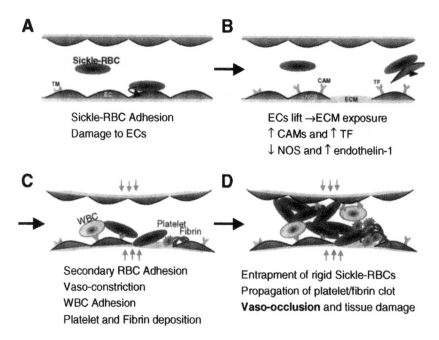

A

Sickle-RBC

TM
EC

Sickle-RBC Adhesion
Damage to ECs

B

CAM   TF
ECM

ECs lift →ECM exposure
↑ CAMs and ↑ TF
↓ NOS and ↑ endothelin-1

C

↓↓↓

WBC   Platelet
Fibrin

↑↑↑

Secondary RBC Adhesion
Vaso-constriction
WBC Adhesion
Platelet and Fibrin deposition

D

↓↓↓

↑↑↑

Entrapment of rigid Sickle-RBCs
Propagation of platelet/fibrin clot
Vaso-occlusion and tissue damage

Figure 1. Hypothetical scenario for the pathogenesis of vaso-occlusion in sickle cell disease. Please see text for description. RBC = red blood cell; EC = endothelial cell; TM = thrombomodulin; ECM = extracellular matrix; CAM = cell adhesion molecule; TF = tissue factor; NOS = nitric oxide synthase; WBC = white blood cell.

For example, Natarajan et al. described a loss of refractility and the typical cobblestone morphology in cultured, cytokine-stimulated endothelial cells after 10 minutes of exposure to sickle erythrocytes under low shear flow conditions;[11] the level of morphological endothelial cell damage correlated with the level of erythrocyte adhesion. Additionally, this group found an increase in endothelial cell ICAM-1 and VCAM-1 expression after 3–6 hours of perfusion with sickle erythrocytes under similar flow conditions.[12] There are also perturbations of vasoregulatory molecules at sites of sickle erythrocyte-induced endothelial damage,[13,14] predisposing to localized sites of vasoconstriction. Furthermore, there is evidence that damaged endothelial cells lift in sickle cell disease, resulting in increased levels of circulating endothelial cells that have increased expression of both proadhesive molecules and the procoagulant molecule tissue factor.[15,16] As a result, the *extracellular matrix*, and its attendant proadhesive and procoagulant components, are also probably exposed at sites of damage. Finally, the combination of entrapment of rigid sickle erythrocytes,[7] the disturbed vasomotor tone, and/or platelet/thrombus plug formation likely results in total occlusion of blood flow, leading to tissue ischemia and infarction in the affected area.

Role of Extracellular Matrix Proteins in Sickle Erythrocyte Adhesion

In order to gain insight into potential interactions of erythrocytes with components of the extracellular matrix, the adhesion of sickle erythrocytes to purified adhesive plasma and extracellular matrix proteins under conditions of controlled flow at a wall shear stress of 1 dyne/cm^2 was studied. These forces are similar to those found in the postcapillary venule, a proposed site of vascular obstruction in sickle cell disease.[6,7,17] The adhesion of sickle erythrocytes to the adhesive ligands thrombospondin-1 (TSP) and laminin was increased more than 15-fold when compared to normal control erythrocytes.[18,19] In contrast, the adhesion of erythrocytes to other purified adhesive extracellular matrix proteins was minimal, including von Willebrand factor, fibronectin, collagen, and vitronectin (<25 erythrocytes/mm^2). In addition, erythrocytes from patients with elevated reticulocyte counts (25–80% reticulocytes) who did not suffer from a hemoglobinopathy did *not* demonstrate increased adhesion to thrombospondin or laminin compared to control erythrocytes.[20] Furthermore, thiazole orange staining of adherent sickle erythrocytes showed minimal adhesion of reticulocytes to TSP or laminin (<5% reticulocytes) compared to examination of unbound washed sickle erythrocytes prior to the flow adhesion assay (range 9–17% reticulocytes). This suggests that the increased adhesion was not due simply to the increased numbers of reticulocytes found in sickle cell disease. This high level of adhesion of erythrocytes to purified immobilized TSP and laminin suggests that binding of erythrocytes to exposed TSP or laminin in the vasculature may play an important role in the evolution of vascular pathology in sickle cell disease.

Thrombospondin Adhesive Domains

Thrombospondin-1 is a 450 kDa, homotrimeric glycoprotein that is present in the extracellular matrix, plasma, and platelet alpha storage granules that can be released in high local concentrations by activated platelets.[21] TSP mediates cell attachment and spreading, stabilizes platelet aggregation, regulates cell growth, and plays a role in angiogenesis, wound healing, cell migration, and phenotypic differentiation. TSP binds to *Plasmodium falciparum*-infected erythrocytes via malarial proteins that are expressed on the surface of the infected erythrocyte and may mediate the adhesion of parasitized erythrocytes to vascular endothelium.[22] In addition to the above data on sickle erythrocytes binding to surface-bound TSP, *soluble* TSP enhances the adhesion of sickle erythrocytes to cultured endothelial cells.[23,24]

TSP has at least 4 domains that mediate cell adhesion: (1) the amino-terminal heparin-binding domain that also binds sulfated glycolipids and heparan sulfate proteoglycans,[25] (2) the CSVTCG sequences within the type 1 repeats that associate with CD36,[26] (3) the RGD integrin-binding site within the last type 3 repeat of the calcium-binding domain,[27] and (4) the carboxy-terminal cell-binding domain that binds to platelets and many transformed cells.[28] The region on TSP that binds sickle erythrocytes has been further mapped using proteolytic fragments of TSP in an in vitro flow adhesion assay at a wall shear stress of 1 dyne/cm[2.29] The purified 25-kDa N-terminal TSP fragment that contains the heparin-binding domain, as well as the 70-kDa and 120-kDa TSP fragments that contain the procollagen-like segment, type 1, type 2, and type 3 repeats did *not* support sickle erythrocyte adhesion. However, the 140-kDa TSP fragment, containing the *C-terminal cell-binding domain* in addition to the type 1, 2, and 3 repeats of TSP, fully supported sickle erythrocyte adhesion under flow conditions.[29] These data indicate that the intact 20-kDa carboxy-terminal segment of TSP, which contains the cell-binding domain, is required for sickle erythrocyte adhesion to surface-bound TSP under flow conditions.

In studies to further map potential adhesive sites within the cell-binding domain of TSP that bind sickle erythrocytes, the anti-TSP monoclonal antibody C6.7, which blocks the binding of platelets and transformed cells to the TSP cell-binding domain, did not significantly inhibit sickle erythrocyte adhesion to TSP.[29] The peptides 4N1K (KRFYVVMWKK) and 7N3 (FIRVVMYEGKK) are 2 well-characterized cell-binding domain adhesive sequences that both inhibit as well as support TSP-mediated adhesion of platelets and transformed cells.[28] However, when the peptides 4N1K or 7N3 were incubated with the sickle erythrocytes during the flow adhesion assay, neither of these peptides significantly inhibited nor supported sickle erythrocyte adhesion to TSP.[29] These data suggest that the 7N3 and 4N1K adhesive epitopes within the TSP cell-binding domain are not involved in the adhesion of sickle erythrocytes to immobilized TSP under flow conditions. The binding characteristics of many adhesive ligands can vary depending on the shear force (e.g., von Willebrand factor) and whether the ligand is in solution phase versus the solid phase (e.g., fibrinogen). While immobilized TSP avidly binds sickle erythrocytes under low shear conditions, *soluble* TSP did not bind sickle erythrocytes as detected by flow cytometry;[29] however, soluble TSP bound to sickle erythrocytes may be detected at low levels by more sensitive methods using

I[125]-TSP.[30] Additionally, soluble TSP did not inhibit sickle erythrocyte adhesion to immobilized TSP.[29] These data suggest that immobilization of TSP on a matrix optimizes the adhesive epitope within TSP that recognizes sickle erythrocytes.

Laminin Adhesive Domains

Laminin, a major structural constituent of the extracellular matrix, is composed of a family of large heterotrimeric glycoproteins that support cellular adhesion and migration and modulate gene expression.[31] Each member of the laminin family of proteins is composed of an α chain, a β chain, and a γ chain.[32] Using known laminin isoforms, adhesive peptide regions, and monoclonal antibodies, Lee et al. found that the laminin alpha5 chain likely recognizes and binds sickle erythrocytes.[33] The alpha5 chain is found in the laminin-10 and laminin-11 isoforms and is widely expressed.[32] Similar to TSP, soluble laminin did not inhibit sickle erythrocyte adhesion to immobilized laminin.[33] Also, peptides from known adhesive regions within laminin neither supported nor inhibited laminin-mediated sickle erythrocyte adhesion under low shear flow conditions.[33] These data suggest a unique adhesive site within the alpha5 chain that recognizes sickle erythrocytes that is optimally exposed only after laminin binds to a surface.

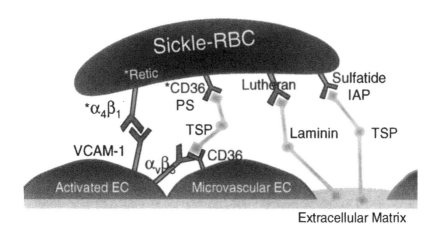

Figure 2. Examples of proposed adhesive interactions between the sickle erythrocyte and the vascular wall. Please see text for description of specific examples. RBC = red blood cell; Retic = reticulocyte; EC = endothelial cell; TSP = thrombospondin-1; IAP = integrin-associated protein; PS = phosphatidylserine.

Adhesion Molecules on the Sickle Erythrocyte Membrane

Potential adhesion molecules on the sickle erythrocyte surface that may mediate interactions with either endothelial cells or the extracellular matrix include CD36 (platelet GP IV),[23,34,35] integrin $\alpha_4\beta_1$,[34,36] the Lutheran antigen,[37] the 50-kDa integrin-associated protein (CD47),[38] sulfated glycolipids,[18] and band 3 (see Figure 2).[39] Other potential adhesion molecules expressed on the erythrocyte surface include the hyaluronan receptor (CD44), ICAM-4 (LW), LFA-3 (CD58), and neurothelin (CD147);[40] however, the role of these molecules in erythrocyte adhesion, including sickle erythrocyte adhesion, is less well understood.

CD36

CD36 is a nonintegrin adhesive receptor that is present on the surface of endothelial cells, platelets, and the reticulocyte subpopulation of normal and sickle erythrocytes.[23,34,35] CD36 binds TSP and collagen and is postulated to play a role in the adhesion of *Plasmodium falciparum*-infected erythrocytes to the vascular endothelium.[41] Sugihara et al. reported that sickle erythrocytes bind to endothelial cells in the presence of soluble TSP and that this adhesion is blocked by anti-CD36 monoclonal antibodies in a static adhesion assay.[23] Brittain et al. reported similar findings under flow conditions.[24] Since CD36 is present primarily on reticulocytes, this data would suggest that reticulocytes are binding in these studies. However, both the blocking anti-CD36 monoclonal antibody, OKM-5, and the blocking TSP peptide, CSVTCG, failed to inhibit the adhesion of sickle erythrocytes to *immobilized* TSP, suggesting a limited role for CD36 in mediating the adhesion of sickle erythrocytes to extracellular matrix TSP under flow conditions.[18,19] Therefore, the exact role of CD36 in erythrocyte adhesion is likely complex and remains unclear.

Integrin $\alpha_4\beta_1$

The integrin $\alpha_4\beta_1$ is a receptor for both fibronectin and endothelial cell VCAM-1 and is present on both normal and sickle reticulocytes.[34,36] Sickle erythrocytes can bind to VCAM-1 on cultured cytokine-stimulated endothelial cells[36] or transfected COS cells[42] as well as to immobilized fibronectin[43] via $\alpha_4\beta_1$. Since $\alpha_4\beta_1$ is present only on reticulocytes, these data again suggest that the reticulocyte subpopulation of sickle erythrocytes is binding.

Lutheran Antigen

The Lutheran antigen (B-CAM/Lu) is a transmembrane glycoprotein that is expressed on the erythrocyte surface as both an 85-kDa (Lu) isoform and a 78-kDa (B-CAM) isoform that differ only by the length of the cytoplasmic domain.[44] B-CAM/Lu is a member of the immunoglobulin superfamily (IgSF) with 5 extracellular disulfide-bonded IgSF domains. Sickle erythrocytes and normal erythrocytes bind laminin, with the level of adhesion correlating with the level of expression of the Lutheran antigen as well as additional affinity seen in sickle erythrocytes.[37,45] Using ligand blot analysis, soluble laminin binds an 80-kDa protein doublet from both sickle and normal erythrocyte membrane preparations, but not Lutheran-negative erythrocyte membrane preparations, suggesting that soluble laminin is binding the Lutheran antigen.[37] In agreement, cells expressing recombinant 85-kDa (Lu) or 78-kDa (B-CAM) Lutheran antigen isoforms specifically bound both soluble and immobilized laminin, giving further evidence for the Lutheran antigen as an adhesive receptor for laminin.[37,45] Using IgSF domain-specific deletion constructs of the Lutheran antigen expressed on the surface of murine erythroleukemia cells, the fifth IgSF domain appears to contain a critical binding site for recognition of laminin.[46] Therefore, the Lutheran antigen is likely an important mediator of sickle erythrocyte adhesion to sites of laminin exposure in the vasculature.

Integrin-Associated Protein

Integrin-associated protein (CD47) is a 50-kDa integral membrane protein found on erythrocytes and other mammalian cells that associate with integrins and bind to the C-terminal cell-binding domain of TSP.[38] Preliminary studies by Brittain et al. suggest that the integrin-associated protein may be involved in sickle erythrocyte adhesion to immobilized TSP.[47]

Sulfated Glycolipids

Sulfated glycolipids are present on the surface of erythrocytes and bind to TSP and laminin with relatively high affinity that is differentially inhibited by anionic polysaccharides.[48] The adhesion of sickle erythrocytes to TSP and laminin is similarly selectively inhibited by the anionic polysaccharides HMW dextran sulfate and chondroitin sulfate A,[18] consistent with a sulfated glycolipid contributing to the sickle erythrocyte adhesive phenotype. In agreement, we identified and purified an acidic erythrocyte membrane lipid that bound both TSP and laminin.[18] This lipid had biochemical properties consistent with a sulfated glycolipid.

Band 3

Band 3 is an abundant erythrocyte anion exchanger (mediates bicarbonate-chloride exchange) that spans the plasma membrane multiple times and is linked to the erythrocyte cytoskeleton. Band 3 mediates the adhesion of malaria-infected erythrocytes to the vascular endothelium via exposure of previously cryptic adhesive sites.[49] Band 3 is abnormally clustered on sickle erythrocytes.[50] Peptides from sites of band 3 that are aberrantly exposed on sickle erythrocytes inhibited their adhesion to cultured endothelial cells.[39] Thus, a conformationally modified band 3 may also contribute to sickle erythrocyte adhesion.

Adhesive Properties of Modified Erythrocytes

Hemoglobin S polymerizes upon deoxygenation and forms long crystals that distort the erythrocyte membrane. In addition, sickle hemoglobin is unstable, resulting in increased amounts of oxidized hemichromes located near the erythrocyte membrane.[51] As a consequence, the sickle erythrocyte manifests many abnormalities that include abnormal cation homeostasis resulting in cellular dehydration,[52] a disruption of the normal phospholipid asymmetry with increased phosphatidylserine exposure,[53] oxidative damage of membrane proteins and lipids,[51] and abnormal clustering of surface proteins.[50]

Several lines of evidence support the thesis that the enhanced adhesive properties of sickle erythrocytes may be due to native erythrocyte membrane lipids or proteins that have been biochemically altered or abnormally exposed in the sickle erythrocyte. This includes the report by Barabino et al. that mechanically injured (sheared) normal erythrocytes bound at higher levels to endothelial cells in an in vitro flow adhesion assay.[5] Also, oxidative treatment of normal erythrocytes, which simulate the auto-oxidative damage of sickle erythrocyte integral membrane proteins and lipids, caused a dose-dependent increase in adhesion to either cultured endothelial cells[54] or immobilized TSP.[55] Furthermore, dehydration of erythrocytes using hypertonic buffers increased their adhesion to both endothelial cells under static conditions[54] and TSP under flow conditions.[55] In converse experiments, rehydration of sickle erythrocytes lessened their adhesive phenotype.[54,55] Finally, treatment of normal erythrocytes with calcium ionophore to disrupt the lipid bilayer and increase the exposure of inner leaflet lipids caused an increase in their adhesion to bound TSP and cultured endothelial cells.[55,56] Annexin V, which binds to phosphatidylserine, reduced the level of ionophore-treated erythrocyte adhesion. This suggests that phosphatidylserine exposure contributes to the observed adhesion of ionophore-treated red cells. Taken together, these data suggest that normal erythrocyte membrane components that have been pathologically modified or exposed on the sickle erythrocyte could play a role in their increased adhesive phenotype.

Adhesion of Sickle Erythrocytes in Live Animal Models

The above data focus on sickle erythrocyte adhesion using in vitro experimental systems. It is also important to test for erythrocyte adhesion in an in vivo model that involves the more complex regional, humoral, and neural factors that may also contribute to vascular obstruction in sickle cell disease. Since cerebrovascular vaso-occlusion, or stroke, is a major cause of morbidity and mortality in sickle cell disease,[57] we developed an in vivo stroke model where surgically placed closed cranial windows were utilized to directly visualize erythrocyte flow and individual erythrocyte adhesive events in the rat cerebral microcirculation. FITC-labeled human erythrocytes were infused intravenously into rats prepared with cranial windows and data were collected by video recording of microvessels from preselected areas following the injection of labeled erythrocytes. We observed erythrocyte adhesion predominately in the capillary network and postcapillary venules for both sickle and control erythrocytes.[8] Human sickle erythrocytes had significantly increased adhesion compared to control erythrocytes.

Nitric oxide is an important regulator of normal vascular tone, cellular adhesion, and thrombosis. When the nitric oxide pathway was inhibited using L-NAME in this sickle erythrocyte-infused rat stroke model, approximately 60% of the animals developed a stroke and died within 30 minutes following the sickle RBC infusion.[58] In contrast, all control groups (sickle erythrocytes infused into rats treated with the control isomer D-NAME, or normal erythrocytes infused into rats treated with either L-NAME or D-NAME) completed the experiment with stable cerebral blood flow and hemodynamics. Therefore, the nitric oxide pathway was essential for maintaining cerebral blood flow in the presence of sickle erythrocytes in this rat model. This suggests that, in addition to the enhanced adhesion of sickle RBCs to the vascular endothelium, abnormal vasomotor tone regulation likely contributes to vaso-occlusion in sickle cell disease.

Since chondroitin sulfate-A (CS-A) inhibited sickle erythrocyte adhesion to TSP and laminin in vitro,[20] we proceeded to test the effect of

CS-A in this same rat stroke model system. We found that pretreatment of the animals with CS-A limited cerebral ischemia and helped maintain cerebral perfusion despite nitric oxide inhibition and sickle erythrocyte infusion.[59] While the mechanism for this effect of CS-A in vivo remains to be elucidated, it is possible that CS-A's inhibition of sickle erythrocyte adhesion observed in vitro may play a key role. Additionally, the potential anticoagulant properties of CS-A may also contribute to its beneficial effect.

Several other studies have shown considerable adhesion of human sickle erythrocytes to the rat ex vivo mesocecum vasculature.[17,60,61] In agreement with in vitro studies, the anionic polysaccharides, CS-A and dextran sulfate, inhibited sickle erythrocyte adhesion in this ex vivo experimental system.[60] Additionally, monoclonal antibodies known to bind human endothelial adhesion molecule $\alpha_V\beta_3$ also inhibited sickle erythrocyte adhesion to the rat mesocecal vasculature following stimulation with platelet-activating factor.[61] These studies suggest strong parallels between in vitro data and mixed human-animal experimental systems.

Recently, transgenic knockout sickle mice that exclusively express human sickle hemoglobin have permitted the study of sickle cell-induced vaso-occlusion in models that closely mimic the pathobiology of severe sickle cell disease in humans.[62,63] Studies using these severely affected sickle mice, as well as less severely affected transgenic sickle mouse models, have demonstrated increased adhesive interactions between murine sickle erythrocytes and murine endothelium.[9,10] Interestingly, these sickle mouse models also have an altered microvascular response to oxygen compared to healthy control mice.[64,65] Finally, washed erythrocytes derived from one of the more severe sickle mouse models[66] showed increased adhesion to immobilized human TSP under flow conditions in vitro.[67]

Conclusion

In summary, there is evidence to suggest that sickle erythrocyte adhesion to the vascular endothelium and extracellular matrix is likely important in the pathogenesis of vascular obstruction in sickle cell disease. Currently, the only proven effective therapies for treatment or prophylaxis of vaso-occlusion in sickle cell disease are transfusion, hydroxyurea, or bone marrow transplantation, each with its own attendant toxicities and limitations. Identification of the relative contributions of the multiple interactions between the sickle erythrocyte and the vascular endothelium and subendothelial matrix will improve our understanding of vaso-occlusive events in sickle cell disease and should result in improved therapy for this disorder.

References

1. Bunn HF. Pathogenesis and treatment of sickle cell disease. *N Engl J Med* 1997;337:762–769.
2. Hebbel RP. Beyond hemoglobin polymerization: The red blood cell membrane and sickle disease pathophysiology. *Blood* 1991;77:214–237.
3. Hillery CA. Potential therapeutic approaches for the treatment of vaso-occlusion in sickle cell disease. *Curr Opin Hematol* 1998;5:151–158.
4. Hebbel RP, Yamada O, Moldow CF, et al. Abnormal adherence of sickle erythrocytes to cultured vascular endothelium: Possible mechanism for microvascular occlusion in sickle cell disease. *J Clin Invest* 1980;65:154–160.
5. Barabino GA, McIntire LV, Eskin SG, et al. Endothelial cell interactions with sickle cell, sickle trait, mechanically injured, and normal erythrocytes under controlled flow. *Blood* 1987;70:152–157.
6. Smith BD, La Celle PL. Erythrocyte-endothelial cell adherence in sickle cell disorders. *Blood* 1986;68:1050–1054.
7. Fabry ME, Rajanayagam V, Fine E, et al. Modeling sickle cell vasoocclusion in the rat leg: Quantification of trapped sickle cells and correlation with 31P metabolic and 1H magnetic resonance imaging changes. *Proc Natl Acad Sci USA* 1989;86:3808–3812.
8. French JA, II, Kenny D, Scott JP, et al. Mechanisms of stroke in sickle cell disease: Sickle erythrocytes decrease cerebral blood flow in rats after nitric oxide synthase inhibition. *Blood* 1997;89:4591–4599.
9. Kaul DK, Fabry ME, Costantini F, et al. In vivo demonstration of red cell-endothelial interaction, sickling and altered microvascular response to oxygen in the sickle transgenic mouse. *J Clin Invest* 1995;96:2845–2853.
10. Embury SH, Mohandas N, Paszty C, et al. In vivo blood flow abnormalities in the transgenic knockout sickle cell mouse. *J Clin Invest* 1999;103:915–920.
11. Natarajan M, Udden MM, McIntire LV. Adhesion of sickle red blood cells and damage to interleukin-1 beta stimulated endothelial cells under flow in vitro. *Blood* 1996;87:4845–4852.
12. Shiu YT, Udden MM, McIntire LV. Perfusion with sickle erythrocytes up-regulates ICAM-1 and VCAM-1 gene expression in cultured human endothelial cells. *Blood* 2000;95:3232–3241.
13. Phelan M, Perrine SP, Brauer M, et al. Sickle erythrocytes, after sickling, regulate the expression of the endothelin-1 gene and protein in human endothelial cells in culture. *J Clin Invest* 1995;96:1145–1151.
14. Phelan M, Perrine SP, Brauer M, Faller DV. Transcriptional regulation of vasoactive genes in human endothelial cells by sickled cell or plasma from patients in crisis. *Blood* 1995;86:418a (abstract).
15. Solovey A, Lin Y, Browne P, et al. Circulating activated endothelial cells in sickle cell anemia. *N Engl J Med* 1997;337:1584–1590.
16. Solovey A, Gui L, Key NS, et al. Tissue factor expression by endothelial cells in sickle cell anemia. *J Clin Invest* 1998;101:1899–1904.
17. Kaul DK, Fabry ME, Nagel RL. Microvascular sites and characteristics of sickle cell adhesion to vascular endothelium in shear flow conditions: Pathophysiological implications. *Proc Natl Acad Sci USA* 1989;86:3356–3360.
18. Hillery CA, Du MC, Montgomery RR, et al. Increased adhesion of erythrocytes to components of the extracellular matrix: Isolation and characterization of a red blood cell lipid that binds thrombospondin and laminin. *Blood* 1996;87:4879–4886.
19. Joneckis CC, Shock DD, Cunningham ML, et al. Glycoprotein IV-

independent adhesion of sickle red blood cells to immobilized thrombo-spondin under flow conditions. *Blood* 1996;87:4862–4870.

20. Hillery CA, Du MC, Montgomery RR, et al. Increased adhesion of eryth-rocytes to components of the extracellular matrix: Isolation and character-ization of a red blood cell lipid that binds thrombospondin and laminin. *Blood* 1996;87:4879–4886.

21. Santoro SA, Frazier WA. Isolation and characterization of thrombospon-din. *Methods Enzymol* 1987;144:438–446.

22. Roberts DD, Sherwood JA, Spitalnik SL, et al. Thrombospondin binds fal-ciparum malaria parasitized erythrocytes and may mediate cytoadher-ence. *Nature* 1985;318:64–66.

23. Sugihara K, Sugihara T, Mohandas N, et al. Thrombospondin mediates adherence of CD36+ sickle reticulocytes to endothelial cells. *Blood* 1992; 80:2634–2642.

24. Brittain HA, Eckman JR, Swerlick RA, et al. Thrombospondin from acti-vated platelets promotes sickle erythrocyte adherence to human micro-vascular endothelium under physiologic flow: A potential role for platelet activation in sickle cell vaso-occlusion. *Blood* 1993;81:2137–2143.

25. Dixit VM, Grant GA, Santoro SA, et al. Isolation and characterization of a heparin-binding domain from the amino terminus of platelet throm-bospondin. *J Biol Chem* 1984;259:10100–10105.

26. Asch AS, Silbiger S, Heimer E, et al. Thrombospondin sequence motif (CSVTCG) is responsible for CD36 binding. *Biochem Biophys Res Commun* 1992;182:1208–1217.

27. Lawler J, Weinstein R, Hynes RO. Cell attachment to thrombospondin: The role of Arg-Gly-Asp, calcium, and integrin receptors. *J Cell Biol* 1988; 107:2351–2361.

28. Kosfeld MD, Frazier WA. Identification of a new cell adhesion motif in two homologous peptides from the COOH-terminal cell-binding domain of human thrombospondin. *J Biol Chem* 1993;268:8808–8814.

29. Hillery CA, Scott JP, Du MC. The carboxy-terminal cell-binding domain of thrombospondin is essential for sickle red blood cell adhesion. *Blood* 1999;94:302–309.

30. Gupta K, Gupta P, Solovey A, et al. Mechanism of interaction of throm-bospondin with human endothelium and inhibition of sickle erythrocyte adhesion to human endothelial cells by heparin. *Biochim Biophys Acta* 1999;1453:63–73.

31. Tryggvason K. The laminin family. *Cell Biol* 1993;5:877–882.

32. Miner JH, Patton BL, Lentz SI, et al. The laminin alpha chains: expression, developmental transitions, and chromosomal locations of alpha1–5, iden-tification of heterotrimeric laminins 8–11, and cloning of a novel alpha3 isoform. *J Cell Biol* 1997;137:685–701.

33. Lee SP, Cunningham ML, Hines PC, et al. Sickle cell adhesion to laminin: Potential role for the alpha5 chain. *Blood* 1998;92:2951–2958.

34. Joneckis CC, Ackley RL, Orringer EP, et al. Integrin $\alpha_4\beta_1$ and glycoprotein IV (CD36) are expressed on circulating reticulocytes in sickle cell anemia. *Blood* 1993;82:3548–3555.

35. Browne PV, Hebbel RP. CD36-positive stress reticulocytosis in sickle cell anemia. *J Lab Clin Med* 1996;127:340–347.

36. Swerlick RA, Eckman JR, Kumar A, et al. $\alpha_4\beta_1$-integrin expression on sickle reticulocytes: Vascular cell adhesion molecule-1-dependent bind-ing to endothelium. *Blood* 1993;82:1891–1899.

37. Udani M, Zen Q, Cottman M, et al. Basal cell adhesion molecule/Lutheran protein: The receptor critical for sickle cell adhesion to laminin. *J Clin Invest* 1998;101:2550–2558.

38. Gao AG, Lindberg FP, Finn MB, et al. Integrin-associated protein is a receptor for the C-terminal domain of thrombospondin. *J Biol Chem* 1996; 271:21–24.

39. Thevenin BM, Crandall I, Ballas SK, et al. Band 3 peptides block the adherence of sickle cells to endothelial cells in vitro. *Blood* 1997;90:4172–4179.

40. Telen MJ. Red blood cell surface adhesion molecules: Their possible roles in normal human physiology and disease. *Semin Hematol* 2000;37:130–142.

41. Barnwell JW, Asch AS, Nachman RL, et al. A human 88-kD membrane glycoprotein (CD36) functions *in vitro* as a receptor for a cytoadherence ligand on *Plasmodium falciparum*-infected erythrocytes. *J Clin Invest* 1989; 84:765–772.

42. Gee BE, Platt OS. Sickle reticulocytes adhere to VCAM-1. *Blood* 1995;85: 268–274.

43. Kasschau MR, Barabino GA, Bridges KR, et al. Adhesion of sickle neutrophils and erythrocytes to fibronectin. *Blood* 1996;87:771–780.

44. Parsons SF, Mallinson G, Holmes CH, et al. The Lutheran blood group glycoprotein, another member of the immunoglobulin superfamily, is widely expressed in human tissues and is developmentally regulated in human liver. *Proc Natl Acad Sci USA* 1995;92:5496–5500.

45. El Nemer W, Gane P, Colin Y, et al. The Lutheran blood group glycoproteins, the erythroid receptors for laminin, are adhesion molecules. *J Biol Chem* 1998;273:16686–16693.

46. Zen Q, Cottman M, Truskey G, et al. Critical factors in basal cell adhesion molecule/Lutheran-mediated adhesion to laminin. *J Biol Chem* 1999;274: 728–734.

47. Brittain JE, Orringer EP, Parise LV. Integrin associated protein is an adhesion receptor on sickle red blood cells for immobilized thrombospondin. *Blood* 1999;94:676a (abstract).

48. Roberts DD, Rao CN, Liotta LA, et al. Comparison of the specificities of laminin, thrombospondin, and von Willebrand factor for binding to sulfated glycolipids. *J Biol Chem* 1986;261:6872–6877.

49. Crandall I, Collins WE, Gysin J, et al. Synthetic peptides based on motifs present in a human band 3 protein inhibit cytoadherence/sequestration of the malaria parasite *Plasmodium falciparum*. *Proc Natl Acad Sci USA* 1993;90:4703–4707.

50. Waugh SM, Willardson BM, Kannan R, et al. Heinz bodies induce clustering of band 3, glycophorin, and ankyrin in sickle cell erythrocytes. *J Clin Invest* 1986;78:1155–1160.

51. Hebbel RP, Morgan WT, Eaton JW, et al. Accelerated autoxidation and heme loss due to instability of sickle hemoglobin. *Proc Natl Acad Sci USA* 1988;85:237–241.

52. Brugnara C, Bunn HF, Tosteson DC. Regulation of erythrocyte cation and water content in sickle cell anemia. *Science* 1986;232:388–390.

53. Kuypers FA, Lewis RA, Hua M, et al. Detection of altered membrane phospholipid asymmetry in subpopulations of human red blood cells using fluorescently labeled Annexin V. *Blood* 1996;87:1179–1187.

54. Hebbel RP, Ney PA, Foker W. Autoxidation, dehydration, and adhesivity may be related abnormalities of sickle erythrocytes. *Am J Physiol* 1989;256: C579–583.

55. Du MC, Scott JP, Hillery CA. Red blood cells treated with phenylhydrazine or calcium ionophore have increased adhesion to thrombospondin, similar to sickle erythrocytes. *Blood* 1995;86:137a (abstract).
56. Manodori AB, Barabino GA, Lubin BH, et al. Adherence of phosphatidylserine-exposing erythrocytes to endothelial matrix thrombospondin. *Blood* 2000;95:1293–1300.
57. Powars D, Wilson B, Imbus C, et al. The natural history of stroke in sickle cell anemia. *Am J Med* 1978;65:461–471.
58. French JA, II, Kenny D, Scott JP, et al. Mechanisms of stroke in sickle cell disease: Sickle erythrocytes decrease cerebral blood flow in rats after nitric oxide synthase inhibition. *Blood* 1997;89:4591–4599.
59. Punzalan RC, Trost BA, Scott JP, et al. Chondroitin sulfate-A limits cerebral ischemia induced by nitric oxide inhibition in sickle erythrocyte-infused rats. *Blood* 1998;92:329a (abstract).
60. Barabino GA, Liu XD, Ewenstein BM, et al. Anionic polysaccharides inhibit adhesion of sickle erythrocytes to the vascular endothelium and result in improved hemodynamic behavior. *Blood* 1999;93:1422–1429.
61. Kaul DK, Tsai HM, Liu XW, et al. Monoclonal antibodies to $\alpha_V\beta_3$ (7E3 and LM609) inhibit sickle red blood cell-endothelium interactions induced by platelet-activating factor. *Blood* 2000;95:368–374.
62. Pàszty C, Brion CM, Manci E, et al. Transgenic knockout mice with exclusively human sickle hemoglobin and sickle cell disease. *Science* 1997; 278:876–878.
63. Ryan TM, Ciavatta DJ, Townes TM. Knockout-transgenic mouse model of sickle cell disease. *Science* 1997;278:873–876.
64. Kaul DK, Fabry ME, Costantini F, et al. In vivo demonstration of red cell-endothelial interaction, sickling and altered microvascular response to oxygen in the sickle transgenic mouse. *J Clin Invest* 1995;96:2845–2853.
65. Embury SH, Mohandas N, Paszty C, et al. In vivo blood flow abnormalities in the transgenic knockout sickle cell mouse. *J Clin Invest* 1999;103:915–920.
66. Pàszty C, Brion CM, Manci E, et al. Transgenic knockout mice with exclusively human sickle hemoglobin and sickle cell disease. *Science* 1997; 278:876–878.
67. Punzalan RC, Holzman SL, Trost BA, et al. Spontaneous stroke and increased erythrocyte adhesion in transgenic knockout sickle cell mice. *Blood* 1999;94:419a (abstract).

Chapter 5

Mechanisms of Monocyte Migration Following Sickle Erythrocyte Adherence to Endothelium

Vijay K. Kalra, PhD, Suresh Selvaraj, PhD, and Cage Johnson, MD

Introduction

The clinical manifestations of sickle cell disease (SCD) include chronic hemolytic anemia, frequent infections, and recurrent episodes of painful crises.[1-6] Vascular occlusion leading to episodes of painful crises and damage to various end organs is the major cause of morbidity and mortality in older children and adults with SCD.[1,3,6] Over long periods of time, the repeated ischemic episodes lead to tissue damage culminating in acute chest syndrome, stroke, and chronic irreversible damage to end organs, resulting in renal failure and aseptic necrosis of bone.[6,7] The pathogenesis of SCD can be attributed to the red cell abnormalities due to the presence of hemoglobin S (HbS). When deoxygenated, HbS has the tendency to form polymers, which induce changes in shape (sickling) and reduce deformability of sickle red blood cells (SS RBCs). When these processes transpire in capillary or postcapillary venules, vaso-occlusion with ensuing local hypoxia and tissue necrosis occurs. Acutely, this generates pain and tissue injury, the hallmarks of the vaso-occlusive crises. However, the cellular and molecular events that initiate vaso-occlusive crises are not well understood.[8] In principle,

This work was supported by National Institutes of Health, Heart, Lung and Blood Institute Grant No. P60-HL-48484.

From: Weir EK, Reeve HL, Reeves JT (eds). *Interactions of Blood and the Pulmonary Circulation.* Armonk, NY: Futura Publishing Company, Inc.; ©2002.

any event that causes impedance in the flow of blood in the microvasculature could be a determinant in the initiation of vascular occlusion. Thus, the adhesion/interaction of SS RBCs, polymorphonuclear neutrophils (PMNs)/monocytes, and platelets with vascular endothelium could modulate the vascular tone, adhesive events, and thus the microcirculatory flow, and might be an important component of the vaso-occlusive process.

Adherence of Sickle Red Blood Cells to Vascular Endothelium

Studies have shown that SS RBCs exhibit abnormal adherence to cultured vascular endothelial cells under both static and flow conditions.[9-13] Moreover, it has been observed that the increased adherence of SS RBCs is dependent on the erythrocyte density as well as on the presence of reticulocytes in an SS RBC population that express adhesion receptors on their cell surface ordinarily absent from the surface of normal RBCs (AA RBCs).[11,12] Additionally, studies have shown that the autologous plasma from SCD patients potentiates the adherence of SS RBCs, presumably due to the presence of adhesive proteins, among which are von Willebrand factor (vWF) and thrombospondin.[9,14] These studies have been confirmed in an animal model system, using the ex vivo mecocecum preparation of the rat, wherein it has been shown that SS RBCs adhered to the venules.[8] It also revealed that, under flow conditions, the light density SS RBC fraction consisting of reticulocytes and discocytes were the most adherent, and subsequently caused the trapping of dense irreversible sickled cells in postcapillary venules, thus contributing to vascular occlusion.[11,12] The early studies of Hebbel and coworkers showed that the extent of adherence of SS RBCs to cultured endothelial cells appears to parallel the clinical severity of vaso-occlusive events in SCD.[15] However, SCD patients with an identical biochemical defect in their β-globin genes show wide variability in the frequency and severity of vaso-occlusive crises and can remain asymptomatic for prolonged periods,[2] indicating phenotypic differences within a given genotype. This could be due to the epistatic effect of co-inherited genes for α-thalassemia, β-globin gene haplotype variability, and expression level of HbF.[8,16-18] However, one finds paradoxical effects of the co-presence of the α-thalassemia gene on the frequency of painful crises.[8] It has been shown that the presence of α-thalassemia decreases polymerization of HbS, though sickle patients with the α-thalassemia gene show increased frequency of painful crises.[19-21] Similarly, the presence of HbF decreases polymerization of Hb SS, yet one does not find a clear protective effect of HbF on sickle cell crises.[22]

Role of Neutrophils and Monocytes in Vaso-Occlusion

Thus, there must be factors other than those directly related to the RBCs in the pathophysiology of vaso-occlusion in SCD. Clinically, it has been noted that infectious episodes, which activate leukocytes, precede development of vaso-occlusive crises. Moreover, a chronically elevated white cell count is a clear indicator of mortality,[23] frequency of acute chest syndrome,[24] and development of stroke[25,26] in SCD. Because PMNs and monocytes are activated during infection and inflammation, we hypothesize they may play a role in the initiation and potentiation of vaso-occlusive episodes. This is supported by the clinical observation wherein treatment with hydroxyurea causes a decrease in white blood cell count, a decrease in myeloperoxidase activity indicative of reduced neutrophil activity, and improvement in the incidence of vaso-occlusive crises.[27-29] That inflammation does play a significant role in the vaso-occlusive crises in SCD is supported by the observation that systemic levels of TNF-α and IL-1β,[30] IL-8 and substance P,[31] and endothelin-1[32] increase during acute painful crises. The cytokines (TNF-α and IL-1β) are known to upregulate the expression of cell adhesion molecules (ICAM-1, VCAM-1, and E-selectin) on vascular endothelium[33,34] and thus can modulate the adhesion of PMNs and monocytes.

PMN Activation in Response to the Adhesion of SS RBCs

SCD is characterized by moderate anemia and leukocytosis, resulting in a higher ratio of PMNs to RBCs. Thus, there is more probability of direct interaction between SS RBCs and PMNs, with concomitant activation of PMNs. The first step of PMN activation by SS RBCs would therefore be the attachment to PMNs. It has been shown that PMNs, even when quiescent, adhere weakly to the microvasculature via the adhesion molecule P-selectin.[35] Under conditions of low shear in the microvasculature, PMNs have a chance to come in contact with RBCs.[36-38] Our recent studies[39] show that SS RBCs but not AA RBCs (normal) adhere to PMNs, and such adherence is augmented by autologous plasma. Furthermore, the dense SS RBC fraction was more adherent than the light density fraction. Because dense SS RBCs express an increased number of IgG molecules on their surface compared to the light density fraction,[40,41] the adhesion of SS RBCs could have occurred via the Fc receptor on PMNs. Studies[39] showed that blocking the Fc receptors on PMNs significantly reduced (>60%) the adherence of SS RBCs to PMNs. The IgG-mediated interaction between

SS RBCs and PMNs was specific for SS RBCs and sickle plasma. ABO-matched sickle plasma did not increase the adhesion of AA RBCs to PMNs. Similarly, the adherence of SS RBCs to PMNs remained unchanged in the presence of normal plasma. Because integrins are involved in the adhesion of SS RBCs to endothelium and such process is blocked by peptides containing the RGD (Arg-Gly-Asp)[42-44] motif, it was determined whether RGD peptides could block the adherence of SS RBCs to PMNs. These studies[39] showed that the RGD peptide, but not a variant peptide GRGESP (Gly-Arg-Gly-Glu-Ser-Pro), blocked approximately 40% attachment of PMNs to SS RBCs. However, saturating concentrations of both RGD and IgG resulted in greater than 75% reduction in the adherence of PMNs to SS RBCs. These results indicate that SS RBCs adhere to the PMNs through IgG-dependent and integrin-mediated mechanisms. Further studies revealed that the interaction of SS RBCs, but not AA RBCs, leads to the generation of respiratory burst in PMNs, indicating that adhesion causes activation of PMNs.

The ability of PMNs to recognize SS RBCs has important clinical significance. Due to the adhesion of SS RBCs or PMNs to vascular endothelium in small capillaries, the flow rate is decreased and thus the probability of adhesion of SS RBCs with PMNs/monocytes increases.[36] As a result of the adhesion of SS RBCs to PMNs, the PMNs become activated, resulting in (a) upregulation of CD11b/CD18 (integrin) on the PMN surface, and (b) release of reactive oxygen species (ROS). The CD11b/CD18 ligand on PMNs mediates adherence to the vascular endothelium via the adhesion molecule E-selectin.[45,46] The release of ROS from activated PMNs can upregulate the expression of VCAM-1 on vascular endothelium, a ligand involved in the adhesion of both sickle reticulocytes and monocytes.[47] These studies suggest that adhesion of SS RBCs to PMNs, particularly in capillaries, can initiate a cascade of events that may promote adherence of PMNs/monocytes and the additional adherence of reticulocytes to the vascular endothelium, conditions which may favor acute vaso-occlusion.

Microvascular Injury in SCD

A number of studies support the contention that SS RBCs not only adhere abnormally to vascular endothelium but can cause injury/activation of endothelium in vivo.[48-50] This is supported by the observation that one finds at least a 10-fold increased number of activated endothelial cells in the circulation of patients with SCD at the onset of acute painful crises,[48,51] when compared to the numbers of circulating endothelial cells in normal blood donors, persons with sickle cell trait (Hb AS), and patients with hemolytic anemias not associated with hemoglobin S. To determine whether circulating endothelial cells were dislodged from microvessels or from large vessels, Solovey et al.[48] utilized the expression of CD36, a marker for endothelial cells from microvascular origin. These studies showed that approximately 75% (78 ± 15%) of circulating endothelial cells in samples from patients with SCD compared to approximately 50% (53 ± 4 %) in samples from normal donors were positive for CD36. However, the absolute number of circulating endothelial cells in the SCD patients was 10-fold normal. Moreover, these circulating endothelial cells were viable[48] and less prone to apoptosis.[51] Additionally, most of the circulating endothelial cells were in the activated state as they expressed cell adhesion molecules ICAM-1, VCAM-1, and E-selectin, markers for the activation state of the endothelium.[48] It is pertinent to note that ICAM-1 is constitutively expressed in small amounts on endothelial cells but its expression and other adhesion molecules, namely VCAM-1, E-selectin, and P-selectin, is substantially upregulated upon activation. These studies showed that the number of circulating endothelial cells tend to increase at the onset of acute painful crises, which may occur as a result of dislodgment of cells from microvessels due to endothelial injury at the time of vaso-occlusion. Overall, these studies suggest that endothelium activation in vivo in SCD patients could be a risk factor for vaso-occlusion. Thus, bacterial infection in SCD patients could aggravate the situation as inflammatory mediators can independently activate endothelial cells.

Endothelium Activation in SCD

Although most investigations have focused on the adhesive events, there is evidence that sickle erythrocyte interaction with vascular endothelium could modulate the vascular tone. Since the overall tone of the vasculature is maintained by homeostasis in the formation of vasoconstrictor and vasodilatory molecules, studies have been undertaken to address the question of how SS RBCs attenuate the normal function of the endothelium. It has been shown that the interaction of deoxygenated SS RBCs with cultured human umbilical vein endothelial cells (HUVECs) caused a several-fold increase in transcriptional induction of the gene coding for endothelin-1 (ET-1), a vasoconstrictor molecule, with a concomitant release of ET-1.[52]

We hypothesized that adhesion/contact of SS RBCs with vascular endothelium may cause generation of intracellular oxidant stress and localized tissue hypoxia. Both of these factors[53,54] can modulate the expression of cell adhesion molecules (e.g., ICAM-1, E-selectin, and VCAM-1) on the endothelium, thereby promoting additional adherence of SS reticulocytes as well as adhesion of PMNs/monocytes to the activated endothelium through counterligands. The adhesion of SS RBCs and/ or leukocytes to injured/activated endothelium can adversely affect the oxygen delivery to tissues and blood flow, thus exacerbating vaso-occlusion and the tissue damage that occurs in vaso-occlusive episodes. Because SS RBCs, as compared to control RBCs (AA RBCs), produce a 2–3-fold greater amount of reactive oxygen species (ROS; superoxide and hydroxide radical) due to the presence of unstable HbS and autoxidation of iron in heme,[55,56] we hypothesized that ROS generated either extracellularly by SS RBCs or intracellularly from endothelial cells may play a role in the activation of the endothelium. The generation of intracellular ROS by endothelial cells could happen as a result of either intracellular signaling mediated by the adhesion of SS RBCs or by soluble factor(s) released from SS RBCs, which then acts on the endothelial cell.

Our studies[44] show that incubation of SS RBCs with HUVECs causes a 3-fold increase in the formation of lipid peroxides over and above those generated in the absence or presence of normal RBCs. However, in the presence of vWF, conditions that potentiate the adherence of SS RBCs, there was an additional 2-fold increase in the formation of ROS. Furthermore, it was observed that interaction of SS RBCs, but not AA RBCs, with HUVECs in the presence of endothelial cell-conditioned medium enriched in multimers of vWF, caused a time-dependent (0.5–4 hour) increase in the activation of transcription factor NF-κB, with maximal activation occurring at 1 hour, as determined by the electrophoretic mobility shift assay (Figure 1). The SS RBC-induced activation of NF-κB in HUVECs was abrogated by an antioxidant (probucol) and by a peptide containing the RGD motif, which blocks vWF-mediated adhesion of SS RBCs to endothelial cells. These studies indicate that adhesion/contact of SS RBCs, mediated by multimers of vWF, localizes the oxidant stimulus from the auto-oxidation of HbS to the plasma membrane of endothelial cells. This process generates intracellular ROS, which activates transcription factor NF-κB, an indicator of oxidant stress.[57–59] Additionally, NADPH oxidase and/or NADH oxido-reductase present in the plasma membrane of endothelial cells[60] may be activated as a result of SS RBC-induced cellular signaling. The generation of cellular oxidant stress is not unique to SS RBCs, as RBCs obtained from diabetic patients also caused increased formation of ROS and the activation of NF-κB.[61,62] In this case, the cellular oxidant stress was generated as a result of interaction of the advanced glycation end products (AGE) present on diabetic RBCs with its receptor (RAGE) expressed on endothelial cells.[61,62] The downstream signaling involved in the activation of NF-κB, upon interaction of SS RBCs with HUVECs, involved activation of tyrosine kinase and p21[ras] as inhibitors of tyrosine kinase (genistein) and ras (HFPA, α-hydroxyfarnesylphosphonic acid) blocked activation of NF-κB (Figure 1).

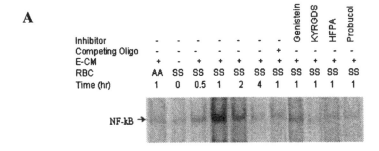

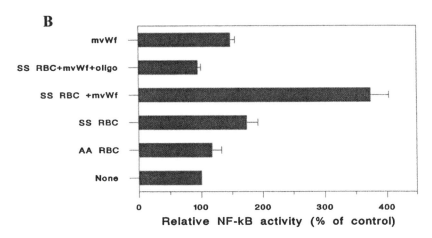

Figure 1. Sickle cell interactions with HUVECs cause activation of transcription factor NF-κB, an indicator of oxidant stress. HUVECs were incubated with normal (AA) or SS RBCs in the presence and absence of endothelial cell-conditioned medium (enriched in multimers of vWF) so as to augment the adherence. Genistein (inhibitor of tyrosine kinase), KYRGDS (inhibits vWF-mediated adherence of SS RBCs), HFPA (inhibitor of p21ras activity) and probucol (antioxidant) were added to HUVECs prior to the addition of RBCs. Nuclear extracts were prepared for assay of NF-κB activity by electrophoretic gel-mobility shift assay. From Sultana et al.,[44] with permission of the American Society of Hematology.

Since the expression of several genes including a subset of cell adhesion molecules (ICAM-1, VCAM-1, and E-selectin) is transcriptionally regulated by the binding of activated NF-κB to the consensus sites in the regulatory regions of DNA,[63,64] we examined whether adhesion of SS RBCs upregulated the expression of these CAMs. As shown in Figure 2, there was a time-dependent increase in the expression of ICAM-1, VCAM-1, and E-selectin upon interaction of SS RBCs with HUVECs under static conditions. The increased expression of CAMs

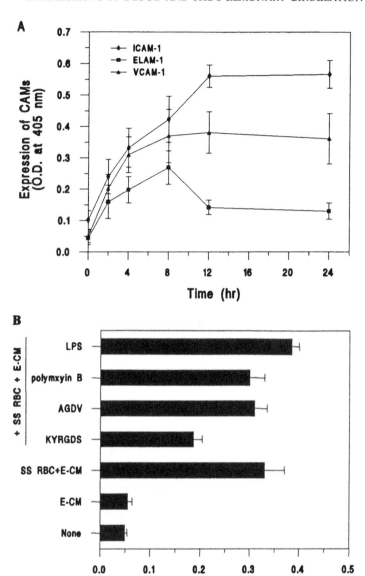

Figure 2. Expression of cell adhesion molecules in HUVECs in response to inter-action with RBCs by ELISA assay. (A) Time course of adhesion molecule ex-pression and (B) effect of inhibitors on VCAM-1 expression. E-CM (endothelial cell-conditioned medium enriched in multimers of vWF augments SS RBC ad-hesion. The peptide KYRGDS containing RGD motif blocks adhesion while vari-ant peptide AGDV does not affect it. The addition of polymyxin B, an endotoxin inhibitor, does not affect SS RBC-induced VCAM-1 expression, while treatment of HUVECs with LPS (a positive control) increases VCAM-1 expression. From Sultana et al.,[44] with permission of the American Society of Hematology.

was abrogated by RGD peptide, but not with a variant peptide AGDV (Arg-Gly-Asp-Gly), indicating that adhesion of SS RBCs to HUVECs was involved in cellular signaling. More recently,[65] it has been shown that under flow conditions, sickle erythrocytes also upregulate the expression of ICAM-1 and VCAM-1 in HUVECs. We suggest that changes in the expression of this subset of cell adhesion molecules, resulting from SS RBC adhesion, may occur by either juxtacrine intercellular signaling[66] or by the autocrine effect of released cytokines.[63]

Sickle RBC Interaction with Endothelium Promotes the Transmigration of Monocytes

Since SS RBC interaction with endothelial cells results in the expression of cell adhesion molecules (ICAM-1, VCAM-1, and E-selectin), which play a role in the adhesion of PMNs and monocytes, we determined whether these events affected the migration of these cells across an endothelial cell monolayer. We studied the transmigration of both monocytic HL-60 cells and peripheral blood monocytes across the HUVEC monolayer in the presence of SS RBCs. However, to distinguish between the migration of monocytes and erythrocytes, the monocytes were first labeled with a fluorescent probe, CellTracker Green BODIPY (Molecular Probes Inc., Eugene, OR). As shown in Figure 3 A, SS RBCs in the presence of endothelial cell-conditioned medium (enriched in multimers of vWF) showed a 2-fold increase in the transmigration of monocyte-like HL-60 cells at 2- and 4-hour time periods. Previous studies[67,68] have shown the role of endothelial cell junction molecule PECAM-1 in the trafficking of PMNs/monocytes across the endothelial cell monolayer. Thus we determined whether PECAM-1 was involved in the transmigration of monocytes. As shown in Figure 3B, antibody to PECAM-1 inhibited by ~75% the SS RBC-induced migration of monocyte-like HL-60 cells, whereas an antibody to ICAM-2, a constitutive molecule expressed on endothelial cells, had no effect on the migration of HL-60 cells. Our previous studies[68] showed that a protein kinase C inhibitor (GF 109203X) reduced the phosphorylation of PECAM-1 and concomitantly inhibited the transmigration of monocytes across a HUVEC monolayer, in response to lipoxygenase metabolites. Here, we observed that protein kinase C inhibitor, which inhibits PECAM-phosphorylation,[44] reduced the migration of monocytes in response to the interaction of SS RBCs with HUVECs. Conversely, the addition of calyculin A, a protein phosphatase inhibitor, which increases the phosphorylation of PECAM-1, augmented the transmigration of monocytes (Figure 3B). Treatment of HUVECs with the antioxidant probucol reduced by ~70% the transmigration of monocytes induced by the interaction of SS RBCs with HUVECs.

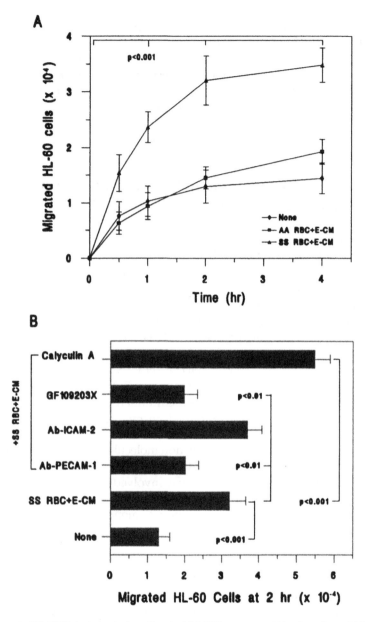

Figure 3. SS RBC-induced signaling in HUVECs causes (A) migration of HL-60 monocyte-like cells across the HUVEC monolayer. (B) Transmigration is inhibited by antibody to PECAM-1, a cell junction molecule. Transmigration is inhibited by protein kinase C inhibitor (GFX) and augmented by protein phosphatase inhibitor (calyculin A), indicating that phosphorylation/dephosphorylation events in HUVECs regulate the trafficking of monocytes in HUVECs in response to SS RBC interaction. From Sultana et al.,[44] with permission of the American Society of Hematology.

The transmigration was not specific for monocyte-like HL-60 cells (a transformed cell line) as studies showed that freshly isolated peripheral blood monocytes (PBMs) and another monocytic cell line (THP-1) behaved in a similar manner. As shown in Figure 4, SS RBC interaction with HUVECs, in the presence of endothelial cell-conditioned medium (E-CM, enriched in multimers of vWF), resulted in a 2-fold increase at the 2-hour time point, in the transmigration of PBMs as was observed with HL-60 cells. Additionally, antibody to PECAM-1 reduced by ~80% the transmigration of PBMs. The addition of synthetic peptide KYRGDS, containing RGD motif, but not a variant peptide AGDV, abrogated by ~70% the transendothelial migration of human PBMs.

These studies indicate that ROS formed by oxygenated SS RBCs and/or SS RBCs ligand-receptor interaction result in the generation of reactive oxygen intermediates in endothelial cells, which activate signaling pathways leading to the activation of the redox-sensitive transcription factor NF-κB[63] and concomitant activation of genes for a subset of adhesion molecules. These adhesion molecules augment the adhesion of PMNs/monocytes, which is then followed by the migra-

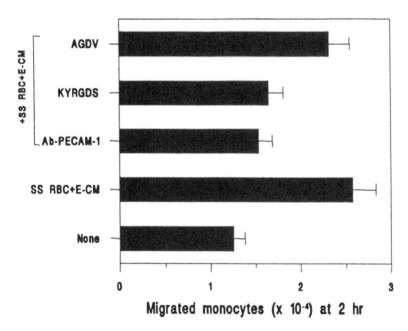

Figure 4. SS RBC-induced signaling in HUVECs causes transmigration of peripheral blood monocytes, which is inhibited by antibody to PECAM-1 (CD31) and by KYRGDS peptide containing RGD motif. From Sultana et al.,[44] with permission of the American Society of Hematology.

tion of PMNs/monocytes across the HUVEC monolayer through cell junction molecules involving PECAM-1 (CD31) molecules.[67,69]

Because SS blood, in vivo, undergoes oxygenation and deoxygenation, and conditioned medium elaborated from deoxygenated SS RBCs has been shown to elicit the formation of endothelin-1[50,52] from HUVECs, we examined the effect of oxygenated and deoxygenated SS RBC-released supernatant/factor(s) on the transmigration of monocytes across the human pulmonary artery endothelial cell (HPAEC) monolayer. We hypothesized that deoxygenated SS RBC-released factor(s) elicits the release of ET-1 from endothelial cells, which then mediates cellular signaling via its autocrine effect. As shown in Figure 5, factor(s) elaborated from deoxygenated SS RBCs (repetitive cycles of deoxygenation and oxygenation for 15 minutes and 5 minutes, respectively, for a period of 2 hours) when added to the HPAEC monolayer for 2 hours,

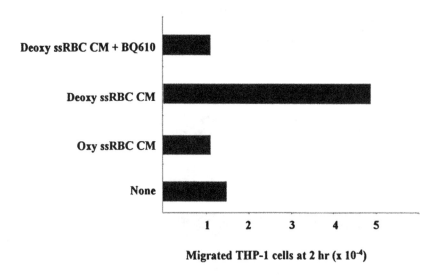

Migrated THP-1 cells at 2 hr (x 10⁻⁴)

Figure 5. Effect of conditioned medium from oxygenated and deoxygenated/oxygenated SS RBCs on the transmigration of monocytes across the human pulmonary aortic endothelial cell monolayer. SS RBCs (10% Hct) suspended in HBSS containing 5 mM glucose were exposed to humidified CO_2 (oxygenated) or nitrogen/CO_2 (15 min/5 min cycle) for a period of 2 hours. The supernatant was collected after centrifugation of RBCs and used immediately. The oxygenated and deoxygenated/oxygenated RBC supernatant was added to the HPAEC monolayer cultivated in fibronectin-coated Transwell chambers (3.0 micron, transendothelial electrical resistance of 85–100 ohms cm²). Where indicated, ETA-receptor antagonist (BQ 610, 100 μM) was added to the HPAECs prior to the addition of SS RBC-conditioned medium. After 1 hour of incubation, THP-1 monocytes (5×10^4 cells) were added to the top compartment of the chamber. At the indicated time points, aliquots were collected from the lower compartment for counting of migrated cells.[44]

A

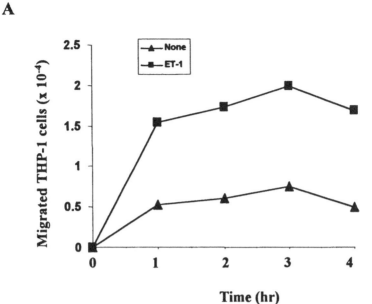

B

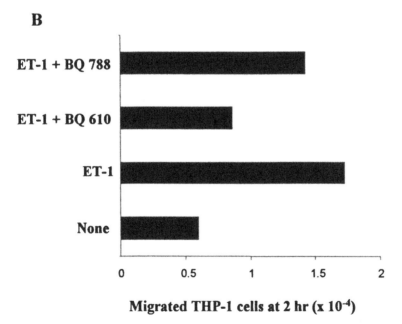

Migrated THP-1 cells at 2 hr (x 10⁻⁴)

Figure 6. Endothelin-1 mediates transmigration of THP-1 monocytes across human pulmonary aortic endothelial cells. (A) Endothelin–1 (100 nM) was added to the upper compartment of the Transwell chamber along with THP-1 monocytes. (B) ET_A-receptor antagonist (BQ 610, 200 nM) and ET_B-receptor antagonist (BQ 788, 200 nM) were added to HPAECs prior to the addition of ET-1.

followed by the addition of monocytes, resulted in a 3-fold increase in the transmigration of human monocytic cells (THP-1). However, factor(s) released from oxygenated SS RBCs did not significantly affect the transmigration of THP-1 monocytes across the HPAEC monolayer. As shown in Figure 5, the addition of BQ 610 (ET_A receptor antagonist), reduced by ~75% the effect of deoxygenated SS RBC-released factor on the transmigration of monocytes. These results suggest that ET-1 released from HPAECs in response to deoxygenated SS RBCs could act in an autocrine manner to induce the transmigration of monocytes. Thus, we examined the effect of ET-1 on the transmigration of monocytes across a HPAEC monolayer. As shown in Figure 6A, ET-1 (100 nM) caused a time-dependent (1–4 hours) increase in the transmigration of THP-1 monocytes across a HPAEC monolayer. There was a 2-fold increase in the transmigration of THP-1 monocytes by ET-1 at 2 hours, over the basal level. As shown in Figure 6B, the ET-1-induced migration of THP-1 monocytes was inhibited by BQ 610 (ET_A receptor antagonist), but not by BQ 788 (ET_B receptor antagonist), indicating that ET-1 utilizes the ET_A receptor for cellular signaling in HPAECs.

These studies indicate that endothelin-1, released as a result of the interaction of deoxygenated SS RBCs with endothelial cells, may modulate the vascular endothelium to cause adhesion of PMNs/monocytes followed by their diapedesis from the intravascular space into the interstitial space, and finally to the alveolar lumen. The migrated PMNs/monocytes may become primed prior to or during migration into the alveolar lumen. These activated PMNs/monocytes may cause alveolar epithelial cell injury through the enhanced release of ROS, thus exacerbating injury to the lung.

Conclusion

The adhesion of SS RBCs to vascular endothelium has long been thought to be an important factor in the pathogenesis of vascular occlusion. However, SCD patients with the same genotype show wide variability in the onset and severity of vaso-occlusive episodes. Thus, factors other than the polymerization of HbS must be important in the pathophysiology of vaso-occlusion. Since erythrocytes in microcirculation come in contact with a host of cells, particularly endothelial cells in the vessel wall and white blood cells including platelets, it is possible that interaction of SS RBCs with vascular endothelium may alter the vascular tone. Alternatively, the interaction of SS RBCs with white blood cells (PMNs/monocytes) may activate these cells to release reactive oxygen species (free radicals), which may cause damage to the endothelium. There is evidence that in SCD the microvascular endothelium is damaged, as one finds an increased number of circulating endothelial cells in SCD patients at the onset of acute painful episodes.

The studies presented here show that the interaction of SS RBCs with vascular endothelium can cause activation/injury of endothelium as the result of generation of intracellular oxidant stress and increased formation of endothelin-1, a vasoconstrictor polypeptide molecule. The cellular signaling emanating from this generation of intracellular ROS in endothelial cells activates the redox-sensitive transcription factor, NF-κB, which plays a major role in regulating the expression of a subset of cell adhesion molecules (CAMs) ICAM-1, E-selectin, and VCAM-1, as well as inflammatory cytokines. The expression of CAMs on endothelium has also been shown to be augmented in response to endotoxin and hypoxia, conditions that are frequently associated with bacterial infection and tissue hypoxemia in SCD patients. These CAMs participate in the adherence of PMNs/monocytes and reticulocytes via counter-receptors. Thus, the adhesion of PMNs/monocytes and reticulocytes to microvessels in which the adhesion of SS RBCs is maximal will adversely affect the flow of blood and thus can lead to tissue hypoxemia. Such sluggish flow conditions will also favor the probability of interaction of SS RBCs with PMNs/monocytes, conditions known to cause activation of PMNs/monocytes and the concomitant generation of reactive oxygen species. Under such conditions damage to the endothelium can occur.

In an environment of tissue hypoxemia, SS RBCs will be deoxygenated and their interaction with endothelium will generate increased amounts of endothelin-1 (ET-I) from endothelial cells. We have seen that the interaction of ET-1 with ET_A receptor expressed on human pulmonary artery endothelial cells causes cellular signaling, which allows monocytes to transmigrate, indicating that a low oxygen tension will favor the diapedesis of PMNs/monocytes across the pulmonary vasculature. We have evidence that monocytes-chemoattractant protein-1 (MCP-1) and IL-8 are formed by HPAECs in response to ET-1, which may then act in a paracrine manner on alveolar epithelium to allow PMNs/monocytes to transmigrate across the alveolar epithelium into the alveolar space. The accumulation of active leukocytes in the alveolar space can also damage the alveolar epithelium, possibly contributing to the pathogenesis of acute chest syndrome and lung injury in SCD.

References

1. Francis RB Jr, Johnson CS. Vascular occlusion in sickle cell disease: Current concepts and unanswered questions. *Blood* 1991;77:1405–1414.
2. Platt OS, Thorington BD, Brambilla DJ, et al. Pain in sickle cell disease: Rates and risk factors [see comments]. *N Engl J Med* 1991;325:11–16.
3. Buchanan GR. Infection. In Embury SH, Hebbel RP, Mohandas N, et al.,

eds: *Sickle Cell Disease: Basic Principles and Clinical Practice*. New York: Raven Press; 1994:567–587.

4. Wong WY, Powars DR, Chan L, et al. Polysaccharide encapsulated bacterial infection in sickle cell anemia: A thirty-year epidemiologic experience. *Am J Hematol* 1992;39:176–182.

5. Embury SH, Hebbel RP, Steinberg MH, et al. Pathogenesis of vasoocclusion. In Embury SH, Hebbel RP, Mohandas N, et al., eds: *Sickle Cell Disease: Basic Principles and Clinical Practice*. New York: Raven Press; 1994:311–326.

6. Powars DR. Sickle cell anemia and major organ failure. *Hemoglobin* 1990; 14:573–598.

7. Powars DR, Elliott-Mills DD, Chan L, et al. Chronic renal failure in sickle cell disease: Risk factors, clinical course, and mortality. *Ann Intern Med* 1991;115:614–620.

8. Kaul DK, Fabry ME, Nagel RL. The pathophysiology of vascular obstruction in the sickle syndromes. *Blood Rev* 1996;10:29–44.

9. Hebbel RP, Yamada O, Moldow CF, et al. Abnormal adherence of sickle erythrocytes to cultured vascular endothelium: Possible mechanism for microvascular occlusion in sickle cell disease. *J Clin Invest* 1980;65:154–160.

10. Mohandas N, Evans E. Sickle erythrocyte adherence to vascular endothelium: Morphologic correlates and the requirement for divalent cations and collagen-binding plasma proteins. *J Clin Invest* 1985;76:1605–1612.

11. Barabino GA, McIntire LV, Eskin SG, et al. Endothelial cell interactions with sickle cell, sickle trait, mechanically injured, and normal erythrocytes under controlled flow. *Blood* 1987;70:152–157.

12. Kaul DK, Fabry ME, Nagel RL. Microvascular sites and characteristics of sickle cell adhesion to vascular endothelium in shear flow conditions: Pathophysiological implications. *Proc Natl Acad Sci USA* 1989;86:3356–3360.

13. Hebbel RP, Mohandas N. Sickle cell adherence. In Embury SH, Hebbel RP, Mohandas N, et al., eds: *Sickle Cell Disease: Basic Principles and Clinical Practice*. New York: Raven Press; 1994:217–230.

14. Brittain HA, Eckman JR, Swerlick RA, et al. Thrombospondin from activated platelets promotes sickle erythrocyte adherence to human microvascular endothelium under physiologic flow: A potential role for platelet activation in sickle cell vaso-occlusion. *Blood* 1993;81:2137–2143.

15. Hebbel RP, Boogaerts MA, Eaton JW, et al. Erythrocyte adherence to endothelium in sickle cell anemia: A possible determinant of disease severity. *N Engl J Med* 1980;302:992–995.

16. Powars DR. Sickle cell anemia: Beta S-gene-cluster haplotypes as prognostic indicators of vital organ failure. *Semin Hematol* 1991;28:202–208.

17. Powars DR, Meiselman HJ, Fisher TC, et al. Beta-S gene cluster haplotypes modulate hematologic and hemorheologic expression in sickle cell anemia: Use in predicting clinical severity. *Am J Pediatr Hematol Oncol* 1994;16:55–61.

18. Nagel RL. Severity, pathobiology, epistatic effects, and genetic markers in sickle cell anemia. *Semin Hematol* 1991;28:180–201.

19. Gill FM, Sleeper LA, Weiner SJ, et al. Clinical events in the first decade in a cohort of infants with sickle cell disease. Cooperative Study of Sickle Cell Disease [see comments]. *Blood* 1995;86:776–783.

20. Billett HH, Kim K, Fabry ME, et al. The percentage of dense red cells does not predict incidence of sickle cell painful crisis. *Blood* 1986;68:301–303.

21. Bailey S, Higgs DR, Morris J, et al. Is the painful crisis of sickle-cell disease due to sickling? [letter]. *Lancet* 1991;337:735.

22. Powars DR, Schroeder WA, Weiss JN, et al. Lack of influence of fetal hemoglobin levels or erythrocyte indices on the severity of sickle cell anemia. J Clin Invest 1980;65:732–740.

23. Platt OS, Brambilla DJ, Rosse WF, et al. Mortality in sickle cell disease: Life expectancy and risk factors for early death [see comments]. *N Engl J Med* 1994;330:1639–1644.

24. Castro O, Brambilla DJ, Thorington B, et al. The acute chest syndrome in sickle cell disease: Incidence and risk factors. The Cooperative Study of Sickle Cell Disease. *Blood* 1994;84:643–649.

25. Gillum RF, Ingram DD, Makuc DM. White blood cell count, coronary heart disease, and death: The NHANES I Epidemiologic Follow-up Study [see comments]. *Am Heart J* 1993;125:855–863.

26. Balkaran B, Char G, Morris JS, et al. Stroke in a cohort of patients with homozygous sickle cell disease. *J Pediatr* 1992;120:360–366.

27. Charache S, Terrin ML, Moore RD, et al. Effect of hydroxyurea on the frequency of painful crises in sickle cell anemia: Investigators of the Multicenter Study of Hydroxyurea in Sickle Cell Anemia [see comments]. *N Engl J Med* 1995;332:1317–1322.

28. Kinney TR, Helms RW, O'Branski EE, et al. Safety of hydroxyurea in children with sickle cell anemia: Results of the HUG-KIDS study, a phase I/II trial. Pediatric Hydroxyurea Group. *Blood* 1999;94:1550–1554.

29. Saleh AW, Hillen HF, Duits AJ. Levels of endothelial, neutrophil and platelet-specific factors in sickle cell anemia patients during hydroxyurea therapy. *Acta Haematol* 1999;102:31–37.

30. Francis RB Jr, Haywood LJ. Elevated immunoreactive tumor necrosis factor and interleukin-1 in sickle cell disease. *J Natl Med Assoc* 1992;84:611–615.

31. Michaels LA, Ohene-Frempong K, Zhao H, et al. Serum levels of substance P are elevated in patients with sickle cell disease and increase further during vaso-occlusive crisis. *Blood* 1998;92:3148–3151.

32. Graido-Gonzalez E, Doherty JC, Bergreen EW, et al. Plasma endothelin-1, cytokine, and prostaglandin E2 levels in sickle cell disease and acute vaso-occlusive sickle crisis. *Blood* 1998;92:2551–2555.

33. Bevilacqua MP. Endothelial-leukocyte adhesion molecules. *Annu Rev Immunol* 1993;11:767–804.

34. Butcher EC. Leukocyte-endothelial cell recognition: Three (or more) steps to specificity and diversity. *Cell* 1991;67:1033–1036.

35. Hammer DA, Apte SM. Simulation of cell rolling and adhesion on surfaces in shear flow: General results and analysis of selectin-mediated neutrophil adhesion. *Biophys J* 1992;63:35–57.

36. Goldsmith HL, Takamura K, Bell D. Shear-induced collisions between human blood cells. *Ann NY Acad Sci* 1983;416:299–318.

37. Goldsmith HL, Spain S. Margination of leukocytes in blood flow through small tubes. *Microvasc Res* 1984;27:204–222.

38. Goldsmith HL, Lichtarge O, Tessier-Lavigne M, et al. Some model experiments in hemodynamics: VI. Two-body collisions between blood cells. *Biorheology* 1981;18:531–555.

39. Hofstra TC, Kalra VK, Meiselman HJ, et al. Sickle erythrocytes adhere to polymorphonuclear neutrophils and activate the neutrophil respiratory burst. *Blood* 1996;87:4440–4447.

40. Green GA, Rehn MM, Kalra VK. Cell-bound autologous immunoglobulin in erythrocyte subpopulations from patients with sickle cell disease. *Blood* 1985;65:1127–1133.

41. Green GA, Kalra VK. Sickling-induced binding of immunoglobulin to sickle erythrocytes. *Blood* 1988;71:636–639.
42. Swerlick RA, Eckman JR, Kumar A, et al. Alpha 4 beta 1-integrin expression on sickle reticulocytes: Vascular cell adhesion molecule-1-dependent binding to endothelium. *Blood* 1993;82:1891–1899.
43. Joneckis CC, Ackley RL, Orringer EP, et al. Integrin alpha 4 beta 1 and glycoprotein IV (CD36) are expressed on circulating reticulocytes in sickle cell anemia. *Blood* 1993;82:3548–3555.
44. Sultana C, Shen Y, Rattan V, et al. Interaction of sickle erythrocytes with endothelial cells in the presence of endothelial cell conditioned medium induces oxidant stress leading to transendothelial migration of monocytes. *Blood* 1998;92:3924–3935.
45. Perry MA, Granger DN. Role of CD11/CD18 in shear rate-dependent leukocyte-endothelial cell interactions in cat mesenteric venules. *J Clin Invest* 1991;87:1798–1804.
46. Lawrence MB, McIntire LV, Eskin SG. Effect of flow on polymorphonuclear leukocyte/endothelial cell adhesion. *Blood* 1987;70:1284–1290.
47. Gee BE, Platt OS. Sickle reticulocytes adhere to VCAM-1. *Blood* 1995;85:268–274.
48. Solovey A, Lin Y, Browne P, et al. Circulating activated endothelial cells in sickle cell anemia. *N Engl J Med* 1997;337:1584–1590.
49. Solovey AA, Solovey AN, Harkness J, Hebbel RP. Modulation of endothelial cell activation in sickle cell disease: A pilot study. *Blood* 2001;97:1937–1941.
50. Faller DV. Vascular modulation. In Embury SH, Hebbel RP, Mohandas N, et al., eds: *Sickle Cell Disease: Basic Principles and Clinical Practice.* New York: Raven Press; 1994:235–246.
51. Sowemimo-Coker SO, Meiselman HJ, Francis RB Jr. Increased circulating endothelial cells in sickle cell crisis. *Am J Hematol* 1989;31:263–265.
52. Phelan M, Perrine SP, Brauer M, et al. Sickle erythrocytes, after sickling, regulate the expression of the endothelin-1 gene and protein in human endothelial cells in culture. *J Clin Invest* 1995;96:1145–1151.
53. Sultana C, Shen Y, Johnson C, et al. Cobalt chloride-induced signaling in endothelium leading to the augmented adherence of sickle red blood cells and transendothelial migration of monocyte-like HL-60 cells is blocked by PAF-receptor antagonist. *J Cell Physiol* 1999;179:67–78.
54. Setty BN, Stuart MJ. Vascular cell adhesion molecule-1 is involved in mediating hypoxia-induced sickle red blood cell adherence to endothelium: Potential role in sickle cell disease. *Blood* 1996;88:2311–2320.
55. Hebbel RP, Morgan WT, Eaton JW, et al. Accelerated autoxidation and heme loss due to instability of sickle hemoglobin. *Proc Natl Acad Sci USA* 1988;85:237–241.
56. Hebbel RP. Membrane-associated iron. In Embury SH, Hebbel RP, Mohandas N, et al., eds: *Sickle Cell Disease: Basic Principles and Clinical Practice.* New York: Raven Press; 1994:163–172.
57. Schreck R, Rieber P, Baeuerle PA. Reactive oxygen intermediates as apparently widely used messengers in the activation of the NF-κB transcription factor and HIV-1. *EMBO J* 1991;10:2247–2258.
58. Henkel T, Machleidt T, Alkalay I, et al. Rapid proteolysis of IκBα is necessary for activation of transcription factor NF-κB. *Nature* 1993;365:182–185.
59. Rattan V, Sultana C, Shen Y, et al. Oxidant stress-induced transendothe-

lial migration of monocytes is linked to phosphorylation of PECAM-1. *Am J Physiol* 1997;273:E453–461.

60. Mohazzab KM, Kaminski PM, Wolin MS. NADH oxidoreductase is a major source of superoxide anion in bovine coronary artery endothelium. *Am J Physiol* 1994;266:H2568–2572.

61. Wautier JL, Wautier MP, Schmidt AM, et al. Advanced glycation end products (AGEs) on the surface of diabetic erythrocytes bind to the vessel wall via a specific receptor inducing oxidant stress in the vasculature: A link between surface-associated AGEs and diabetic complications. *Proc Natl Acad Sci USA* 1994;91:7742–7746.

62. Rattan V, Shen Y, Sultana C, et al. Diabetic RBC-induced oxidant stress leads to transendothelial migration of monocyte-like HL-60 cells. *Am J Physiol* 1997;273:E369–375.

63. Baeuerle PA, Henkel T. Function and activation of NF-κB in the immune system. *Annu Rev Immunol* 1994;12:141–179.

64. Marui N, Offermann MK, Swerlick R, et al. Vascular cell adhesion molecule-1 (VCAM-1) gene transcription and expression are regulated through an antioxidant-sensitive mechanism in human vascular endothelial cells. *J Clin Invest* 1993;92:1866–1874.

65. Shiu YT, Udden MM, McIntire LV. Perfusion with sickle erythrocytes up-regulates ICAM-1 and VCAM-1 gene expression in cultured human endothelial cells. *Blood* 2000;95:3232–3241.

66. Zimmerman GA, Lorant DE, McIntyre TM, et al. Juxtacrine intercellular signaling: Another way to do it. *Am J Respir Cell Mol Biol* 1993;9:573–577.

67. Vaporciyan AA, DeLisser HM, Yan HC, et al. Involvement of platelet-endothelial cell adhesion molecule-1 in neutrophil recruitment in vivo. *Science* 1993;262:1580–1582.

68. Sultana C, Shen Y, Rattan V, et al. Lipoxygenase metabolites induced expression of adhesion molecules and transendothelial migration of monocyte-like HL-60 cells is linked to protein kinase C activation. *J Cell Physiol* 1996;167:477–487.

69. Shen Y, Rattan V, Sultana C, et al. Cigarette smoke condensate-induced adhesion molecule expression and transendothelial migration of monocytes. *Am J Physiol* 1996;270:H1624–1633.

Chapter 6

Inflammation Causing Adhesion of Sickle Erythrocytes to Endothelium

Timothy M. Wick, PhD

Introduction

Vascular complications arising from homozygous inheritance of hemoglobin β_s in patients with sickle cell anemia are multifactorial, complex, and involve both large vessels and microvessels.[1,2] Microvascular complications include pain episodes (vaso-occlusive crises) resulting from polymerization of deoxygenated hemoglobin S to form rigid (sickled) erythrocytes that occlude capillaries, leading to intermittent tissue ischemia and pain. However, red cell sickling alone does not account for the diverse pathophysiology-associated vaso-occlusive episodes. Platelets, leukocytes, plasma factors, and erythrocyte-endothelial interactions all appear to contribute to initiation and propagation of vaso-occlusion.[1,2]

The kinetics of hemoglobin polymerization vary widely and are a strong function of intracellular hemoglobin S concentration and the presence of polymer nuclei.[3] Hemoglobin polymerization is delayed following deoxygenation in the microvasculature and delay times are long enough to allow most erythrocytes to traverse the microcirculation prior to morphological sickling.[4] This observation forms the basis of the kinetic hypothesis of vaso-occlusion,[5] which compares the time required for hemoglobin gelation (or erythrocyte sickling) following deoxygenation to the time required for the red cell to traverse the microcirculation. If the erythrocyte gelation (or sickling) time is longer than the red cell capillary transit time, red cells should not sickle and become trapped in the microcirculation. That the majority of red cells traverse the microcirculation without sickling suggests that patients

This work was supported by HL-44960.

From: Weir EK, Reeve HL, Reeves JT (eds). *Interactions of Blood and the Pulmonary Circulation*. Armonk, NY: Futura Publishing Company, Inc.; ©2002.

not in crisis experience an unstable flow equilibrium, and pain episodes may result from changes in the polymerization rate or capillary transit time that lead to microvascular flow disruption and vaso-occlusion. Thus, factors that increase the hemoglobin polymerization rate or delay erythrocyte microvascular transit will initiate intracapillary sickling, microvascular occlusion, and pain crisis.

Abnormal adherence of sickle erythrocytes to endothelium is one factor hypothesized to delay red cell microcirculatory transit and initiate or propagate microvascular occlusion in sickle cell anemia.[6,7] This is supported by the observation that erythrocyte-endothelial adherence in vitro correlates with one measure of disease severity for sickle patients.[7] Further support for abnormal sickle cell adherence initiating vaso-occlusion comes from ex vivo perfusion models demonstrating that microvascular obstruction appears to be a 2-step process. Vaso-occlusion is initiated by adherence of sickle erythrocytes to microvascular endothelium. Subsequent entrapment of dense and irreversibly sickled red cells leads to complete occlusion.[8,9]

Sickle red cells exhibit an intrinsic ability to bind to endothelium[10] and adherence is elevated by sickle plasma.[11] Patient plasma collected during pain episodes contains more adhesive factors than patient plasma collected during asymptomatic periods.[11] Fibrinogen,[11] von Willebrand factor,[12–14] (vWF) (particularly the unusually large multimers[12]), and thrombospondin[15,16] are specific adhesive plasma proteins shown to promote sickle (but not normal) erythrocyte adherence to endothelium.

Sickle erythrocyte membranes exhibit significant abnormalities compared to normal red cell membranes. Altered membrane charge distribution,[17] abnormal exposure of phosphatidylserine,[18,19] aggregated band 3,[20] or sulfated glycolipids[21] on sickle erythrocytes may facilitate endothelial adherence.[22] Some sickle reticulocytes also express adhesion receptors $\alpha_4\beta_1$,[23,24] CD36,[15,24] and possibly others[25,26] that can mediate adherence to endothelium.

Sickle cell adherence is thought to predominate in postcapillary venules[8] where the wall shear stress is on the order of 1.0 dyne/cm^2.[27] Studies in parallel-plate flow chambers demonstrate that sickle erythrocytes adhere to endothelium under dynamic flow at 1.0 dyne/cm^2 shear stress. However, this may not be the flow condition that dominates in postcapillary venules of sickle patients. Oscillatory, intermittent, and reduced blood flow is observed in sickle microvasculature for patients at steady state[28,29] (e.g., not in crisis) and in the microcirculation of transgenic mice.[30]

Microvascular flow conditions promoting sickle cell adherence in vivo are not well understood and arguments can be made for both low flow[31] or unperturbed flow[32] as the prevailing condition when adherence initiates the vaso-occlusive cascade. Low or intermittent flow provides increased opportunities for adherence to occur since endothelial contact times are increased and shear forces opposing adherence are decreased compared to flow in uncompromised microvasculature. On the other hand, if adherence initiates vaso-occlusion,[31] the prevailing hemodynamics may be steady, unobstructed flow. Thus, identifying conditions promoting extensive and strong sickle cell adherence under in vivo flow conditions will provide important insights into vascular perturbations that disturb unstable flow equilibrium in sickle microvasculature.

Inflammation, Adhesion, and Vaso-Occlusion

Reports that a subfraction of sickle reticulocytes express $\alpha_4\beta_1$ integrin[21,23] initiated investigations to identify endothelial cell adhesion molecules that promote sickle cell adherence via $\alpha_4\beta_1$. Three different interactions have been described for $\alpha_4\beta_1$: binding to vascular cell adhesion molecule-1 (VCAM-1) on cytokine-activated endothelium,[33] binding to the CS-1 domain of plasma fibronectin when $\alpha_4\beta_1$ is activated by phorbol ester or chemokine,[34] and mediation of homotypic leukocyte aggregation by specific monoclonal antibodies.[35] These binding events are independent and regulatable,[36] raising the possibility that cell adhesion via $\alpha_4\beta_1$ may occur by multiple pathways.

Initial investigations of sickle cell adherence via $\alpha_4\beta_1$ focused on binding to VCAM-1. In dynamic adhesion assays under continuous flow at a shear stress of 1.0 dyne/cm², sickle erythrocytes adhered to endothelium stimulated for 6 hours with 500 units/mL tissue necrosis factor-α (TNF-α), but did not adhere to unstimulated endothelium.[23] Erythrocytes containing hemoglobin AA did not adhere to cytokine-stimulated endothelium. Blocking studies with monoclonal antibodies confirmed sickle erythrocyte/endothelial adhesion was via $\alpha_4\beta_1$/VCAM-1, since pretreating TNF-α-stimulated endothelium with anti-VCAM-1 antibody or sickle erythrocytes with anti-CD49d antibody inhibited sickle cell adherence by 75% (Figure 1). Control antibodies did not inhibit sickle cell binding to TNF-α-stimulated endothelium.[23]

The data of Figure 1 suggest a link between inflammation, endothelial activation, and sickle cell adherence. In sickle patients, pain episodes are precipitated or coincide with bacterial or viral infection[37–41] and cytokines are elevated in blood of sickle patients,[42,43] especially during crisis.[44] Many pathogenic viruses, including influenza, rhinovirus, flavivirus, and Coxsackie virus, possess a double-stranded genome or replicate through double-stranded RNA intermediates.[45] Endothelial response to infection with double-stranded RNA includes

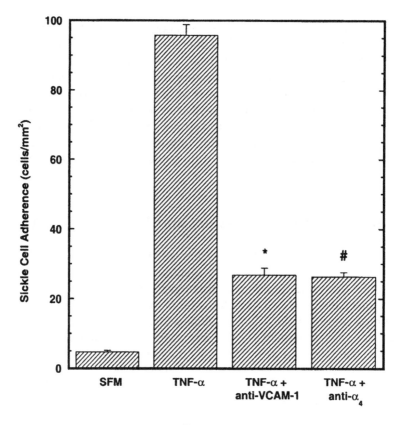

Figure 1. TNF-α-induced sickle cell adherence is via $\alpha_4\beta_1$/VCAM-1. Data are mean ±SEM (n=7) sickle cell adherence to unstimulated (SFM) or TNF-α-stimulated HUVEC at 1.0 dyne/cm^2 shear stress. Incubation of *TNF-α-stimulated HUVEC with anti-VCAM-1 antibody (n=7, P=0.004) or #sickle erythrocytes with anti-α_4 antibody (n=6, P=0.005) inhibited sickle cell adherence to TNF-α-stimulated endothelium. Adapted from Swerlick et al.,[23] and reprinted with permission by The American Society of Hematology.

expression of VCAM-1.[46] This suggests that certain types of viral infection increase sickle cell adherence via $\alpha_4\beta_1$/VCAM-1 providing a mechanism by which infection and inflammation can initiate vaso-occlusion.

In order to establish a more direct link between infection in sickle cell patients and adhesive vaso-occlusion, erythrocyte adherence to endothelium infected with virus was studied. In these experiments, endothelial cells were incubated with parainfluenza-1 virus for 1 hour, washed, and then cultured for 20 additional hours. Following viral infection, endothelial cells expressed significant VCAM-1[47] and supported sickle erythrocyte adherence under flow at a shear stress of 1.0 dyne/cm^2 (Figure 2).

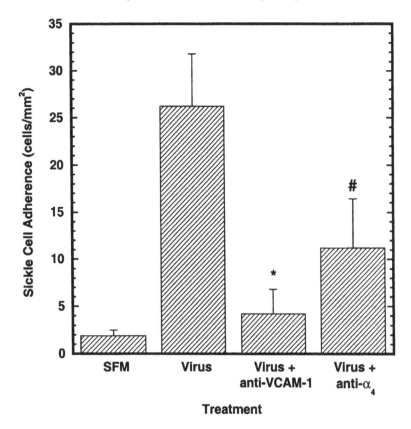

Figure 2. Endothelial infection with virus induces sickle cell adherence via $\alpha_4\beta_1$/VCAM-1. Data are mean ±SEM (n=4) sickle cell adherence to endothelium infected with parainfluenza virus A (Sendai virus) quantified at 1.0 dyne/cm^2 shear stress. Incubation of *virus-stimulated HUVEC with anti-VCAM-1 antibody (P=<0.009, n=4) or #sickle erythrocytes with anti-α_4 antibody (p<0.002) inhibits sickle cell adherence induced by virus by 92% or 63%, respectively, to TNF-α-stimulated endothelium. Adapted from Smolinski et al.,[47] and reprinted with permission by The American Society of Hematology.

Anti-VCAM-1 antibody on virus-infected endothelium or anti-CD49d on sickle erythrocytes inhibited 92% or 63%, respectively, of the sickle cell adherence induced by parainfluenza-1 virus (Figure 2). These studies suggest that direct activation of endothelium by virus and sickle cell adherence via $\alpha_4\beta_1$/VCAM-1 may be an important initiator of vaso-occlusion for sickle patients infected with virus.

In addition to sickle cell adherence induced by double-stranded RNA virus, a previous study has shown that endothelial infection with Herpes simplex type 1 virus (a DNA virus) also activates endothelium and induces sickle cell adherence.[48] In those studies, virus-induced glycoprotein on infected endothelium provided binding sites for sickle erythrocyte immunoglobulin.[48,49] Sickle cells bind abnormal amounts of IgG[50] and show preferential adherence to endothelium infected with herpes simplex type 1 virus.[51] Those adherence studies were done under static incubation conditions and it is not clear whether the adhesive interactions observed are strong enough to withstand microvascular shear forces opposing adherence. In any event, those studies demonstrate that endothelial response to viral infection can vary widely and can induce sickle cell adhesion via diverse interactions.

Activation of integrin $\alpha_4\beta_1$ with phorbol ester,[52] activating antibodies,[53] or proinflammatory chemokines[54] exposes epitopes on $\alpha_4\beta_1$ that promote binding to the CS-1 domain of plasma fibronectin[34] in addition to VCAM-1. Activation of sickle erythrocytes with phorbol ester or chemokines (such as IL-8) was hypothesized to induce sickle cell adherence via $\alpha_4\beta_1$ binding to fibronectin.[55] To test this, sickle erythrocytes were incubated with IL-8 and endothelial adherence was measured under flow conditions at 1.0 dyne/cm^2 shear stress. In those experiments, IL-8 promoted sickle erythrocyte adherence to unactivated endothelium.[55] In contrast, IL-8-stimulated erythrocytes containing hemoglobin AA were not adhesive to endothelium.[55] Pretreatment of endothelium (and not sickle erythrocytes) with IL-8 did not promote sickle erythrocyte adherence,[55] confirming that the effect of IL-8 was localized to sickle cells. Endothelial incubation with anti-VCAM-1 antibody did not inhibit sickle cell adherence induced by IL-8 stimulation,[55] suggesting that IL-8-activated sickle red cells did not bind to VCAM-1 on endothelium. In contrast, incubation of IL-8-stimulated sickle erythrocytes with soluble fibronectin inhibited by 97% the sickle erythrocyte adherence induced by IL-8 treatment (Figure 3). Similarly, incubation of endothelium with anti-fibronectin antibody inhibited IL-8-induced sickle cell binding to endothelium by 96% (Figure 3). Sickle cell adhesion to endothelium induced by IL-8 is also inhibited by incubation of IL-8-treated sickle cells with a blocking anti-α_4 antibody or a synthetic peptide containing the CS-1 domain of fibronectin.[55]

Taken together, these data suggest that IL-8 exerts its proadhesive effect on sickle erythrocyte epitopes. Blocking with soluble fibronectin, anti-α_4 antibody, or fibronectin CS-1 fragment peptide all support the notion that IL-8-activated $\alpha_4\beta_1$ on sickle erythrocytes binds to fibronectin on the endothelial cell surface. Immunohistochemical analysis revealed significant amounts of fibronectin associated with the surface of *washed* endothelium under conditions where vWF binding to endothelium was unremarkable.[55] This implies that fibronectin forms firm associations or bonds with endothelium, at least in vitro. That soluble fibronectin inhibits IL-8-induced sickle cell adherence to endothelium further supports the conclusion that activated $\alpha_4\beta_1$ can bind fibronectin. Presumably, soluble fibronectin binds to IL-8-activated $\alpha_4\beta_1$ in a way

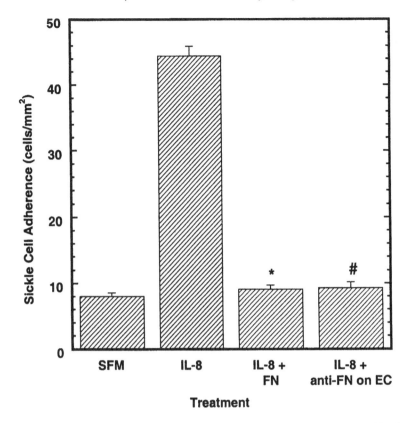

Figure 3. Endothelial fibronectin mediates sickle cell adherence induced by IL-8. Data are mean ±SEM (n=5) sickle cell adherence at 1.0 dyne/cm² shear stress following treatment with interleukin-8 (IL-8). Preincubation of sickle erythrocytes with soluble fibronectin (IL-8 + FN, *P=0.01) or endothelial cells with anti-fibronectin antibody (IL-8 + anti-FN on HUVEC, #P=0.007) completely inhibits sickle cell adherence induced by IL-8. Adapted from Kumar et al.,[55] and reprinted with permission by The American Society of Hematology.

that inhibits the activated $\alpha_4\beta_1$ from binding to fibronectin on the endothelial cell surface. Clearly, additional studies are necessary to confirm the presence of endothelial-associated fibronectin in vasculature.

The data of Figures 1–3 demonstrate a link between infection, inflammation, sickle cell adherence to endothelium, and vaso-occlusion. TNF-α[42,56] and circulating soluble VCAM-1 (sVCAM-1)[57,58] are both elevated in sickle plasma, particularly during pain crises. Serum IL-8 levels are also elevated during sickle pain episodes in some[44,59] (but not all[60,61]) studies. Thus, inflammation leading to endothelial and sickle cell activation may promote sickle cell adherence to endothelium via both activated $\alpha_4\beta_1$/fibronectin or $\alpha_4\beta_1$/VCAM-1 interactions in vivo. That the data in Figures 1–3 were generated under flow conditions thought to prevail in venules suggests that sickle cell adherence can occur in the absence of prior vascular obstruction. Thus, adherence via these mechanisms during tissue inflammation may initiate the vaso-occlusive cascade of microvascular flow sludging and red cell sickling leading to complete occlusion.

Strength of Sickle Cell Adherence Mediated by High-Affinity Pathways

The mechanism(s) of sickle cell adherence to endothelium described to date include (1) adherence mediated by unusually large molecular weight vWF (ULvWF) multimers bridging GPIb-like and integrin receptors on sickle cells and similar receptors on endothelial cells[12,25]; (2) plasma thrombospondin bridging CD36 on sickle reticulocytes and the $\alpha_v\beta_3$ integrin on large-vessel endothelium[15] or $\alpha_v\beta_3$ and CD36 on microvascular endothelium[16]; (3) binding of sickle reticulocyte $\alpha_4\beta_1$ receptors to VCAM-1 expressed on endothelial cells stimulated by cytokine[23] or virus[47]; (4) binding of sickle reticulocyte $\alpha_4\beta_1$ activated by phorbol ester or IL-8 to endothelial cell-associated fibronectin[55]; (5) sickle red cell binding to E-selectin on cytokine-activated endothelium[26]; and (6) sickle erythrocyte immunoglobulin binding to viral glycoprotein expressed by endothelial cells infected with herpes virus.[48] Aggregated band 3[20] or sulfated glycolipids[21,22] on sickle erythrocytes can also promote abnormal sickle cell adherence. Subendothelial matrix proteins expressed following vascular injury may also support sickle cell adherence[21] in addition to endothelial cells.[22] Adhesive interactions between sickle erythrocytes and extracellular matrix proteins are reviewed in a subsequent chapter.

Most studies of sickle erythrocyte adherence to endothelium have been under conditions where only one adherence pathway is active. Studies of this nature are useful to identify specific receptors and ligands involved in adherence. In vivo, erythrocyte/endothelial adherence via more than one pathway is plausible. For example, inflammation and cytokine release in vivo raise the possibility that endothelial cells express VCAM-1 and integrin $\alpha_4\beta_1$ is activated on sickle reticulocytes to induce binding to both endothelial-associated fibronectin and VCAM-1. To test whether adherence via multiple pathways is possible, studies were undertaken to test whether simultaneous binding via $\alpha_4\beta_1$/VCAM-1 and activated $\alpha_4\beta_1$/fibronectin enhances sickle cell adherence compared to either pathway alone. For these experiments, endothelial cells were treated with TNF-α (to upregulate VCAM-1) and sickle cells were treated with IL-8 (to activate $\alpha_4\beta_1$). Adherence assays were performed under continuous flow at a shear stress of 1.0 dyne/cm^2 and adherence was compared to that measured when either pathway was activated separately.

Two parameters were identified to characterize adherence via an individual pathway or the combined pathways: initial adherence and adherence strength. To compare which, if any, pathway(s) promoted higher adherence (under otherwise identical conditions, e.g., endothelial cells from the same harvest and red cells from the same donor), the initial adherence, defined as that measured following 10 minutes of red cell perfusion at 1.0 dyne/cm^2, was quantified. In addition, the strength of adherence promoted by different pathways was measured in detachment assays by sequentially increasing fluid shear force (in 0.5 dyne/cm^2 increments) after initial adherence was measured. Adherence strength of a bound population of erythrocytes was defined as the shear stress required to remove 50% of the initially adherent red cells.[62] Adherence strength is presented as τ_{50} (dynes/cm^2). Again, to directly compare adherence strength promoted by different pathways, a series of detachment experiments testing individual or multiple pathways was performed using endothelial cells from the same harvest and erythrocytes from the same sickle donor.[63,64] The adherence pathways investigated are summarized in Table 1.

For adherence promoted by a single pathway, initial adherence at 1.0

Table 1

Description of Sickle Cell-Endothelial Adherence Pathways Studied

Pathway Designation	Erythrocyte Ligand	Bridging Molecule	Endothelial Ligand(s)	Comments
Unusually large vWF (ULvWF)[12,25]	Integrin	ULvWF	Integrin, GP-Ib (?)	ULvWF multimers collected from endothelial cell supernatants[12]
Thrombospondin (TSP)[15,16]	CD36	TSP	$\alpha_v\beta_3$	Large vessel endothelium[16]
$\alpha_4\beta_1$/VCAM-1[23,76]	$\alpha_4\beta_1$	None	VCAM-1	Cytokine-activated endothelium
Activated $\alpha_4\beta_1$/ Fibronectin[55]	$\alpha_4\beta_1$	None	Fibronectin	Integrin $\alpha_4\beta_1$ activated by chemokine
$\alpha_4\beta_1$/VCAM-1 and $\alpha_4\beta_1$/fibronectin	$\alpha_4\beta_1$	None	VCAM-1 and fibronectin	Endothelium activated with TNF-α and sickle cells treated with IL-8

ULvWF = unusually large von Willebrand factor.

dyne/cm^2 is generally equivalent for the 4 individual pathways described in Table 1.[64] This varies with patient[63] and suggests that under some conditions, certain pathways may promote more extensive erythrocyte/ endothelial cell adherence in vivo. The right shift of the detachment curves for sickle cell adherence via $\alpha_4\beta_1$/VCAM-1 or $\alpha_4\beta_1$/FN (Figure 4) demonstrates that adherence promoted by either pathway involving sickle reticulocyte $\alpha_4\beta_1$ is stronger than adherence promoted by adhesive plasma proteins thrombospondin or ULvWF. Adherence strength quantified as τ_{50} confirms that adherence via either sickle cell $\alpha_4\beta_1$ pathway is

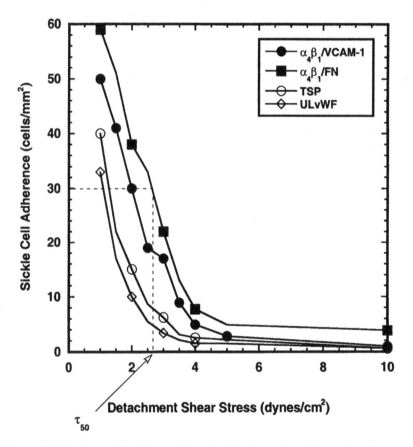

Figure 4. Detachment of sickle erythrocytes by increasing shear stress for endothelial adherence via individual pathways. Sickle erythrocytes attached to endothelium under flow at a shear stress of 1.0 dyne/cm^2 via the indicated pathway. Adherent erythrocytes were detached from endothelium by sequentially increasing shear stress. The dashed lines illustrate how the shear stress required to remove 50% of the originally adherent red cells (τ_{50}) is determined for the activated $\alpha_4\beta_1$/VCAM-1 pathway. Data are mean sickle cell adherence to endothelium for 1 representative experiment from Smolinski.[63,64]

approximately 50% stronger than endothelial adherence promoted by TSP or ULvWF[63] (Table 2[64]).

To test whether adherence via multiple pathways increases the level or strength of sickle cell adherence to endothelium, experiments were conducted for conditions where more than one pathway is invoked simultaneously.[63] For example, adherence promoted by both $\alpha_4\beta_1$/VCAM-1 and $\alpha_4\beta_1$/FN is higher and stronger than adherence promoted by either pathway alone[63] (Figure 5[64]). Adherence strength (τ_{50}) measured when both pathways are involved is 5.9 ± 1.1 dyne/cm^2 and significantly greater than adherence strength measured for either pathway alone (τ_{50} = 2.8 ± 0.4 and 2.4 ± 0.1 for $\alpha_4\beta_1$/VCAM-1 and $\alpha_4\beta_1$/FN, respectively[64]). In addition, when adherence is promoted by both $\alpha_4\beta_1$/VCAM-1 and $\alpha_4\beta_1$/FN, more than 30% of the initially adherent sickle erythrocytes remain attached to the endothelium at a detachment shear stress of 10 dynes/cm^2.[63] Additional experiments testing the potential synergy between sickle cell/endothelial cell adherence via the TSP pathway and $\alpha_4\beta_1$/VCAM-1 or $\alpha_4\beta_1$/FN pathways show that thrombospondin does not appear to increase the sickle cell adherence level or strength compared to $\alpha_4\beta_1$/VCAM-1 or $\alpha_4\beta_1$/FN alone (Table 3).

These data suggest that sickle cells that adhere to endothelium via $\alpha_4\beta_1$/VCAM-1 or $\alpha_4\beta_1$/FN under physiological flow (e.g., 1.0 dyne/cm^2) are firmly attached to the endothelium and many of the adherent red cells are able to resist detachment shear stress more than twice the physiological flow (Table 2).[63,64] Adherence occurring via both $\alpha_4\beta_1$/VCAM-1 and $\alpha_4\beta_1$/FN simultaneously is very strong. Fully one-third of the sickle cells binding to endothelium at 1.0 dyne/cm^2 via both pathways are able to resist shear forces *more than ten times* those normally existing in postcapillary venules.[63] These cells are not likely to be dislodged simply by increasing blood flow (or pressure drop) through the occluded vessel(s). Thus, blood flow through tissues where occlusion includes red cell adherence via reticulocyte $\alpha_4\beta_1$ may be restored only reluctantly.

Table 2

Adherence Strength for Individual Pathways

	Adherence Pathway			
	$\alpha_4\beta_1$/VCAM-1	$\alpha_4\beta_1$/FN	TSP	ULvWF
Adhesion strength τ_{50} (dynes/cm^2)	2.2	2.7	1.6	1.5

Data are adherence strength measured in one experiment when blood was from the same sickle donor and endothelial cells were from the same harvest and are representative of experiments performed with blood from several donors. Adapted from Smolinski, 1996.[63]

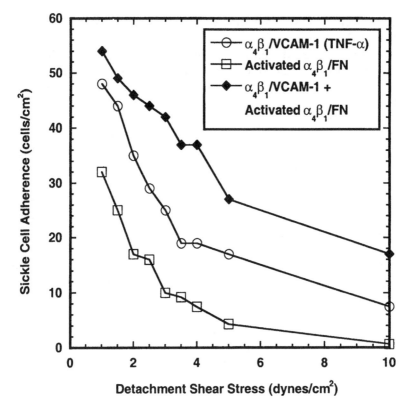

Figure 5. Sickle cell adherence mediated simultaneously by both $\alpha_4\beta_1$ pathways. Sickle erythrocytes attached to endothelium under flow at a shear stress of 1.0 dyne/cm². Adherence was by $\alpha_4\beta_1$/VCAM-1 alone (endothelium activated by TNF-α[23]), activated $\alpha_4\beta_1$/fibronectin alone (sickle erythrocytes activated by IL-8[55]), or both pathways simultaneously. Adherent erythrocytes were detached from endothelium by sequentially increasing shear stress. Data are mean sickle cell adherence to endothelium for 1 representative experiment from Smolinski.[63,64]

Sickle cell adherence to endothelium via TSP or ULvWF appears weaker than adherence promoted by $\alpha_4\beta_1$/VCAM-1 or $\alpha_4\beta_1$/FN[64] (Figure 4). Adherence via TSP or ULvWF occurs by these adhesive plasma proteins bridging receptors on sickle erythrocytes and endothelial cells[12,15,16] in so-called series bonds.[65] In contrast, sickle cell adherence mediated by reticulocyte $\alpha_4\beta_1$ involves direct binding of the sickle erythrocyte integrin to an endothelial counterligand[23,55] (referred to as a single bond[65]). This is consistent with recent investigations showing that cell adhesion mediated by single bonds is stronger than adherence mediated by bonds in series, regardless of the relative strength of the individual receptor-ligand interactions in the series bond.[66] Those ob-

Table 3

Effect of Multiple Adhesion Pathways on Sickle Cell Adherence Strength

	Adherence Pathway						
	$\alpha_4\beta_1$/VCAM-1	$\alpha_4\beta_1$/FN	TSP	$\alpha_4\beta_1$/VCAM-1 + $\alpha_4\beta_1$/FN	$\alpha_4\beta_1$/VCAM-1 + TSP	$\alpha_4\beta_1$/FN + TSP	$\alpha_4\beta_1$/VCAM-1 + $\alpha_4\beta_1$/FN + TSP
Initial adherence (cells/mm^2)	69.5	33.8	26.5	74.5	27.4	18.2	24.9
Adhesion strength τ_{50} (dynes/cm^2)	2.8	2.8	1.7	9.6	3.2	2.4	6.8

Data are adherence strength measured in one experiment when blood was from the same sickle donor and endothelial cells were from the same harvest. Adapted from Smolinski, 1996.[63]

servations plus the present data provide evidence that sickle cell adherence in vivo via single bonds (e.g., $\alpha_4\beta_1$/VCAM-1 or $\alpha_4\beta_1$/FN) may be stronger than sickle cell adherence utilizing several bonds in series such as TSP or ULvWF-mediated adherence.

In summary, sickle erythrocyte adherence to endothelium via reticulocyte $\alpha_4\beta_1$ integrin can occur in a dynamic flow environment under shear forces present in postcapillary venules where adherence may dominate.[8] Adherence via $\alpha_4\beta_1$/VCAM-1 or $\alpha_4\beta_1$/FN (or both) is strong enough to resist elevated detachment forces (Tables 2 and 3) resulting from increased perfusion pressure in response to the partial occlusion. These data imply that adherence under physiological flow conditions can persist in the microcirculation and suggest that inflammation leading to sickle cell adherence promoted by integrin $\alpha_4\beta_1$ may provide a "trigger" that disrupts microvascular blood flow and initiates vaso-occlusion.

Significance

Although intravascular sickling of hemoglobin SS remains the dominant pathological feature of sickle cell anemia, hemoglobin polymerization kinetics are delayed following deoxygenation. Erythrocytes traverse the microcirculation without sickling unless the dynamic between capillary transit time and hemoglobin polymerization delay time is disturbed,[5] for example, when sickle red cells adhere to endothelium and increase microvascular transit time. That the level of sickle cell adherence to endothelium in vitro correlates with a clinical severity score[7] that measures the frequency, intensity, and duration of patient pain episodes provides the most direct evidence that sickle cell adherence is related to sickle patient clinical complications. Perturbations that could initiate adherence of sickle erythrocytes via known pathways have been documented during acute vaso-occlusive complications. These acute events include endothelial damage,[13,21,22,25,67-69] thrombin formation or platelet activation,[15,16,70-75] and inflammation or infection,[23,26,42,44,47,55,76,77] which, among other things, can initiate sickle cell adherence to endothelium.

The focus of this chapter has been sickle cell adherence to endothelium related to inflammation. Cytokines, chemokines, and other vasoactive substances released during inflammation are hypothesized to activate endothelium and sickle erythrocytes leading to a proadhesive condition. Sickle cell adherence to endothelium via $\alpha_4\beta_1$/VCAM-1 or $\alpha_4\beta_1$/FN (or both) can occur under flow conditions (Figures 1–3) that predominate in postcapillary venules and is strong enough to withstand elevated shear forces (Figures 4 and 5) that may arise to reperfuse occluded vessels. Thus, adherence via reticulocyte $\alpha_4\beta_1$ induced by cytokines and chemokines during inflammation has characteristics appropriate to initiate or propagate microvascular occlusion, tissue ischemia, and pain.

However, steady flow may not be the condition that dominates in postcapillary venules of sickle patients where oscillatory[28] and intermittent[29] blood flow have been observed in sickle patients during steady state (e.g., not in crisis). Blood flow is significantly reduced in sickle microvessels compared to HbAA controls and flow stasis is a frequent observation in sickle microcirculation.[29] Both reduced and oscillatory microvascular blood flow occur in transgenic sickle mice under normoxic conditions,[30] further supporting the hypothesis that blood flow is compromised in sickle cell microvasculature.

Reduced flow or flow stasis provide a less stringent environment for adherence to occur since contact time between red cells and endothelium is increased and shear forces opposing adherence are lessened. Thus, decreased or intermittent blood flow or transient erythrostasis can enhance adherence by prolonging contact between erythrocytes and endothelium. Under these conditions, adherence may not require high-affinity sickle cell-endothelial cell interactions. Indeed, in static adhesion assays, sickle erythrocytes demonstrate significant intrinsic adhesivity without addition of plasma adhesive factors or adhesion-promoting cell agonists.[6,7,10,78–81] However, adherence occurring under static conditions in vitro is relatively weak.[64] This is consistent with the observation that sickle erythrocyte adherence occurring in capillaries during periods of incipient flow stasis (induced by a pressure cuff) is rapidly diminished upon removal of the pressure cuff and restoration of blood flow.[29,82] Although adherence may be favored in sickle microcirculation by low flow rates and intimate sickle erythrocyte/endothelial contacts,[83] in tissues with adequate perfusion, only high-affinity sickle cell-endothelial cell adhesion can resist detachment by physiological shear and pressure forces. Thus, conditions favoring strong adherence via specific receptor-ligand interactions, such as $\alpha_4\beta_1$/VCAM-1 or $\alpha_4\beta_1$/FN following inflammation, appear capable of *initiating* the 2-step cascade of adhesion and entrapment.

Conclusion

Painful vaso-occlusive crises cause significant morbidity in patients with sickle cell anemia. Although deoxyhemoglobin S polymerization is the dominant pathology, red cell sickling only partially accounts for vaso-occlusion. Research over decades has identified roles for platelets, leukocytes, endothelium, inflammatory mediators, clotting factors, and sickle erythrocyte membrane proteins in pain episodes. Recent data suggest that vaso-occlusion exhibits features of ischemia-reperfusion injury[84,85] and confirm a proinflammatory phenotype for patients with sickle cell anemia. The studies reviewed here demonstrating that sickle cell adherence to endothelium is induced by proinflammatory cytokines and chemokines provide a plausible mechanism linking inflammation and vaso-occlusion.

References

1. Bunn HF. Pathogenesis and treatment of sickle cell disease. *N Engl J Med* 1997;337:762–769.
2. Steinberg MH. Management of sickle cell disease. *N Engl J Med* 1999;340: 1021–1030.
3. Eaton WA, Hofrichter J. Sickle hemoglobin polymerization. In Embury SH, Hebbel RP, Mohandas N, et al., eds: *Sickle Cell Disease: Basic Principles and Clinical Practice*. New York: Raven Press; 1994:53–87.
4. Mozzarelli A, Hofrichter J, Eaton WA. Delay times of hemoglobin S gelation prevent most cells from sickling in vivo. *Science* 1987;237:104–113.
5. Hofrichter J, Ross PD, Eaton WA. Kinetics and mechanism of deoxyhemoglobin S gelation: A new approach to understanding sickle cell disease. *Proc Natl Acad Sci USA* 1974;71:4864–4868.
6. Hoover R, Rubin R, Wise G, et al. Adhesion of normal and sickle erythrocytes to endothelial monolayer cultures. *Blood* 1979;54:872–876.
7. Hebbel RP, Boogaerts MAB, Eaton JW, et al. Erythrocyte adherence to endothelium in sickle cell anemia: A possible determinant of disease severity. *N Engl J Med* 1980;302:992–995.
8. Kaul DK, Fabry ME, Nagel RL. Microvascular sites and characteristics of sickle cell adhesion to vascular endothelium in shear flow conditions: Pathophysiological implications. *Proc Natl Acad Sci USA* 1989;86:3356–3360.
9. Fabry ME, Fine E, Rajanayagam V, et al. Demonstration of endothelial adhesion of sickle cells in vivo: A distinct role for deformable sickle cell discocytes. *Blood* 1992;79:1602–1611.
10. Hebbel RP, Eaton JW, Steinberg MH, et al. Erythrocyte/endothelial interactions in the pathogenesis of sickle cell disease: A "real logical" assessment. *Blood Cells* 1982;8:163–173.
11. Hebbel RP, Moldow CF, Steinberg MH. Modulation of erythrocyte-endothelial interactions and the vaso-occlusive severity of sickling disorders. *Blood* 1981;58:947–952.
12. Wick TM, Moake JL, Udden MM, et al. Unusually large von Willebrand factor multimers increase adhesion of sickle erythrocytes to human endothelial cells under controlled flow. *J Clin Invest* 1987;80:905–910.
13. Kaul DK, Nagel RL, Chen D, et al. Sickle erythrocyte-endothelial interactions in microcirculation: The role of von Willebrand factor and implications for vaso-occlusion. *Blood* 1993;81:2429–2438.
14. Patel VP, Ciechanover A, Platt O, et al. Mammalian reticulocytes lose adhesion to fibronectin during maturation to erythrocytes. *Proc Natl Acad Sci USA* 1985;82:440–444.
15. Sugihara K, Sugihara T, Mohandas N, et al. Thrombospondin mediates adherence of CD36+ sickle reticulocytes to endothelial cells. *Blood* 1992; 80:2634–2642.
16. Brittain HA, Eckman JR, Swerlick RA, et al. Thrombospondin from activated platelets promotes sickle erythrocyte adherence to human micro-

vascular endothelium under physiologic flow: A potential role for platelet activation in sickle cell vaso-occlusion. *Blood* 1993;81:2137–2143.

17. Hebbel RP, Yamada O, Moldow CF, et al. Abnormal adherence of sickle erythrocytes to cultured vascular endothelium: Possible mechanism for microvascular occlusion in sickle cell disease. *J Clin Invest* 1980;65:154–160.

18. Zwaal RF, Bevers EM, Comfurius P, et al. Loss of membrane phospholipid asymmetry during activation of blood platelets and sickled red cells: Mechanisms and physiological significance. *Mol Cell Biochem* 1989;91:23–31.

19. Tomer A, Harker LA, Casey S, Eckman JR. Dietary n-3 fatty acid treatment reduces the frequency of pain episodes and the prothrombotic state in sickle cell anemia. *Blood* 1997;90(Suppl 1):445a.

20. Thevenin BJM, Crandall I, Ballas SK, et al. Band 3 peptides block the adherence of sickle cells to endothelial cells in vitro. *Blood* 1997;90:4172–4179.

21. Joneckis CC, Shock DD, Cunningham ML, et al. Glycoprotein IV-independent adhesion of sickle red blood cells to immobilized thrombospondin under flow conditions. *Blood* 1996;87:7865–7870.

22. Hillery CA, Du MC, Montgomery RR, et al. Increased adhesion of erythrocytes to components of the extracellular matrix: Isolation and characterization of a red blood cell lipid that binds thrombospondin and laminin. *Blood* 1996;87:4879–4886.

23. Swerlick RA, Eckman JR, Kumar A, et al. $\alpha_4\beta_1$-integrin expression on sickle reticulocytes: Vascular cell adhesion molecule-1-dependent binding to endothelium. *Blood* 1993;82:1891–1899.

24. Joneckis CC, Ackley RL, Orringer EP, et al. Integrin alpha 4 beta 1 and glycoprotein IV (CD36) are expressed on circulating reticulocytes in sickle cell anemia. *Blood* 1993;82:3548–3555.

25. Wick TM, Moake JL, Udden MM, et al. Unusually large von Willebrand factor multimers preferentially promote young sickle and nonsickle erythrocyte adhesion to endothelial cells. *Am J Hematol* 1993;42:284–292.

26. Natarajan M, Udden MM, McIntire LV. Adhesion of sickle red blood cells and damage to interleukin-1β-stimulated endothelial cells under flow in vitro. *Blood* 1996;87:4845–4852.

27. Turitto VT. Blood viscosity, mass transport, and thrombogenesis. *Prog Hemost Thromb* 1982;6:139–177.

28. Rodgers GP, Schechter AN, Noguchi CT, et al. Periodic microcirculatory flow in patients with sickle cell disease. *N Engl J Med* 1984;311:1534–1538.

29. Lipowsky HH, Sheikh NU, Katz DM. Intravital microscopy of capillary hemodynamics in sickle cell disease. *J Clin Invest* 1987;80:117–127.

30. Embury SH, Mohandas N, Paszty C, et al. In vivo blood flow abnormalities in the transgenic knockout sickle cell mouse. *J Clin Invest* 1999;103:915–920.

31. Hebbel RP. Blockade of adhesion of sickle cells to endothelium by monoclonal antibodies. *N Engl J Med* 2000;342:1910–1912.

32. Barabino GA, McIntire LV, Eskin SG, et al. Endothelial cell interactions with sickle cell, sickle trait, mechanically injured, and normal erythrocytes under controlled flow. *Blood* 1987;70:152–157.

33. Elices MJ, Osborn L, Takada Y, et al. VCAM-1 on activated endothelium interacts with the leukocyte integrin VLA-4 at a site distinct from the VLA-4/fibronectin binding site. *Cell* 1990;60:577–584.

34. Wayner EA, Garcia-Pardo A, Humphries MJ, et al. Identification and characterization of the T lymphocyte adhesion receptor for an alternative cell attachment domain (CS-1) in plasma fibronectin. *J Cell Biol* 1989;109:1321–1330.

35. Bednarczyk JL, McIntyre BW. A monoclonal antibody to VLA-4 alpha-

chain (CDw49d) induces homotypic lymphocyte aggregation. *J Immunol* 1990;144:777–784.

36. Pulido R, Elices MJ, Campanero MR, et al. Functional evidence for three distinct and independently inhibitable adhesion activities mediated by the human integrin VLA-4:. Correlation with distinct alpha 4 epitopes. *J Biol Chem* 1991;266:10241–10245.

37. Barrett-Connor E. Bacterial infection and sickle cell anemia: An analysis of 250 infections in 166 patients and a review of the literature. *Medicine* 1971;50:97–112.

38. Lachant NA, Oseas RS. Vaso-occlusive crisis-associated neutrophil dysfunction in patients with sickle cell disease. *Am J Med Sci* 1987;294:253–257.

39. Winkelstein JA. Pneumococcal infections in sickle cell disease. *J Pediatr* 1977;91:521–522.

40. Powars D, Overturf G, Turner E. Is there an increased risk of Haemophilus influenzae septicemia in children with sickle cell anemia? *Pediatrics* 1983; 71:927–931.

41. Goldstein AR, Anderson MJ, Serjeant GR. Parvovirus-associated aplastic crisis in homozygous sickle cell disease. *Arch Dis Child* 1987;62:585–588.

42. Francis RB Jr, Haywood LJ. Elevated immunoreactive tumor necrosis factor and interleukin-1 in sickle cell disease. *J Natl Med Assoc* 1992;84:611–615.

43. Taylor SC, Shacks SJ, Mitchell RA, et al. Serum interleukin-6 levels in the steady state of sickle cell disease. *J Interferon Cytokine Res* 1995;15:1061–1064.

44. Duits AJ, Schnog JB, Lard LR, et al. Elevated IL-8 levels during sickle cell crisis. *Eur J Haematol* 1998;61:302–305.

45. Murphy FA, Kingsbury D. Virus taxonomy. In Fields BS, Knipe DM, Chanock RM, et al., eds: *Virology*, 1st ed. New York: Raven Press; 1990:9–40.

46. Offermann MK, Zimring J, Mellits KH, et al. Activation of the double-stranded RNA-activated protein kinase and induction of vascular cell adhesion molecule-1 by poly (I):poly (C) in endothelial cells. *Eur J Biochem* 1995;232:28–36.

47. Smolinski PA, Offermann MK, Eckman JR et al. Double-stranded RNA induces sickle erythrocyte adherence to endothelium: A potential role for viral infection in vaso-occlusive pain episodes in sickle cell anemia. *Blood* 1995;85:2945–2950.

48. Hebbel RP, Visser MR, Goodman JL, et al. Potentiated adherence of sickle erythrocytes to endothelium infected by virus. *J Clin Invest* 1987;80:1503–1506.

49. Hebbel RP, Mohandas N. Sickle cell adherence. In Embury SH, Hebbel RP, Mohandas N, Steinberg MH, eds: *Sickle Cell Disease: Basic Principles and Clinical Practice.* New York: Raven Press; 1994:217–230.

50. Petz LD, Yam P, Wilkinson L, et al. Increased IgG molecules bound to the surface of red blood cells of patients with sickle cell anemia. *Blood* 1984;64: 301–304.

51. Hebbel RP. Blockade of adherence of sickle cells to endothelium by monoclonal bodies. *N Engl J Med* 2000;342:1910–1912.

52. Wilkins JA, Stupack D, Stewart S, et al. Beta 1 integrin-mediated lymphocyte adherence to extracellular matrix is enhanced by phorbol ester treatment. *Eur J Immunol* 1991;21:517–522.

53. Masumoto A, Hemler ME. Multiple activation states of VLA-4: Mechanistic differences between adhesion to CS1/fibronectin and to vascular cell adhesion molecule-1. *J Biol Chem* 1993;268:228–234.

54. Nathan C, Sporn M. Cytokines in context. *J Cell Biol* 1991;113:981–986.

55. Kumar A, Eckman JR, Swerlick RA, et al. Phorbol ester stimulation increases sickle erythrocyte adherence to endothelium: A novel pathway involving $\alpha_4\beta_1$ integrin receptors on sickle reticulocytes and fibronectin. *Blood* 1996;88:4348–4358.

56. Kuvibidila S, Gardner R, Ode D, et al. Tumor necrosis factor alpha in children with sickle cell disease in stable condition [see comments]. *J Natl Med Assoc* 1997;89:609–615.

57. Duits AJ, Pieters RC, Saleh AW, et al. Enhanced levels of soluble VCAM-1 in sickle cell patients and their specific increment during vaso-occlusive crisis. *Clin Immunol Immunopathol* 1996;81:96–98.

58. Saleh AW, Hillen HF, Duits AJ. Levels of endothelial, neutrophil and platelet-specific factors in sickle cell anemia patients during hydroxyurea therapy. *Acta Haematol* 1999;102:31–37.

59. Michaels LA, Ohene-Frempong K, Zhao H, et al. Serum levels of substance P are elevated in patients with sickle cell disease and increase further during vaso-occlusive crisis. *Blood* 1998;92:3148–3151.

60. Graido-Gonzalez E, Doherty JC, Bergreen EW, et al. Plasma endothelin-1, cytokine, and prostaglandin E2 levels in sickle cell disease and acute vaso-occlusive sickle crisis. *Blood* 1998;92:2551–2555.

61. Fadlon E, Vordermeier S, Pearson TC, et al. Blood polymorphonuclear leukocytes from the majority of sickle cell patients in the crisis phase of the disease show enhanced adhesion to vascular endothelium and increased expression of CD64. *Blood* 1998;91:266–274.

62. Saterbak A, Kuo SC, Lauffenburger DA. Heterogeneity and probabilistic binding contributions to receptor-mediated cell detachment kinetics. *Biophys J* 1993;65:243–252.

63. Smolinski PA. Biophysical analysis of receptor-mediated erythrocyte adherence in sickle cell anemia: Involvement of infection and hemodynamics. PhD thesis, Georgia Institute of Technology. 1996:148–161.

64. Smolinski PA, Eckman JR, Wick TM. Tenacity of sickle red blood cell-endothelial cell adherence is augmented under hemodynamic shear and by involvement of multiple adhesion pathways. Blood 1996;88(Suppl 1), 649a.

65. Saterbak A, Lauffenburger DA. Adhesion mediated by bonds in series. *Biotechnol Prog* 1996;12:682–699.

66. Lauffenburger DA, Wells A. Getting a grip: New insights for cell adhesion and traction. *Nat Cell Biol* 2001;3:E110–112.

67. Klug PP, Lessin LS, Radice P. Rheological aspects of sickle cell disease. *Arch Intern Med* 1974;133:577–590.

68. Sowemimo-Coker SO, Meiselman HJ, Francis RP Jr. Increased circulating endothelial cells in sickle cell crisis. *Am J Hematol* 1989;31:263–265.

69. Solovey A, Lin Y, Browne PV, et al. Circulating activated endothelial cells in sickle cell anemia. *N Engl J Med* 1997;337:1590.

70. Browne PV, Mosher DF, Steinberg MH, et al. Disturbance of plasma and platelet thrombospondin levels in sickle cell disease. *Am J Hematol* 1996; 51:296–301.

71. Setty BN, Chen D, O'Neal P, et al. Eicosanoids in sickle cell disease: Potential relevance of 12(S)-hydroxy-5,8,10,14-eicosatetraenoic acid to the pathophysiology of vaso-occlusion. *J Lab Clin Med* 1998;131:344–353.

72. Wun T, Paglieroni T, Rangaswami A, et al. Platelet activation in patients with sickle cell disease. *Br J Haematol* 1998;100:741–749.

73. Wun T, Paglieroni T, Tablin F, et al. Platelet activation and platelet-

erythrocyte aggregates in patients with sickle cell anemia. *J Lab Clin Med* 1997;129:507–516.

74. Francis RB Jr. Platelets, coagulation, and fibrinolysis in sickle cell disease: Their possible role in vascular occlusion. *Blood Coagul Fibrinolysis* 1991;2: 341–353.

75. Beurling-Harbury C, Schade SG. Platelet activation during pain crisis in sickle cell anemia patients. *Am J Hematol* 1989;31:237–241.

76. Gee BE, Platt OS. Sickle reticulocytes adhere to VCAM-1. *Blood* 1995;85: 268–274.

77. Belcher JD, Marker PH, Weber JP, et al. Activated monocytes in sickle cell disease: Potential role in the activation of vascular endothelium and vaso-occlusion. *Blood* 2000;96:2451–2459.

78. Smith CM, II, Hebbel RP, Tukey DP, et al. Pluronic F-68 reduces the endothelial adherence and improves rheology of liganded sickle erythrocytes. *Blood* 1987;69:1631–1636.

79. Stone PCW, Stuart J, Nash GB. Effects of density and dehydration of sickle cells on their adhesion to cultured endothelial cells. *Am J Hematol* 1996;52: 135–143.

80. Mohandas N, Evans E. Sickle erythrocyte adherence to endothelium. *J Clin Invest* 1985;76:1605–1612.

81. Mohandas N, Evans E. Adherence of sickle erythrocytes to vascular endothelial cells: Requirements for both cell membrane changes and plasma factors. *Blood* 1984;64:282–287.

82. Lipowsky HH, Williams ME. Shear rate dependency of red cell sequestration in skin capillaries in sickle cell disease and its variation with vaso-occlusive crisis. *Microcirculation* 1997;4:289–301.

83. Hebbel RP. Adhesive interactions of sickle erythrocytes with endothelium. *J Clin Invest* 1997;99:2561–2564.

84. Osarogiagbon UR, Choong S, Belcher JD, et al. Reperfusion injury pathophysiology in sickle transgenic mice. *Blood* 2000;96:314–320.

85. Kaul DK, Hebbel RP. Hypoxia/reoxygenation causes inflammatory response in transgenic sickle mice but not in normal mice. *J Clin Invest* 2000;106:411–420.

Chapter 7

Phospholipid Products from Activated Polymorphonuclear Cells:
Potential Role in Sickle Red Blood Cell Microvascular Occlusion

Johnson Haynes Jr, MD, and
Boniface Obiako, MS

Introduction

Central to microvascular occlusion in sickle cell disease (SCD) is the polymerization of deoxyhemoglobin S, which results in increased rigidity of the sickle red blood cell (SRBC). Because hemoglobin polymerization does not occur immediately after deoxygenation, most SR-BCs pass through the capillary bed before sickling, thus making microvascular occlusion uncommon.[1,2] Based on this observation, hemoglobin S polymerization is not likely the exclusive cause of microvascular occlusion and suggests that factors that increase the capillary transit time are also operative. Factors demonstrated in experimental models to increase transit time of the SRBCs through the microcirculation are random precapillary obstruction by rigid dense SRBCs (irreversible SRBCs) and increased adhesion of SRBCs to vascular endothelium.[3–5] Hebbel and colleagues found that SRBCs, particularly reticulocytes, have an increased tendency to adhere to vascular

Supported by the Comprehensive Sickle Cell Program Grant P60 HL-38639 from the National Heart, Lung and Blood Institute and the Florence Foundation Research Career Development Grant.

From: Weir EK, Reeve HL, Reeves JT (eds). *Interactions of Blood and the Pulmonary Circulation.* Armonk, NY: Futura Publishing Company, Inc.; ©2002.

endothelial cells[6] and that increased adherence can be correlated with clinical severity of vaso-occlusion.[7] Unlike sickle reticulocytes, the correlation of dense SRBCs to clinical severity of vaso-occlusion is divergent. For example, Ballas[8] has described a subset of patients with sickle cell anemia and increased numbers of rigid, dense SRBCs who have mild disease as related to pain, leg ulcers, and lower mortality, when compared to patients with highly deformable SRBCs and low numbers of dense SRBCs. In contrast, Powars et al.[9] have shown that sickle cell patients with the most severe disease produce twice the number of dense SRBCs as compared to patients with disease of minimal severity. Nonetheless, dense SRBCs and reticulocytes are present during steady-state conditions and during clinical disease. This raises an interesting question as to whether or not other blood cells, such as polymorphonuclear leukoocytes (PMNs), play a role in the initiation of microvascular occlusion. Indeed, PMN activation has been implicated in the pathophysiology of SCD.[10,11]

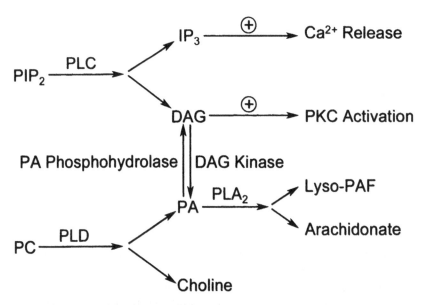

Figure 1. Generation of phospholipid products in activated human polymorphonuclear leukocytes. Phosphatidic acid (PA) can be formed indirectly from phosphatidylinositol 4,5-biphosphate (PIP_2) through hydrolysis by phospholipase C (PLC) and diacylglycerol (DAG) phosphorylation by DAG kinase or directly from phosphatidylcholine (PC) through phospholipase D (PLD). Lyso-platelet-activating factor (lyso-PAF) and arachidonate can be generated from PA by phospholipase A_2 (PLA_2).

Phospholipid Products of Activated Polymorphonuclear Cells

Arachidonic acid, lyso-platelet-activating factor and other metabolites are released from membrane phospholipids of stimulated PMNs by phospholipases (PL) C, D, and A$_2$ (Figure 1). PMN activation[12] is initiated by the binding of a chemotactic agonist to its receptor. Activated chemotactic receptors couple to GTP-binding proteins. This is followed by the activation of PLC, which hydrolyzes phosphatidylinositol 4,5-biphosphate (PIP$_2$) to generate the second messengers, 1,4,5-inositoltriphosphate (IP$_3$), and diacylglycerol (DAG). IP$_3$ diffuses into the cytosol and induces the release of Ca^{++} from intracellular stores leading to a transient increase in cytosolic Ca^{++}. DAG remains membrane-associated where it participates in the activation of protein kinase C. Phosphatidic acid (PA) is formed either directly from phosphatidylcholine through PLD or from DAG phosphorylation by DAG kinase. PA hydrolysis by PLA$_2$ generates free arachidonate acid (AA) and lyso-platelet-activating factor.[12] Acetylation of lyso-platelet-activating factor produces active platelet-activating factor (PAF).[13] PA, lyso-PAF, and AA are all capable of activating NADPH oxidase in a cell-free activation system and may function as physiological activators of the respiratory burst in intact PMNs.[12]

Polymorphonuclear Cell Activation in Sickle Cell Vaso-Occlusion

During crisis, sickle PMNs are often more adherent to vascular endothelium than during steady state.[14,15] This suggests that activated PMNs may play a role in microvascular occlusion. There is indeed an increasing body of evidence that supports the suggestion that PMN activation is important and could play a role in the initiation and propagation of vaso-occlusive processes in SCD.[10,15] Lard et al.[10] have demonstrated that during steady-state and vaso-occlusive crisis, the sickle PMN is activated compared to healthy normal (HbAA) controls. This was exemplified by decreased L-selectin expression, enhanced expression of CD64 on the sickle PMN, and the presence of increased levels of soluble (s) markers such as sCD16, elastase, and sL-selectin. During PMN activation, phospholipase A$_2$ (PLA$_2$) and 5-lipoxygenase (5-LO) activities are also increased.[11,16] Mollapour et al. have demonstrated that resting levels of PMN PLA$_2$ activity in steady-state SCD are elevated relative to normal controls.[11] AA and lyso-PAF are released from membrane phospholipids of activated PMN by PLA$_2$.[12,17] Of the potential products of AA metabolism secreted by human PMNs, the 5-LO product, leukotriene B_4 (LTB_4), is the principal product.[18] Acetylation of the lyso-PAF acether by acetyltransferase results in the metabolically active product, PAF.[13] Both LTB_4 and PAF are inflammatory mediators and influence vascular permeability, cell infiltration, and PMN adhesion.[19-22] While the specific roles of LTB_4 and PAF in SCD are not clear, Ibe et al.[23] have demonstrated a higher urinary excretion of LTB_4 and plasma levels of LTC_4 in sickle cell patients as compared to normal controls. Also Oh et al.[24] found during steady state, PAF was ~2X higher in individuals with SCD than observed in age-matched normal controls. In an ex vivo rat mesocecum vasculature preparation, Kaul et al.[25] demonstrated that PAF increased SRBC adhesion to venules accompanied by frequent postcapillary blockage and increased peripheral resistance units. Pretreatment of the vasculature with the monoclonal antibody, LM609, which selectively inhibits $\alpha_V\beta_3$, almost completely inhibited SRBC adhesion to postcapillary venules. This study further supports a potential role for PAF in the pathophysiology of SCD and suggests blockade of $\alpha_V\beta_3$ as a potential therapeutic approach to the prevention of SRBC-endothelium interactions.

Recently, we have demonstrated that in isolated rat lungs perfused with SRBC suspensions (Hct 10%) ± PMN, PMN activation was required to increase the retention of SRBCs in the microcirculation.[26-28] SRBC retention in lungs perfused with unstimulated PMNs did not differ from lungs perfused with SRBCs alone. We further demonstrated that the addition of PAF and LTB_4 in tandem to perfusate not containing PMNs increased SRBC retention significantly as compared with the SRBC control. Increased SRBC retention was partially reversed, as compared with controls, in lungs pretreated with the PAF antagonist, WEB 2170 BS, followed by perfusion with PAF + LTB_4. In lungs pretreated with WEB 2170 BS prior to the addition of activated PMNs, a significant decrease in SRBC retention was also observed. Pretreatment of PMNs with the 5-lipoxygenase inhibitor, zileuton, prior to activation with phorbol myristate acetate also attenuated activated PMN-mediated SRBC retention. These findings, coupled with the findings that neither PAF nor LTB_4, when individually perfused, had any effect on decreased SRBC retention in the pulmonary circulation, provide convincing evidence that when both of the soluble lipid products, PAF and LTB_4, are secreted by the activated PMNs, increased SRBC retention/adherence occurs in the pulmonary circulation of the isolated-perfused rat lung model. While these findings had not been reported previously, Setty et al.[29] have reported in a static incubation system that AA metabolites are involved in mediating basal adhesion of normal and SRBCs to endothelium via lipoxygenase metabolites. In subsequent studies, Setty et al.[30,31] found that SRBCs stimulate endothelial cell production of AA and diacylglycerol and that the lipoxygenase product, 12(s)-

hydroxy-5,8,10,14-eicosatetraenoic acid (12-HETE), increased hypoxia-induced SRBC-endothelial adherence via the upregulation of VCAM-1 on endothelial cells. These studies are similar to ours in that products of membrane phospholipids, related in part to the lipoxygenase enzyme system, appear to be involved in mediating SRBC retention/adherence. The studies differ in that Setty et al. analyzed RBC-endothelial cell interaction in a static system, while our study investigated PMN-SRBC-endothelial cell interactions in a dynamic flow model.

Potential Clinical Importance

While the role of PMNs in the initiation of vaso-occlusion by SRBCs is unclear, clinical studies show that elevated total white blood cell counts are common in SCD[32,33] and that a white blood cell count greater than 15,000 cells/mL is associated with an increased risk of early death.[34] Other clinical observations of importance stem from studies on hydroxyurea (HU). While HU has been reported to decrease sickle vaso-occlusive crisis through the induction of fetal hemoglobin in F cells, this effect is variable and correlates poorly with clinical response.[35] What does seem to be associated with a lower crisis rate in patients treated with HU is a consistent lowering of the PMN count.[36] Furthermore, Saleh et al.[36] reported a decrease in PMN myeloperoxidase activity in patients treated with HU and suggested that decreased PMN activity rather than the white blood cell count may attenuate PMN initiation of vaso-occlusive crisis.

PLA$_2$ has been implicated in the pathophysiology of vaso-occlusive crisis[37,38] and acute chest syndrome (ACS).[39] In vaso-occlusive crisis, intravenous steroids have been reported to shorten the hospital stay of children and adolescents. This effect was attributed to the inhibitory effect of steroids on PLA$_2$ and possibly the suppression of inflammatory cytokines.[37,38] Styles et al.[39] reported elevated levels of secretory PLA$_2$ in ACS but not in vaso-occlusive crisis or non-SCD patients with pneumonia, and suggested a role for secretory PLA$_2$ in ACS. These studies suggest that PMN activation and the release of inflammatory mediators may prove to be a vital link in further understanding the pathophysiology of microvascular occlusion in SCD.

Potential Role for Anti-inflammatory Therapy in SCD

There is a growing body of evidence that inflammation plays a role(s) in the initiation of sickle cell vaso-occlusion. Anti-inflammatory interventions targeting a decrease in the PMN count and/or activity may prove to

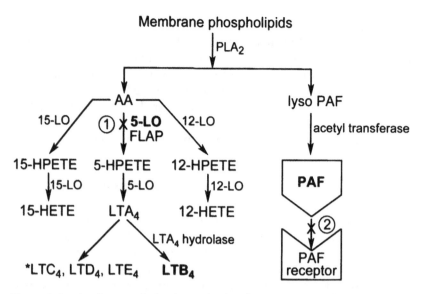

Figure 2. Leukotriene and platelet-activating factor synthesis in human poly-morphonuclear leukocytes. PLA_2 = phospholipase A_2; AA = arachidonate; PAF = platelet-activating factor; LO = lipoxygenase; FLAP = 5-lipoxygenase-activating protein; HETE = eicosatetraenoic acid; HPETE = hydroperoxye-icosatetraenoic acid; LT = leukotriene; *very little produced by human poly-morphonuclear leukocytes. 1 and 2 denote sites for potential therapeutic interventions with selective 5-LO inhibitors and/or PAF receptor antagonist, respectively.

be clinically beneficial in the prevention and treatment of vaso-occlusive crisis and ACS. To date, there are no selective inhibitors of PLA_2. There are, however, selective PAF receptor antagonists[40,41] and 5-lipoxygenase inhibitors.[42–46] Based on the data presented above, therapies that inhibit the inflammatory effects of PAF and LTB_4 may prove to be useful adjuncts to analgesics, antibiotics, bronchodilators, and transfusions in the treatment of vaso-occlusive crisis and ACS (Figure 2).

Acknowledgments: Many thanks to Marilyn Chancellor for the preparation of this manuscript.

References

1. Hofrichter J, Ross PD, Eaton WA. Kinetics and mechanism of deoxyhe-moglobin S gelation: A new approach to understanding sickle cell disease. *Proc Natl Acad Sci USA* 1974;71:4864–4868.
2. Mozzarelli A, Hofrichter J, Eaton WA. Delay time of hemoglobin S poly-merization prevents most cells from sickling in vivo. *Science* 1987;237: 500–506.

3. Kaul DK, Chen D, Zhan J. Adhesion of sickle cells to vascular endothelium is critically dependent on changes in density and shape of the cells. *Blood* 1994;83:3006–3017.

4. Kaul DK, Fabry ME, Nagel RL. Microvascular sites and characteristics of sickle cell adhesion to vascular endothelium in shear flow conditions: Pathophysiological implications. *Proc Natl Acad Sci USA* 1989;86:3356–3360.

5. Kaul DK, Fabry ME, Nagel RL. Vaso-occlusion by sickle cells: Evidence for selective trapping of dense red cells. *Blood* 1986;68:1162–1166.

6. Hebbel RP, Yamada O, Moldow CF, et al. Abnormal adherence of sickle erythrocytes to cultured vascular endothelium: A possible mechanism for microvascular occlusion in sickle cell disease. *J Clin Invest* 1980;65:154–160.

7. Hebbel RP, Boogaerts MAB, Eaton JW, et al. Erythrocyte adherence to endothelium in sickle cell anemia: Possible determinant of disease severity. *N Engl J Med* 1980;302:992–995.

8. Ballas SK. Sickle cell anemia with few painful crises is characterized by decreased red cell deformability and increased number of dense cells. *Am J Hematol* 1991;36(2):122–130.

9. Powars DR, Meiselman JH, Fishter TC, et al. Beta-S gene cluster haplotypes modulate hematologic and hemorheologic expression in sickle cell anemia: Use in predicting clinical severity. *Am J Pediatr Hematol Oncol* 1994;16(1):55–61.

10. Lard LR, Mul FP, de Haas M, et al. Neutrophil activation in sickle cell disease. *J Leukoc Biol* 1999;66(3):411–415.

11. Mollapour E, Porter JB, Kaczmarski R, et al. Raised neutrophil phospholipase A2 activity and defective priming of NADPH oxidase and phospholipase A2 in sickle cell disease. *Blood* 1998;91(9):3423–3429.

12. Baggiolini M, Boulay F, Badwey JA, et al. Activation of neutrophil leukocytes: Chemoattractant receptors and respiratory burst. *FASEB J* 1993;7:1004–1010.

13. Snyder F. Metabolism of platelet-activating factor and related ether lipids: Enzymatic pathways, subcellular sites, regulation, and membrane processing. *Prog Clin Biol Res* 1988;282:57–72.

14. Fadlon E, Vordermeier S, Pearson TC, et al. Blood polymorphonuclear leukocytes from the majority of sickle cell patients in the crisis phase of the disease show enhanced adhesion to vascular endothelium and increased expression of CD64. *Blood* 1998;91:266–274.

15. Boghossian SH, Nash G, Dormandy J, et al. Abnormal neutrophil adhesion in sickle cell anaemia and crisis: Relationship to blood rheology. *Br J Haematol* 1991;78:437–441.

16. Pouliot M, McDonald PP, Krump E, et al. Colocalization of cytosolic phospholipase A_2, 5-lipoxygenase and 5-lipoxygenase-activating protein at the nuclear membrane of A23187-stimulated human neutrophils. *Eur J Biochem* 1996;238:250–258.

17. Benveniste J, Chignard M. A role for PAF-acether (platelet-activating factor) in platelet-dependent vascular disease? *Circulation* 1985;72:713–717.

18. Guidot DM, Repine MJ, Westcott JY, et al. Intrinsic 5-lipoxygenase activity is required for neutrophil responsivity. *Proc Natl Acad Sci USA* 1994;91:8156–8159.

19. Lindström P, Lerner R, Palmblad J, et al. Rapid adhesive responses of endothelial cells and of neutrophils induced by leukotriene B_4 are mediated by leucocytic adhesion protein CD18. *Scand J Immunol* 1990;31:737–744.

20. Minamiya V, Tozawa K, Kitamura M, et al. Platelet-activating factor medi-

ates intercellular adhesion molecule-1-dependent radical production in the nonhypoxic ischemia rat lung. *Am J Respir Cell Mol Biol* 1998;19:150–157.

21. Kubes P, Suzuki M, Granger N. Platelet-activating factor-induced microvascular dysfunction: Role of adherent leukocytes. *Am J Physiol* 1990; 258:G158–G163.

22. Lewis RE, Granger HJ. Diapedesis and permeability of venous microvessels to protein macromolecules: The impact of leukotriene B$_4$ (LTB$_4$). *Microvasc Res* 1988;35:27–47.

23. Ibe BO, Kurantsin-Mills J, Raj JU, et al. Plasma and urinary leukotrienes in sickle cell disease: Possible role in the inflammatory process. *Eur J Clin Invest* 1994;24:57–64.

24. Oh SO, Johnson C, Kurantsin-Mills J, et al. Platelet-activating factor in plasma with sickle cell disease in steady state. *J Lab Clin Med* 1997;130(2): 191–196.

25. Kaul DK, Tsai HM, Liu XD, et al. Monoclonal antibodies to αVβ3 (7E3 and LM609) inhibit sickle red blood cell-endothelium interactions induced by platelet-activating factor. *Blood* 2000;95(2):368–374.

26. Haynes J, Obiako B. Platelet activating factor with leukotriene B$_4$ enhances sickle red blood cell retention in the lung circulation. 1999; 26th National Sickle Cell Program Meeting.

27. Dixon B, Pace B, Obiako B, et al. Zileuton: A potential new treatment approach for acute chest syndrome (ACS). *Blood* 2000;96(11):A29.

28. Haynes J, Obiako B. WEB 2170: A potential new treatment approach for acute chest syndrome. *Am J Respir Crit Care Med* 2001;163(3):A39.

29. Setty BNY, Dampier CD, Stuart MJ. Arachidonic acid metabolites are involved in mediating red blood cell adherence to endothelium. *J Lab Clin Med* 1995;125:608–617.

30. Setty BN, Chen D, O'Neal P, et al. Eicosanoids in sickle cell disease: Potential relevance of 12(S)-hydroxy-5,8,10,14-eicosatraenoic acid to the pathophysiology of vaso-occlusion. *J Lab Clin Med* 1998;131:344–353.

31. Setty BN, Chen D, Stuart MJ. Sickle red blood cells stimulate endothelial cell production of eicosanoids and diacylglycerol. *J Lab Clin Med* 1996;128: 313–321.

32. Diggs LW. The blood picture in sickle cell anemia. *South Med J* 1932;25: 615–620.

33. Boggs DR, Hyde F, Srodes C. An unusual pattern of neutrophil kinetics in sickle cell anemia. *Blood* 1973;41:59–65.

34. Platt OS, Brambilla DJ, Rosse WF, et al. Mortality in sickle cell disease: Life expectancy and risk factors for early death. *N Engl J Med* 1994;330:1639–1644.

35. Charache S. Mechanism of action of hydroxyurea in the management of sickle cell anemia in adults. *Semin Hematol* 1997;34(Suppl 3):15–21.

36. Saleh AW, Hillen HF, Duits AJ. Levels of endothelial, neutrophil and platelet-specific factors in sickle cell anemia patients during hydroxyurea therapy. *Acta Haematol* 1999;102(1):31–37.

37. Griffin TC, McIntire D, Buchanan GR. High-dose intravenous methylprednisolone therapy for pain in children and adolescents with sickle cell disease. *N Engl J Med* 1994;330(11):733–737.

38. Bernini JC, Rogers ZR, Sandler ES, et al. Beneficial effect of intravenous dexamethasone in children with mild to moderately severe acute chest syndrome complicating sickle cell disease. *Blood* 1998;92(9):3082–3089.

39. Styles LA, Schalkwijk CG, Aarsman AJ, et al. Phospholipase A$_2$ levels in acute chest syndrome of sickle cell disease. *Blood* 1996;87(6):2573–2578.

40. Heuer H, Birke FW, Casals-Stenzel J, et al. Inhibition of the binding and aggregation to PAF in vitro in comparison with PAF-antagonists in vivo: An investigation using different types of PAF-antagonists. *Prostaglandins* 1988;35:838.
41. Weber KH, Heuer H. Structure-activity relationships and effects of PAF-antagonists in the hetrazepine series. *Int Arch Allergy Appl Immunol* 1989;88:82.
42. Wenzel SE, Trudeau JB, Kaminsky DA, et al. Effect of 5-lipoxygenase inhibition on bronchoconstriction and airway inflammation in nocturnal asthma. *Am J Respir Crit Care Med* 1995;152(3):897–905.
43. Dube LM, Swanson LJ, Awni W. Zileuton, a leukotriene synthesis inhibitor in the management of chronic asthma: Clinical pharmacokinetics and safety. *Clin Rev Allergy Immunol* 1999;17(1–2):213–21.
44. Drazen J. Clinical pharmacology of leukotriene receptor antagonists and 5-lipoxygenase inhibitors. *Am J Respir Crit Care Med* 1998;157:S233–S237.
45. Bell RL, Young PR, Albert D, et al. The discovery and development of zileuton: An orally active 5-lipoxygenase inhibitor. *Int J Immunopharmacol* 1992;14:505–510.
46. Bell RL, Bouska JB, Malo PE, et al. Optimization of the potency and duration of action of N-hydroxyurea 5-lipoxygenase inhibitors. *J PET* 1995;272:724.

Chapter 8

Potential New Approaches to the Treatment of Sickle Cell Disease

John V. Weil, MD, and Peter A. Lane, MD

Introduction

Sickle cell disease is caused by a well-characterized molecular abnormality in the structure and function of hemoglobin and is thus considered a hemoglobinopathy. Yet most of the morbidity and mortality in patients with this disorder are the result of vascular injury and occlusion (Figure 1).

Thus, in clinical terms, sickle cell disease is a vascular disease. Considerable investigation has generated several hypotheses concerning the nature of the linkage of the sickle hemoglobin abnormality with vascular injury and obstruction. These proposed mechanisms share common features with vascular injury in other vasculopathic states, which suggests the potential utility of several agents currently used to protect blood vessels in other disorders. In this chapter, the evidence that deficient production of nitric oxide (NO), increased endothelin, and inflammatory and oxidant activity contribute to the genesis of the vascular complications of sickle cell disease will be explored, as well as the implications for potential new practical therapeutic strategies for prevention and amelioration of vascular events in sickle cell disease.

Processes thought to contribute to vascular complications of sickle cell disease include the early idea of obstruction of small vessels by a logjam of rigid, sickled cells. Subsequent observations have also emphasized the importance of avid adherence of sickle red cells to vascular endothelium as a potential early step in the vaso-occlusive process.[1–3] Vasoconstriction promoted by sickle cells may contribute to stasis and obstruction.[4,5] Finally, there are findings that support a role for inflam-

From: Weir EK, Reeve HL, Reeves JT (eds). *Interactions of Blood and the Pulmonary Circulation*. Armonk, NY: Futura Publishing Company, Inc.; ©2002.

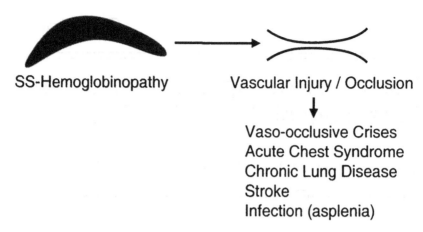

Figure 1. Schematic illustration showing how the interaction of sickle erythrocytes and vessels ultimately leads to several vasculopathic complications, which account for the major portion of morbidity and mortality of sickle cell disease.

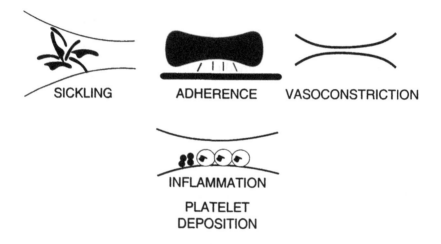

Figure 2. Processes thought to cause vascular injury and occlusion in sickle cell disease.

mation[6] and platelet activation[7] in the vascular features of sickle cell disease (Figure 2).

Sickle Cell Disease and the Lung

The lung circulation is a major target of these processes, perhaps because the low perfusion pressure and intermittent flow conditions in pulmonary vessels promote accumulation and adhesion of abnormal and activated blood-formed elements and because the lung receives the deoxygenated venous effluent of the systemic circulation.

Pulmonary complications of sickle cell disease fall mainly into 2 categories: the acute chest syndrome and chronic lung disease. The acute chest syndrome has been broadly defined as the development of new chest symptoms such as cough or chest pain, associated with a new infiltrate on chest radiograph with occasional progression to diffuse pulmonary edema and multisystem organ failure.[6,8,9] Causes of the syndrome are often uncertain but are thought to include pneumonia, especially in children, and infarction, which is often suspected, but rarely proven. Pulmonary vascular injury due to fat embolism is thought to be a common cause of the syndrome because of a frequent association with antecedent or coincident bone pain and appearance of fat in bronchoalveolar lavagate.[10–12] Treatment of the syndrome consists mainly of supportive measures: fluid, oxygen, and antibiotics. In moderate and severe cases, red blood cell transfusion is often followed by prompt and dramatic improvement in oxygenation through mechanisms that remain unclear. Preventive measures include chronic administration of hydroxyurea, which was initially thought to act by increasing hemoglobin F levels. However, recent findings suggest its effects may be related to decreased leukocytosis,[13] augmentation of nitric oxide activity,[14,15] or decreased red cell/endothelial adherence.[16] Chronic transfusion and bone marrow transplantation are also used for prevention of the syndrome.

Chronic lung disease is a common complication and major cause of mortality in patients with sickle cell disease who survive to adulthood. Manifested as pulmonary hypertension and restrictive lung disease, the etiology of the syndrome is largely unknown.[17–19] Repeated episodes of the acute chest syndrome may contribute to its development, but the disorder is occasionally seen in patients without such history. There are no studies of measures aimed at prevention or treatment of the syndrome.

Potential Therapeutic Strategies

Nitric Oxide-Based Approaches

Several lines of evidence suggest that NO activity could inhibit most of the proposed mechanisms of vascular injury and obstruction in sickle cell disease (Figure 3). These include an increase in sickle red cell oxygen affinity[20] and decreased sickling,[21] although the effect on oxygen affinity was not confirmed in another report.[22] Nitric oxide is known to suppress endothelial adherence molecules, such as VCAM-1, which have been im-

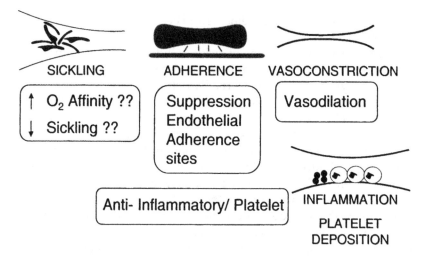

Figure 3. Actions of nitric oxide, which may ameliorate vascular injury and occlusion in sickle cell disease.

plicated in endothelial adherence of sickle red cells.[23] In vitro studies show that inhibitors of NO synthase augment adherence of normal red cells to cultured endothelium and that NO donors inhibit endothelial adherence of normal and sickle red cells [24] (Figure 4). In rats infused with sickle red cells, an inhibitor of NO synthase (L-NAME) markedly increased cerebral red cell retention, attenuated cerebral blood flow, and increased stroke and mortality.[25] In addition, the well-known vasodilator effect of NO could act to enhance microvascular blood flow and thus reduce stasis and adherence and plugging by sickle red cells. Finally, the anti-inflammatory and antiplatelet effects of NO[26,27] could quench the suspected contributions of leukocytes and platelets to sickle-associated vascular injury and obstruction.

Studies in patients provide circumstantial support for a possible beneficial role of endogenous NO activity in sickle cell disease. Low levels of stable NO metabolites (NOx), interpreted as indicating decreased NO activity, are associated with increased severity and duration of painful crises.[28,29] A recent report showed that NOx levels in patients with clinically stable sickle cell disease were similar to those in normal subjects, but levels were decreased in patients with vaso-occlusive crisis or acute chest syndrome.[30] Further, low NOx levels were associated with increases in circulating soluble VCAM-1, suggesting a linkage of decreased NO activity with vascular injury[30] (Figure 5).

Reasons for, and implications of, reduced NOx levels in sickle cell disease patients with vascular complications are unclear. It is possible that endothelial injury, which may be an early feature of vascular complica-

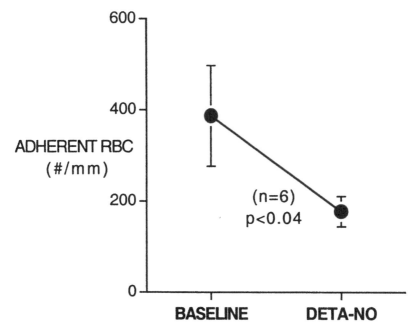

Figure 4. A nitric oxide donor (DETA-NO) reduces adherence of sickle red blood cells to cultured endothelium. Drawn from data of Space et al.[24]

tions, impairs NO generation. Alternatively, antecedent decreases in NO activity may predispose to vascular complications in sickle patients.

Substrate limitation is a potential contributor to decreased NO generation in sickle cell disease. Two studies indicate that circulating levels of L-arginine, the sole substrate for NO synthase, are decreased in patients with the stable disorder.[31,32] A balance study suggests that this is attributable to increased L-arginine consumption,[31] although aminoaciduria, a feature of sickle cell disease, and insufficient diet may also contribute. It is possible that increased arginine consumption could reflect augmentation of vascular shear, a classic stimulus to NO generation, by endothelial contact with stiff, adherent sickle red cells. The resulting increased NO generation might consume arginine, lower levels, and limit NO activity.

The general concept that L-arginine availability may limit endothelial NO function is broadly evident in numerous reports that indicate that impaired NO-mediated vasodilator function is corrected by administration of exogenous L-arginine in several cardiovascular disorders such as coronary artery disease, hypertension, and heart failure and in risk conditions such as hyperlipidemia, diabetes, and smoking.[33,34] This is a surprising finding in view of the biochemical predictions that circulating arginine levels, together with active transport, generate intracellular lev-

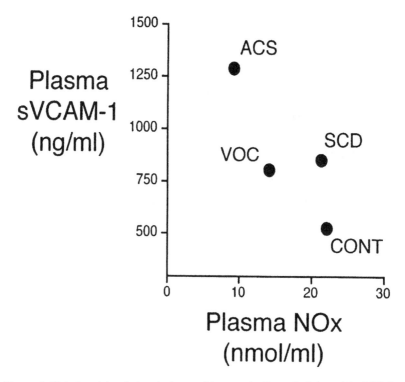

Figure 5. Relationship of circulating stable metabolites of nitric oxide (NOx) to a soluble VCAM-1 (sVCAM), a putative marker of inflammation. Patients with the acute chest syndrome (ACS) and vaso-occlusive crisis (VOC) show an association of lower NOx levels with increased circulating sVCAM. Drawn from data of Stuart and Setty.[30]

els vastly in excess of those required for maximal NO synthase requirements. Reasons for these unexpected responses to exogenous L-arginine, the arginine paradox, are uncertain. Possible explanations include the presence of competitive inhibition by endogenous arginine analogs, defects in cellular arginine transport, disrupted co-localization of arginine transporter and NO synthase, or some undefined nonsubstrate action of arginine.[33,34]

A recent preliminary report suggests that administration of L-arginine to patients with sickle cell disease may increase circulating levels of NOx during sickle vaso-occlusive crisis, but not in steady-state sickle cell disease.[35] Thus, it is possible that substrate availability may be rate-limiting during crises.

As outlined below, sickle cell disease is characterized by increased oxidant activity. This could limit NO activity by accelerated degradation of NO itself or by oxidant degradation and depletion of tetrahydrobiopterin, a critical cofactor for NO synthase.[36]

Potential Applications of Nitric Oxide-Based Therapy

Thus, both theoretical considerations and experimental evidence suggest that NO-based therapeutic strategies might be useful and practical approaches to treatment and prevention of vascular complications of sickle cell disease.

Acute interventions during sickle crises (vaso-occlusive crisis or acute chest syndrome) might include use of inhaled NO, administration of NO donors such as nitroglycerin or nitroprusside, or infusion of L-arginine. Of these, the only reports to date are 2 accounts of beneficial responses to inhaled NO during episodes of acute chest syndrome.[37,38] The rationale for this approach was similar to that for the use of inhaled NO in other types of lung injury (respiratory distress syndromes) where the agent acts as an inhaled pulmonary vasodilator, delivered preferentially to the ventilated lung, which improves matching of perfusion to ventilation and reduces pulmonary hypertension. Similar findings were evident in patients with the sickle acute chest syndrome in both reports. Whether inhaled NO might have additional beneficial effects on vascular injury and obstruction attributable to NO's anti-red cell adherence, anti-inflammatory, and antiplatelet actions in patient sickle crises is unexplored.

Chronic prophylaxis of sickle-associated vascular events based on augmentation of NO activity might be addressed by dietary supplementation with L-arginine. Administration of antioxidants such as vitamins E and C may augment NO activity by protection of NO against oxidant degradation, enhanced release of bound NO, and recycling of metabolites such as nitrite to NO.[39] Another practical approach to chronic augmentation of NO activity in sickle cell disease might be with the use of angiotensin-converting enzyme inhibitors. These agents, which have been shown to improve proteinuria in sickle cell disease, are known to augment NO activity due largely to decreased degradation of bradykinin–stimulator of NO generation.[40] The extent to which angiotensin-converting enzyme inhibitors might ameliorate the vascular occlusion and injury of sickle cell disease remains unexplored.

Augmentation of NO activity in sickle cell disease, while theoretically appealing, must be approached with some caution. The most commonly cited risk of such an approach is a possible oxidant injury resulting from the conversion of NO to its toxic oxidant metabolite peroxynitrite. In support of this possibility, evidence of peroxynitrite activity has been evident in the kidneys of transgenic sickle cell disease mice and the associated nephropathy has been reduced by inhibition of NO synthase.[41] It is possible that co-administration of antioxidants such as vitamins E and C might protect against such injury.

Endothelin

Several observations indicate that endothelin activity is increased in stable sickle cell disease[42] and circulating endothelin levels are markedly increased in patients with the acute chest syndrome or vaso-occlusive crisis[43,44] (Figure 6).

In vitro exposure of cultured endothelial cells to sickled red cells or sickled red cell ghosts elicits an increase in endothelin-1 expression.[44,45] Similar responses are seen when endothelium is exposed to media conditioned by sickle cells or ghosts, or exposed to plasma from patients with the acute chest syndrome. These findings suggest that the response is mediated by a soluble factor.[45] The nature of the factor remains unknown. One study suggests that it may be an oxidant,[46] while another suggests otherwise.[45] Sickle-induced increases in endothelin activity also decrease NO activity[5,46] and the augmentation of endothelin expression is blocked by NO donors and is mimicked by inhibitors of NO synthase.[45] Thus, sickle-induced increases in endothelial endothelin expression might be related to decreased NO activity.

In addition to its potent vasoconstrictor action, endothelin-1 is known to promote proliferation of vascular myocytes and fibroblasts[47,48] and the activation of neutrophils[49] and platelets.[50-52] Information presented by Dr. Kalra elsewhere in this book suggests that endothelin-1 mediates the endothelial adherence and transmigration of monocytes induced by exposure of endothelium to sickle red cells. To date there are

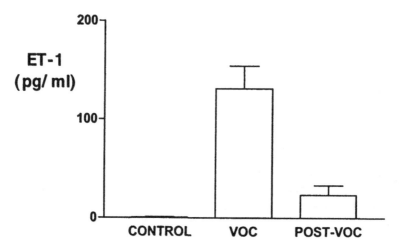

Figure 6. Marked elevations in circulating levels of endothelin-1 (ET-1) in patients with sickle vaso-occlusive crises when compared with levels in normal (control) subjects. Levels in sickle patients decline following the crises. Drawn from data in Graido-Gonzalez.[43]

no reports that indicate whether endothelin influences the endothelial adherence of sickle red cells to endothelium.

Thus, it is possible that endothelin-1 via vasoconstriction, cellular activation, and proliferation effects might contribute to the development of the acute and chronic vascular complications of sickle cell disease. Because decreased NO activity may contribute sickle-associated increased endothelin activity, measures that increase NO activity may have useful endothelin suppressant effects. In addition, several endothelin-blocking agents are in clinical trials for other disorders and may have therapeutic utility in sickle cell disease.

Inflammation

Clinical observations suggest an association of inflammatory activity with vascular complications of sickle cell disease.[6] Inflammatory illness is a common precipitant of vaso-occlusive events, and leukocytosis during clinically stable intervals is a risk factor for increased frequency of vascular crises and mortality.[6,53] Reduction of leukocytosis correlates with the extent to which hydroxyurea reduces vascular complications of sickle cell disease and is considered a possible mechanism of its protective effect.[13,54] Further, recent experimental evidence for an inflammatory contribution to the vasculopathy of sickle cell disease is a report that hypoxia followed by reoxygenation produces vascular inflammation in transgenic sickle cell disease mice but not in wild-type animals.[55]

These considerations suggest that existing anti-inflammatory agents might be capable of preventing or ameliorating vascular complications of sickle cell disease, but this idea remains largely untested by adequate clinical trials. An exception is a study of the effect of acute administration of glucorticoids, which shortened hospital stay for sickle vaso-occlusive crisis but was associated with a possible increase in recurrence.[56]

Aspirin has the potential advantage of both anti-inflammatory and antiplatelet activity. Low-dose aspirin has been tested in only 2 small placebo-controlled trials of 29 and 49 patients, lasting 5 and 21 months. Both failed to show an effect on vascular events.[57,58] There are no reports of trials of higher doses, which might confirm anti-inflammatory as well as antiplatelet actions. The potential preventive actions of other common anti-inflammatory agents such as nonsteroidal anti-inflammatory agents and COX-2 inhibitors also remain untested.

Initial, brief clinical protocols could determine whether anti-inflammatory agents reduce sickle cell disease-associated inflammatory activity measured as white blood cell count, C-reactive protein, and circulating levels of soluble adhesion molecules. Agents with actions at this level could be selected for longer, larger clinical trials for prevention and early treatment of vascular complications.

Oxidants

Considerable evidence indicates that augmented oxidant activity is a prominent feature of sickle cell disease as recently reviewed by Aslan[59] (Figure 7). Iron is thought to be among the central contributors reflecting the translocation of iron from sickle hemoglobin to the red cell surface[60] and transfusion-induced iron overload. Some but not all studies also indicate increased levels of homocysteine in patients with sickle cell disease,[61] which may represent a pro-oxidant state.[62] Finally, as mentioned earlier, oxidant degradation limits NO activity and promotes generation of the toxic product peroxynitrite (ONOO-), which has been implicated in the nephropathy of sickle cell disease mice.[41]

Considering the low risk and modest expense of antioxidant interventions, the absence of clinical trials of these agents in sickle cell disease is remarkable. Of particular potential interest are the possible effects of vitamin C. Ascorbate has several actions that could potentiate the possible useful effects of NO. These include protection of NO from oxidant degradation, recycling of nitrite to NO, enhanced release of NO from thio-compounds, potentiation of endothelial NO synthase activity, and augmentation of the NO synthase cofactor tetrahydrobiopterin.[39]

Because antioxidant vitamins may work best in combination as an electron, or oxidant, transport system,[63] clinical trials of combined treatment with vitamins E and C might be appropriate.

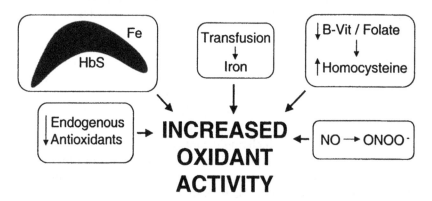

Figure 7. Sources of oxidant activity in sickle cell disease: contributions of sickle hemoglobin, iron translocated to the surface of the erythrocyte as a consequence of transfusion, insufficient levels of folate and possibly vitamin B_{12}, and conversion of nitric oxide to peroxynitrite.

Chronic Lung Disease

As mentioned, this complication, manifested as pulmonary hypertension and restrictive lung disease, becomes a major source of morbidity and mortality in patients with sickle cell disease who survive to early adulthood.[17,19] There are no thorough studies of the natural history of the disorder or of therapeutic approaches, and pathophysiological mechanisms remain unclear.

Noninvasive echocardiographic estimation of pulmonary arterial pressure in young adult sickle cell disease patients could be useful in early detection, in monitoring progression, and as an objective end-point in therapeutic clinical trials. Unlike other forms of pulmonary hypertension that are typically detected late in their course, pulmonary hypertension in young adults with sickle cell disease seems sufficiently common that screening could yield a substantial number of cases at an early stage. Detection of early pulmonary hypertension might be greatly be augmented by use of stress echocardiography, during exercise or dobutamine infusion, in patients with normal resting pressures.

Agents, mentioned above, that potentiate NO activity and/or reduce inflammatory or platelet activity or have antiproliferative actions might reduce incidence or blunt the progression of the chronic syndrome. Of special interest might be the endothelin-blocking agents for which there is preliminary indication of potential benefit in treatment of other forms of pulmonary hypertension.[64]

Conclusion

Current ideas concerning the mechanisms linking the sickle hemoglobinopathy to vascular obstruction and injury include obstruction by sickled rigid cells, endothelial adherence of red cells, vasoconstriction, platelet activation and deposition, inflammation, and oxidant activity. There exist drugs in common use in other conditions with the potential to inhibit these processes that are well tolerated and inexpensive. These include agents that enhance NO activity, have anti-inflammatory, antiplatelet, or antioxidant activity, and investigational drugs that block endothelin action. However, the utility of these approaches remains untested by appropriate investigation.

It would seem that the time is long overdue for initiation of clinical trials to evaluate the possible ability of some of these agents to prevent or ameliorate the vascular complications of sickle cell disease that account for such high proportion of morbidity and mortality of the disorder. What is needed is a multicenter consortium dedicated to therapeutic clinical trials that might best be organized and funded by the National Institutes of Health and involve the Blood, Heart, and Lung Institutes.

References

1. Hebbel RP. Perspectives series. Cell adhesion in vascular biology: Adhesive interactions of sickle erythrocytes with endothelium. *J Clin Invest* 1997;99:2561–2564.
2. Hebbel RP, Boogaerts MA, Eaton JW, Steinberg MH. Erythrocyte adherence to endothelium in sickle-cell anemia: A possible determinant of disease severity. *N Engl J Med* 1980;302:992–995.
3. Telen MJ. Red blood cell surface adhesion molecules: Their possible roles in normal human physiology and disease. *Semin Hematol* 2000;37:130–142.
4. Faller DV. Vascular modulation in sickle cell anemia. In Embury SH, Hebbel RP, Mohandas N, eds: *Sickle Cell Disease: Basic Principles and Clinical Practice.* New York, NY: Raven Press, 1994:235.
5. Mosseri M, Bartlett-Pandite AN, Wenc K, Isner JM, et al. Inhibition of endothelium-dependent vasorelaxation by sickle erythrocytes. *Am Heart J* 1993;126:338–346.
6. Platt OS. The acute chest syndrome of sickle cell disease [editorial; comment]. *N Engl J Med* 2000;342:1904–1907.
7. Wun T, Paglieroni T, Rangaswami A, et al. Platelet activation in patients with sickle cell disease. *Br J Haematol* 1998;100:741–749.
8. Quinn CT, Buchanan GR. The acute chest syndrome of sickle cell disease. *J Pediatr* 1999;135:416–422.
9. Hassell KL, Eckman JR, Lane PA. Acute multiorgan failure syndrome: A potentially catastrophic complication of severe sickle cell pain episodes. *Am J Med* 1994;96:155–162.
10. Godeau B, Schaeffer A, Bachir D, et al. Bronchoalveolar lavage in adult sickle cell patients with acute chest syndrome: Value for diagnostic assessment of fat embolism. *Am J Respir Crit Care Med* 1996;153:1691–1696.
11. Vichinsky EP, Neumayr LD, Earles AN, et al. Causes and outcomes of the acute chest syndrome in sickle cell disease. National Acute Chest Syndrome Study Group [see comments]. *N Engl J Med* 2000;342:1855–1865.
12. Maitre B, Habibi A, Roudot-Thoraval F, et al. Acute chest syndrome in adults with sickle cell disease. *Chest* 2000;117:1386–1392.
13. Charache S, Barton FB, Moore RD, et al. Hydroxyurea and sickle cell anemia: Clinical utility of a myelosuppressive "switching" agent. The Multicenter Study of Hydroxyurea in Sickle Cell Anemia. *Medicine* (Baltimore) 1996;75:300–326.
14. Glover RE, Ivy ED, Orringer EP, et al. Detection of nitrosyl hemoglobin in venous blood in the treatment of sickle cell anemia with hydroxyurea. *Mol Pharmacol* 1999;55:1006–1010.
15. Jiang J, Jordan SJ, Barr DP, et al. In vivo production of nitric oxide in rats after administration of hydroxyurea. *Mol Pharmacol* 1997;52:1081–1086.
16. Hillery CA, Du MC, Wang WC, Scott JP. Hydroxyurea therapy decreases the in vitro adhesion of sickle erythrocytes to thrombospondin and laminin. *Br J Haematol* 2000;109:322–327.
17. Collins FS, Orringer EP. Pulmonary hypertension and cor pulmonale in the sickle hemoglobinopathies. *Am J Med* 1982;73:814–821.
18. Simmons BE, Santhanam V, Castaner A, et al. Sickle cell heart disease: Two-dimensional echo and Doppler ultrasonographic findings in the hearts of adult patients with sickle cell anemia. *Arch Intern Med* 1988;148:1526–1528.
19. Sutton LL, Castro O, Cross DJ, et al. Pulmonary hypertension in sickle cell disease. *Am J Cardiol* 1994;74:626–628.

20. Head CA, Brugnara C, Martinez-Ruiz R, et al. Low concentrations of nitric oxide increase oxygen affinity of sickle erythrocytes in vitro and in vivo [see comments]. *J Clin Invest* 1997;100:1193–1198.
21. McDade WA. Nitric oxide increases the solubility of deoxyhemoglobin S solutions and promotes unsickling of sickled cells [abstract]. Proceedings of national annual meeting. *Sickle Cell Prog* 1997:252.
22. Gladwin MT, Schechter AN, Shelhamer JH, et al. Inhaled nitric oxide augments nitric oxide transport of sickle cell hemoglobin without affecting oxygen affinity [see comments]. *J Clin Invest* 1999;104:937–945.
23. Khan BV, Harrison DG, Olbrych MT, et al. Nitric oxide regulates vascular cell adhesion molecule 1 gene expression and redox-sensitive transcriptional events in human vascular endothelial cells. *Proc Natl Acad Sci USA* 1996;93:9114–9119.
24. Space SL, Lane PA, Pickett CK, Weil JV. Nitric oxide attenuates normal and sickle red blood cell adherence to pulmonary endothelium. *Am J Hematol* 2000;63:200–204.
25. French JA, 2nd, Kenny D, Scott JP, et al. Mechanisms of stroke in sickle cell disease: Sickle erythrocytes decrease cerebral blood flow in rats after nitric oxide synthase inhibition. *Blood* 1997;89:4591–4599.
26. Moncada S, Radomski MW, Palmer RM. Endothelium-derived relaxing factor: Identification as nitric oxide and role in the control of vascular tone and platelet function. *Biochem Pharmacol* 1988;37:2495–2501.
27. Kubes P, Suzuki M, Granger DN. Nitric oxide: An endogenous modulator of leukocyte adhesion. *Proc Natl Acad Sci USA* 1991;88:4651–4655.
28. Lopez BL, Barnett J, Ballas SK, et al. Nitric oxide metabolite levels in acute vaso-occlusive sickle cell crisis. *Acad Emerg Med* 1996;3:1098–1103.
29. Lopez BL, Davis-Moon L, Ballas SK, Ma XL. Sequential nitric oxide measurements during the emergency department treatment of acute vaso-occlusive sickle cell crisis. *Am J Hematol* 2000;64:15–19.
30. Stuart MJ, Setty BN. Sickle cell acute chest syndrome: Pathogenesis and rationale for treatment. *Blood* 1999;94:1555–1560.
31. Enwonwu CO. Increased metabolic demand for arginine in sickle cell anaemia. *Med Sci Res* 1989;17:997–998.
32. Lowenthal E, Thornley-Brown D, Rutledge L, et al. Correlation of nitric oxide (NO) metabolites with plasma L-arginine in adults with sickle cell disease (SCD). *Blood* 1996;88(Suppl 1):35 (abstract).
33. Maxwell AJ, Cooke JP. Cardiovascular effects of L-arginine. *Curr Opin Nephrol Hypertens* 1998;7:63–70.
34. Tenenbaum A, Fisman EZ, Motro M. L-Arginine: Rediscovery in progress. *Cardiology* 1998;90:153–159.
35. Morris C, Vichinsky E, Styles LA, et al. Arginine: A new therapy for sickle cell disease? Workshop on Nitric Oxide as a Potential Therapeutic Agent for Sickle Cell Disease and other Vascular Diseases. Bethesda, MD, 2000.
36. Cosentino F, Luscher TF. Tetrahydrobiopterin and endothelial nitric oxide synthase activity [editorial]. *Cardiovasc Res* 1999;43:274–278.
37. Atz AM, Wessel DL. Inhaled nitric oxide in sickle cell disease with acute chest syndrome. *Anesthesiology* 1997;87:988–990.
38. Sullivan KJ, Goodwin SR, Evangelist J, et al. Nitric oxide successfully used to treat acute chest syndrome of sickle cell disease in a young adolescent. *Crit Care Med* 1999;27:2563–2568.
39. May JM. How does ascorbic acid prevent endothelial dysfunction? *Free Radic Biol Med* 2000;28:1421–1429.

40. Cannon RO III. Potential mechanisms for the effect of angiotensin-converting enzyme inhibitors on endothelial dysfunction: The role of nitric oxide. *Am J Cardiol* 1998;82:8S–10S.
41. Bank N, Kiroycheva M, Singhal PC, et al. Cell biology-immunology-pathology: Inhibition of nitric oxide synthase ameliorates cellular injury in sickle cell mouse kidneys. *Kidney Int* 2000;58:82–89.
42. Werdehoff SG, Moore RB, Hoff CJ, et al. Elevated plasma endothelin-1 levels in sickle cell anemia: Relationships to oxygen saturation and left ventricular hypertrophy. *Am J Hematol* 1998;58:195–199.
43. Graido-Gonzalez E, Doherty JC, Bergreen EW, et al. Plasma endothelin-1, cytokine, and prostaglandin E2 levels in sickle cell disease and acute vaso-occlusive sickle crisis. *Blood* 1998;92:2551–2555.
44. Hammerman SI, Kourembanas S, Conca TJ, et al. Endothelin-1 production during the acute chest syndrome in sickle cell disease. *Am J Respir Crit Care Med* 1997;156:280–285.
45. Phelan M, Perrine SP, Brauer M, Faller DV. Sickle erythrocytes, after sickling, regulate the expression of the endothelin-1 gene and protein in human endothelial cells in culture. *J Clin Invest* 1995;96:1145–1151.
46. Hammerman SI, Klings ES, Hendra KP, et al. Endothelial cell nitric oxide production in acute chest syndrome. *Am J Physiol* 1999;277:H1579–1592.
47. Takuwa Y, Yanagisawa M, Takuwa N, Masaki T. Endothelin, its diverse biological activities and mechanisms of action. *Prog Growth Factor Res* 1989;1:195–206.
48. Mumtaz FH, Khan MA, Sullivan ME, et al. Potential role of endothelin and nitric oxide in physiology and pathophysiology of the lower urinary tract. *Endothelium* 1999;7:1–9.
49. Caramelo C, Lopez Farre A, Riesco A, Casado S. Role of endothelin-1 in the activation of polymorphonuclear leukocytes. *Kidney Int Suppl* 1997;61:S56–59.
50. Tanner FC, Boulanger CM, Luscher TF. Endothelium-derived nitric oxide, endothelin, and platelet vessel wall interaction: Alterations in hypercholesterolemia and atherosclerosis. *Semin Thromb Hemost* 1993;19:167–175.
51. Warner TD. Relationships between the endothelin and nitric oxide pathways. *Clin Exp Pharmacol Physiol* 1999;26:247–252.
52. Luscher TF, Wenzel RR. Endothelin and endothelin antagonists: Pharmacology and clinical implications. *Agents Actions Suppl* 1995;45:237–253.
53. Miller ST, Sleeper LA, Pegelow CH, et al. Prediction of adverse outcomes in children with sickle cell disease. *N Engl J Med* 2000;342:83–89.
54. Castro O. Management of sickle cell disease: Recent advances and controversies. *Br J Haematol* 1999;107:2–11.
55. Kaul DK, Hebbel RP. Hypoxia/reoxygenation causes inflammatory response in transgenic sickle mice but not in normal mice [see comments]. *J Clin Invest* 2000;106:411–420.
56. Griffin TC, McIntire D, Buchanan GR. High-dose intravenous methylprednisolone therapy for pain in children and adolescents with sickle cell disease [see comments]. *N Engl J Med* 1994;330:733–737.
57. Greenberg J, Ohene-Frempong K, Halus J, et al. Trial of low doses of aspirin as prophylaxis in sickle cell disease. *J Pediatr* 1983;102:781–784.
58. Zago MA, Costa FF, Ismael SJ, et al. Treatment of sickle cell diseases with aspirin. *Acta Haematol* 1984;72:61–64.
59. Aslan M, Thornley-Brown D, Freeman BA. Reactive species in sickle cell disease. *Ann NY Acad Sci* 2000;899:375–391.

60. Hebbel RP. Auto-oxidation and a membrane-associated Fenton reagent: A possible explanation for development of membrane lesions in sickle erythrocytes. *Clin Haematol* 1985;14:129–140.
61. Lowenthal EA, Mayo MS, Cornwell PE, Thornley-Brown D. Homocysteine elevation in sickle cell disease. *J Am Coll Nutr* 2000;19:608–612.
62. van Guldener C, Stehouwer CD. Hyperhomocysteinemia, vascular pathology, and endothelial dysfunction. *Semin Thromb Hemost* 2000;26:281–289.
63. Carr AC, Zhu BZ, Frei B. Potential antiatherogenic mechanisms of ascorbate (vitamin C) and alpha-tocopherol (vitamin E). *Circ Res* 2000;87:349–354.
64. Williamson DJ, Wallman LL, Jones R, et al. Hemodynamic effects of bosentan, an endothelin receptor antagonist, in patients with pulmonary hypertension. *Circulation* 2000;102:411–418.

Chapter 9

Red Blood Cell-Derived ATP Is a Determinant of Nitric Oxide Synthesis in the Pulmonary Circulation

Randy S. Sprague, MD, Mary L. Ellsworth, PhD, Alan H. Stephenson, PhD, and Andrew J. Lonigro, MD

Introduction

In contradistinction to other vascular beds, the pulmonary circulation must, at all times, accept the entire cardiac output. In spite of highly variable flow rates, pulmonary vascular resistance is maintained at a relatively low level, i.e., one-tenth that of the systemic circulation. Vascular resistance in the lung is considered to be determined both by the physical properties of the lungs and by active vasomotion, the latter related to nervous as well as humoral influences. In addition to the regulation of resistance to blood flow, mechanisms within the lung participate in the intrapulmonary distribution of that flow such that ventilation-perfusion relationships are maintained. These adjustments of intrapulmonary blood flow distribution are mediated, in part, by the response of resistance vessels to alveolar hypoxia, i.e., hypoxic pulmonary vasoconstriction. The controls of pulmonary vascular resistance as well as the intrapulmonary

This work was supported by NIH NHLBI grants HL51298, HL52675, HL64180, and HL56249.

We thank Jo Schreiweis and Kristy Mcdowell for technical assistance. We also thank Drs. S. Sutera and H. Meiselman for the use of their St. George's filtrometers. Finally, we thank J L. Sprague for her inspiration.

From: Weir EK, Reeve HL, Reeves JT (eds). *Interactions of Blood and the Pulmonary Circulation.* Armonk, NY: Futura Publishing Company, Inc.; ©2002.

distribution of blood flow appear to be locally mediated events; thus, neither central nervous nor circulating humoral influences are required for the maintenance of low vascular resistance or for the matching of ventilation with perfusion.

The finding that the endothelium produces factors that are capable of relaxing the underlying vascular smooth muscle has stimulated efforts to define a role for these endothelium-derived relaxing factors (EDRFs) in the control of pulmonary vascular resistance. The best-characterized EDRFs are prostacyclin and nitric oxide (NO). Both pulmonary arteries and veins produce NO.[1] Moreover, in isolated pulmonary artery rings from several species, NO mediates the relaxation initiated by the application of a variety of substances including bradykinin,[2] vasoactive intestinal polypeptide,[2] and the calcium ionophore, A23187.[1] Although these studies demonstrate that NO is synthesized by the pulmonary endothelium and is capable of relaxing isolated pulmonary vessels, they do not demonstrate a role for endogenous NO in the regulation of pulmonary vascular resistance in the intact lung. To address this issue, a number of studies have been performed both in intact animals and in isolated perfused lungs.

The Contribution of Endogenous NO to Pulmonary Vascular Resistance in the Presence of Alveolar Hypoxia

A physiological role for NO in the regulation of pulmonary vascular resistance was suggested by several studies in which endogenous NO was shown to oppose hypoxic pulmonary vasoconstriction (HPV) in isolated lungs ventilated with a gas mixture containing a reduced oxygen tension.[3–5] In these studies, administration of agents that inhibit the synthesis of NO[3] or the generation of cGMP,[5] a second messenger that mediates several effects of NO, resulted in augmentation of the increase in pulmonary arterial pressure that occurred when the lungs were ventilated bilaterally with a hypoxic gas mixture. In addition, the administration of either dissolved NO or the active cGMP analog, 8-bromo-cGMP, resulted in vasodilation in isolated rat lungs preconstricted by alveolar hypoxia.[4] Although these studies demonstrate that NO, either synthesized endogenously or administered exogenously, acts to oppose the marked increase in pulmonary perfusion pressure in response to global alveolar hypoxia, this model may not reflect the physiological role of HPV in the pulmonary circulation. In the intact lung, HPV is responsible for the redistribution of blood flow away from poorly ventilated (hypoxic) alveoli to well-ventilated (well-oxygenated) lung units. Moreover, in the healthy lung, an increase in pulmonary arterial pressure is not required for redistribution of blood flow to occur.

The Contribution of Endogenous NO to the Intrapulmonary Distribution of Blood Flow Between Well-Oxygenated and Hypoxic Lung Units

To examine the contribution of endogenous NO to the intrapulmonary distribution of blood flow, we performed experiments in intact anesthetized rabbits in which the lungs were individually cannulated such that they could be ventilated simultaneously, but independently, with gases of similar or dissimilar composition.[6] Mean pulmonary arterial pressure was measured via a catheter placed into the pulmonary artery. Total pulmonary blood flow and blood flow to the left lung were determined using ultrasonic flow probes placed around the aorta and left main pulmonary artery, respectively. Blood flow to the right lung was determined as total pulmonary blood flow (cardiac output) less the blood flow to the left lung. Ventilation of the right lung with 100% oxygen and the left lung with 100% nitrogen (unilateral alveolar hypoxia) resulted in redistribution of blood flow from the hypoxic left lung to the well-oxygenated right lung.[6] To determine the contribution of endogenous NO to the intrapulmonary distribution of blood flow, an inhibitor of NO synthesis, N^{ω}-nitro-L-arginine methyl ester (L-NAME), was administered during unilateral alveolar hypoxia. The administration of L-NAME resulted in dose-dependent reductions in blood flow to the hypoxic lung and concomitant increases in arterial oxygen tension.[6] The effects of L-NAME were prevented by an excess of L-arginine, a substrate for nitric oxide synthase.[6] These studies demonstrate that, in the intact animal, endogenous NO is present in areas of alveolar hypoxia and that this potent vasodilator can influence the intrapulmonary distribution of blood flow by opposing hypoxic pulmonary vasoconstriction. Importantly, this redistribution of blood flow did not require an increase in pulmonary arterial pressure. Finally, the redistribution of blood flow away from hypoxic lung units to well-oxygenated alveoli in response to L-NAME administration was accompanied by an increase in arterial oxygen tension, i.e., the redistribution of blood flow had a functional consequence.

The Contribution of Endogenous NO to Pulmonary Vascular Resistance in the Absence of Alveolar Hypoxia

Although the studies described above demonstrate a role for endogenous NO in opposing the vasoconstriction associated with either global or localized alveolar hypoxia, they do not address the contribution of NO to pulmonary vascular resistance under resting conditions in the healthy lung when alveolar hypoxia is minimal. Several studies in isolated lungs perfused with a physiological salt solution have yielded conflicting results. Thus, although the administration of inhibitors of NO synthesis augmented hypoxic pulmonary vasoconstriction, these agents were reported to have had little or no effect on pulmonary artery pressure in lungs ventilated with room air.[3,4] However, these studies did not include a comprehensive assessment of the contribution of NO to vascular resistance over a wide range of flow rates, i.e., the effect of inhibition of NO synthesis on pressure-flow relationships was not determined.

In contrast to studies in isolated lungs, we reported that, in intact anesthetized rabbits ventilated with room air, administration of L-NAME resulted in increases in resting pulmonary arterial pressure.[6] Although this study suggested that, in the intact animal, NO is synthesized endogenously and contributes to vascular resistance in the pulmonary circulation under resting conditions, the increase in pulmonary arterial pressure was accompanied by a fall in cardiac output (total pulmonary blood flow).[6] Thus, the observed changes in pulmonary vascular resistance could have been related, in part, to the de-recruitment of vessels in the lung and not to active vasomotion. To address this important issue, studies were performed in isolated perfused lungs in which flow rate could be varied and pressure-flow relationships determined.

Rabbit lungs were isolated and placed in a heated humidified box and perfused with a physiological salt solution (PSS) of the following composition (in mM); 118.3 NaCl, 4.7 KCl, 2.5 $CaCl_2$, 1.2 $MgSO_4$, 1.2 KH_2PO_4, 25.0 $NaHCO_3$, 0.026 Na-EDTA and 11.1 glucose to which bovine serum albumin (3%) was added. The lungs were ventilated with gas containing 15% oxygen, 6% carbon dioxide, and 79% nitrogen. Ventilation with this gas mixture resulted in perfusate oxygen and carbon dioxide tension of 136.9 ± 3.0 and 30.3 ± 0.7 mm Hg, respectively, with a pH of 7.44 ± 0.02. Lungs were perfused under zone 3 conditions via a roller pump at a basal flow rate of 10–12 mL $\cdot$ g lung $wt^{-1} \cdot min^{-1}$. Mean pulmonary arterial pressure (Ppa) and left atrial pressure (Pla) were measured continuously. Pressure-flow curves were generated in the absence and presence of L-NAME (100 μM) by recording the pressure drop across the pulmonary circulation (Ppa-Pla) at flow rates over the range of 50 to 350 mL/min. Estimates of microvascular pressure (Pmv) were made with the double occlusion technique at each flow rate. It was anticipated that if NO were a determinant of pulmonary vascular resistance, then the administration of an inhibitor of endogenous NO synthesis would result in a shift in the pressure-flow relationship such that the pressure drop across the lung would be greater over the flow rates studied and the slope of the pressure-flow relationship would increase.

In contradistinction to our findings implicating endogenous NO in the maintenance of basal pulmonary vascular resistance in intact rabbits,[6] in lungs perfused with PSS, L-NAME was without effect on pressure-flow relationships[7] (Figure 1 A). However, a major difference between these studies was that, in the intact animal, the lungs were not perfused with PSS, but rather with blood. To determine if the failure to demonstrate a role for endogenous NO in the isolated perfused lung was related to the nature of the perfusate used, we performed additional studies in which the lungs were perfused with whole rabbit blood. In blood-perfused lungs, the addition of L-NAME to the perfusate resulted in a significant shift in the pressure-flow relationship consistent with a decrease in vascular caliber, i.e., in the presence of blood, the response to L-NAME was consistent with that in the intact animal (Figure 1 B). Thus, when isolated lungs are perfused with blood, NO is a determinant of pulmonary vascular resistance in the absence of alveolar hypoxia. The finding that blood was required to demonstrate endogenous NO synthesis in the lung does not appear to be unique to the rabbit because similar findings were reported in studies with isolated perfused rat lungs.[8,9]

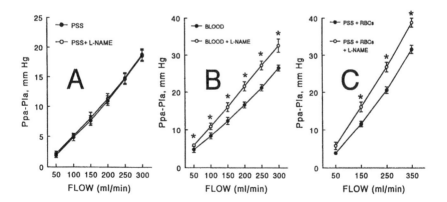

Figure 1. Effect of Nω-nitro-L-arginine methyl ester (L-NAME, 100 μM) on the relationship between flow rate and the pressure difference across the pulmonary circulation in isolated rabbit lungs perfused with physiological salt solution (PSS, panel A), rabbit blood (panel B) or PSS to which rabbit RBCs were added (hematocrit 20% ± 1%) . Ppa = mean pulmonary arterial pressure; Pla = mean left atrial pressure; *different from values in the absence of L-NAME.

The Role of Shear Stress as a Stimulus
for Endogenous NO Synthesis
in the Isolated Perfused Lung

The mechanism responsible for the stimulation of endogenous NO synthesis would be anticipated to be a local one. An example of such a local control mechanism is the increase in endothelial NO synthesis associated with the application of shear stress to the endothelium.[10–14] Flow-induced increases in shear stress have been reported to stimulate NO synthesis in cultured endothelial cells,[10] in isolated arteries,[11] in isolated hearts,[12] in arteries perfused in situ,[13] and in microvessels.[14] Shear stress applied to the endothelium of a blood vessel can be defined mathematically as:

$$\tau = 4 \mu Q / \pi r^3$$

where τ represents shear stress, μ the viscosity of a fluid, Q the flow rate of a fluid, and r the radius of the vessel that is perfused. Thus, in the isolated perfused rabbit lung, in addition to alterations in perfusate flow rate, manipulation of viscosity and vascular radius can be used to investigate the contribution of shear stress applied to the endothelium to the synthesis and/or activity of NO.

To determine if the mechanism by which blood, but not PSS, stimulated endogenous NO synthesis in isolated perfused lungs was related to the viscosity of the perfusate, we performed studies in isolated rabbit lungs in which the viscosity of PSS was increased to that of blood with dextran (70,000 mol wt). In these experiments, the addition of L-NAME was without effect on pressure-flow relationships, suggesting that the property of blood that stimulated NO synthesis in the isolated rabbit lung could not be related to viscosity per se.[7]

A second possible explanation for the stimulation of NO synthesis solely in lungs perfused with blood was that vascular resistance was greater in lungs perfused with blood than in those perfused with PSS, i.e., vascular radius was smaller. Indeed, it was reported that isolated lungs perfused with salt solutions lack the capacity to increase vascular resistance under some conditions.[15] This issue was addressed in 2 ways. First, we performed studies in which the pulmonary vasoconstrictor prostaglandin $F_{2\alpha}$ ($PGF_{2\alpha}$) was added to the perfusate of lungs perfused with either PSS or blood. The increase in perfusion pressure produced by $PGF_{2\alpha}$ administration was not different in either preparation.[7] Second, we generated pressure-flow curves in the absence and presence of L-NAME in lungs perfused with PSS in which vascular resistance was increased with potassium chloride. In the latter studies, L-NAME was again without effect on pressure-flow relationships.[7]

These data demonstrate that lungs perfused with PSS are capable of increasing vascular resistance in response to a vasoconstrictor and that in the presence of increased vascular tone, but in the absence of blood, the synthesis of endogenous NO is not stimulated. Taken together, these findings suggest that the failure of L-NAME to increase vascular resistance in rabbit lungs perfused with PSS cannot be attributed to a general loss of the ability to increase vascular resistance.

The results of the above studies suggested that some property of blood not related to an effect on shear stress alone is responsible for the stimulation of NO synthesis in the isolated perfused rabbit lung. To determine what component(s) of blood are responsible for the stimulation of endogenous NO synthesis, additional studies were performed in which the effect of L-NAME on pressure-flow relationships was determined in isolated rabbit lungs perfused with either plasma (containing normal numbers of platelets and white blood cells)[7] or PSS to which washed red blood cells (RBCs) were added. In lungs perfused with plasma and non-RBC-formed elements of blood, L-NAME was without effect on pressure-flow relationships. In contrast, in lungs perfused with PSS to which washed RBCs were added, L-NAME administration resulted in a shift in pressure-flow relationships (Figure 1 C) similar to that seen in lungs perfused with blood (Figure 1 B). Moreover, the increase in vascular resistance was confined to upstream (arterial) vascular segments. Although the results of these studies demonstrated that the RBC is a required component of the perfusate of isolated rabbit lungs for the effects of L-NAME on pressure-flow relationships to be observed, they did not reveal the mechanism by which the RBC stimulated endogenous NO synthesis.

RBC-Derived Adenosine Triphosphate as a Stimulus for Endogenous NO Synthesis

The results of the studies described above demonstrate that, in the absence of RBCs, alterations in shear stress alone do not stimulate NO release in the isolated rabbit lung. The application of agents such as acetylcholine, bradykinin, and adenosine triphosphate (ATP) to endothelial cells results in the synthesis and release of NO.[16] ATP is of particular interest because it is present in millimolar concentrations in RBCs[17,18] and is the major adenine nucleotide present in that cell (ratios for intracellular concentrations of ATP, adenosine diphosphate (ADP), and adenosine monophosphate (AMP) are 100:10:1, respectively).[18] Multiple receptors for ATP have been identified and partially characterized.[19] In the vasculature, the P_{2x} purinergic receptor is present primarily on vascular smooth muscle cells and its activation results in contraction of that cell.[19]

In contrast, the P_{2y} receptor is found primarily on the endothelium.[19] The binding of ATP to the endothelial P_{2y} receptor results in the synthesis of NO.[16,20] Thus, ATP applied directly to the VSM of an intact vessel, e.g., that released from nerve terminals, would be expected to produce vasoconstriction via activation of P_{2x} receptors. In contrast, ATP applied to the luminal side of a vessel, e.g., that released within the circulation from RBCs, would be expected to produce endothelium-dependent vasodilation through interaction with the P_{2y} receptor present on the endothelial cell and the subsequent release of NO.[16,19,20]

Recently, it was reported that ATP present in the vascular lumen may act in concert with shear stress to augment NO synthesis.[21,22] Indeed, it was reported that endothelial cells in culture showed little change in intracellular Ca^{+2} ($[Ca^{+2}]_i$), a stimulus for NO synthesis, when the cells were exposed to increases in shear stress in the absence of ATP.[21] In contrast, in the presence of 1 μM ATP, identical increases in shear stress resulted in increases in $[Ca^{+2}]_i$. Similarly, it was reported that, in endothelial cells grown in flow chambers, increases in flow rate did not alter $[Ca^{+2}]_i$ in the absence of ATP.[22] However, in the presence of 500 nM to 1 μM ATP, changes in $[Ca^{+2}]_i$ were related to changes in flow rate. Thus, as flow rate was increased or decreased, $[Ca^{+2}]_i$ increased or decreased, respectively.[21] Finally, increments in flow were reported to result in increased cGMP levels in endothelial cells in the presence, but not in the absence, of 1 μM ATP.[22] This increase in cGMP was prevented by an inhibitor of NO synthesis. Although these studies provide strong support for the hypothesis that ATP is a requisite for shear stress-induced release of NO, such a requirement for ATP has not been reported by others.[10–14] This discrepancy may be related to differences in experimental conditions, such as the degree of shear stress applied or the unintentional use of medium containing ATP.[21,22] One interpretation of this discrepancy is that, although shear stress alone may stimulate some NO synthesis in buffer-perfused systems, ATP potentiates that response.

If ATP is an important regulator of pulmonary NO synthesis and, thereby, pulmonary vascular resistance, in vivo, a hemodynamic response to ATP should be demonstrable in the intact circulation of that organ. Hassessian and Burnstock[23] reported that, in isolated PSS-perfused rat lungs, the addition of ATP to the perfusate resulted in a decrease in perfusion pressure. Following L-NAME, the same concentration of ATP evoked an increase in pressure, presumably via activation of P_{2x} receptors present on the vascular smooth muscle and unopposed by the synthesis of NO. These results suggest that intraluminal ATP produces vasodilation via stimulation of endothelial P_{2y} receptors resulting in NO synthesis.[23] Although these studies demonstrate that ATP administered into the lumen of the blood vessels of the lung results in vasodilation and that NO may mediate this response, an endogenous source of ATP was not defined.

To address this issue we quantified the amount of ATP present in perfusate of isolated rabbit lungs perfused with either PSS or PSS to which washed rabbit RBCs were added. ATP was measured by the luciferin-luciferase technique[17,24] in which the amount of light generated by the reaction of ATP with firefly tail extract is dependent on the ATP concentration. Sensitivity was augmented by addition of synthetic D-luciferin to the crude firefly tail extract. A 200 μL sample of RBC-containing solution was injected into a cuvette containing 100 μL crude firefly tail extract (5 mg/5 mL distilled water, FLE 50, Sigma, St. Louis, MO) and 100 μL of a solution of synthetic D-luciferin (50 mg/100 mL distilled water, Sigma, St. Louis, MO). The peak light efflux from cuvettes to which either known ATP standards or samples are added was determined using a luminometer. An ATP standard curve was obtained on the day of each experiment. To exclude the presence of significant he-

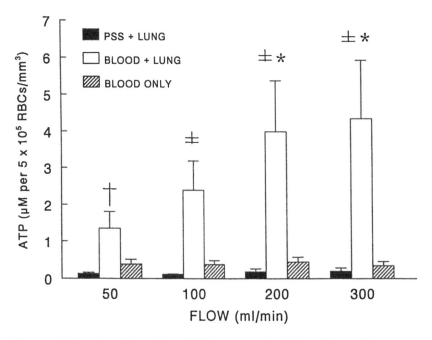

Figure 2. Adenosine triphosphate (ATP) concentration in the effluent of lungs perfused with either physiological salt solution (PSS, solid bars) or PSS containing rabbit RBCs (hematocrit 20% ± 1%, open bars) and the concentration of ATP in the perfusion circuit in the presence of PSS containing rabbit RBCs (hematocrit 22% ± 2%) but in the absence of a lung (cross-hatched bars).*$P<0.05$ different from respective 50 mL/min value; + = different from values in lungs perfused with PSS; ± = different from values in lungs perfused with PSS and PSS containing RBCs in the absence of a lung in the perfusion circuit.

molysis, after ATP determinations, RBC suspensions were centrifuged at 500 × g at 4°C for 10 minutes and the presence of hemoglobin in the supernatant was determined by light absorption at wavelengths of 385, 405, 560, 577, and 630 nm. This technique for hemoglobin determination is sufficiently sensitive to detect hemolysis of 0.5% of RBCs studied. The amount of ATP released in association with this level of hemolysis was not detectable in the luciferin-luciferase assay. Finally, in all experiments, ATP content of RBCs was determined by measurement of ATP in solution following lysis of a known number of RBCs in distilled water.

Minimal amounts of ATP were detected in the effluent of lungs perfused with PSS and these values did not change in response to increases in flow rate (Figure 2). In contrast, in lungs perfused with PSS containing washed rabbit RBCs at a hematocrit of 20 ± 1%, ATP was detected in the lung effluent and the concentration increased *pari passu* with flow rate (Figure 2). Importantly, the passage of RBCs through the perfusion circuit in the absence of a lung did not result in release of ATP from these cells (Figure 2). These studies demonstrate that RBC-derived ATP is released in the intact pulmonary circulation and that amounts of ATP released increased with increments in flow rate.[25] This finding is consistent with the hypothesis that RBC-derived ATP could stimulate endogenous NO synthesis in the intact lung and, thereby, contribute to the maintenance of low levels of vascular resistance in the circulation of that organ. However, these studies did not identify the stimulus for ATP release from the RBCs.

The Stimulus for ATP Release from RBCs

If RBC-derived ATP is an important determinant of endogenous NO synthesis in the lung, then ATP should be released in response to physiological stimuli. Indeed, it was reported that exposure of RBCs to reduced oxygen tension and reduced pH resulted in the release of ATP.[17,26] These stimuli for ATP release from RBCs were suggested to be of importance for ATP release from RBCs in the skeletal muscle circulation.[26] However, in the lungs, the oxygen tension and pH of mixed venous blood (the blood perfusing the lung via the pulmonary artery) would not be expected to fall to values required for the release of ATP.[17,26] Thus, if ATP release from RBCs is the mechanism responsible for the stimulation of NO synthesis in the intact pulmonary circulation, then some additional mechanism for ATP release must be present in these cells. We postulated that such a stimulus was the mechanical deformation that RBCs are subjected to as they traverse the microcirculation of the lung.

To address this important issue, we performed experiments in which RBCs of healthy humans, rabbits, and dogs were deformed by passage through filters of decreasing pore size, i.e., increasing mechanical deformation. These species were chosen because in both rabbits and humans, NO *is* a determinant of pulmonary vascular resistance, whereas, in the dog, NO *does not* subserve this role in the pulmonary circulation.[27] RBCs were subjected to mechanical deformation using the St. George's Blood Filtrometer (Carri-Med Ltd., Dorking, UK).[28] This device develops a calibrated pressure gradient across a vertically mounted filter. A 13-mm diameter polycarbonate filter (Nucleopore) with a 9.53-mm exposed surface diameter and average pore size of either 12, 8, or 5 μm was placed in the filter chamber and the outflow channel was filled with PSS. Flow was prevented by an outflow channel tap. For calibration, proximal to the filter, an open-ended capillary tube was filled with PSS. The time taken for the PSS to pass 4 fiberoptic detectors was recorded with a computer. This process was repeated until coefficients of variance between runs were 1% or less.

Deformation of RBCs was achieved by passing cells suspended in PSS at a hematocrit of 10% through the filters. The filtration rate of the RBC suspension relative to PSS alone, the red cell transit time (RCTT), was calculated as described previously.[28,29] The RCTT is dependent on the deformability of the RBCs, the hematocrit, and the size of the filter pores relative to the size of the RBCs studied. Thus, the St. George's Blood Filtrometer can be used to determine the deformability of RBCs[28] as well as ATP released in response to increasing deformation (decreasing pore size).[29] The concentration of ATP present in the effluent from the various filters or under basal conditions was measured by the luciferin-luciferase technique and was normalized to that released from 2×10^5 RBCs/mm^3.

Using this technique, we determined that mechanical deformation of RBCs of rabbits and healthy humans resulted in the release of ATP (Figure 3 B).[29] Moreover, the amount of ATP released increased in a stimulus-dependent fashion, i.e., as the degree of deformation applied to the RBCs increased, reflected by the increase in RCTT with decreasing average pore size (Figure 3 A), amounts of ATP released increased. In contrast, RBCs of dogs *did not* release ATP in response to mechanical deformation (Figure 3 B).

To demonstrate that the ability of RBCs to release ATP in response to mechanical deformation was associated with the stimulation of endogenous NO synthesis in the pulmonary circulation, we performed experiments in which RBCs of either humans or dogs were added to the perfusate (PSS) of isolated rabbit lungs. The addition of the NO synthase inhibitor, L-NAME, was without effect on pressure-flow relationships in lungs perfused with RBCs of dogs (Figure 4 A).[29] In contrast, in lungs perfused with RBCs of humans, L-NAME administration resulted in a shift in pressure-flow relationships (Figure 4 B), demon-

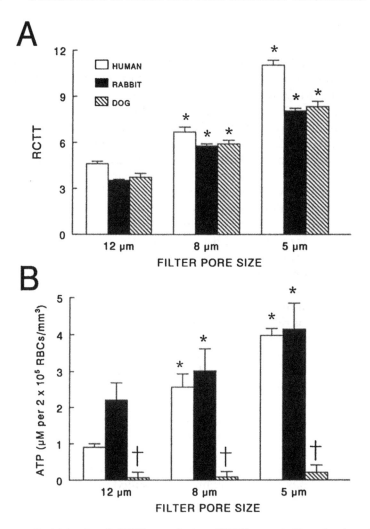

Figure 3. Red blood cell (RBC) transit time (RCTT, panel A) and adenosine triphosphate (ATP) release (concentration in filter effluent, panel B) in response to passage RBCs of humans (open bars), rabbits (solid bars) or dogs (cross-hatched bars) through filters with decreasing average pore size. *Different from values for respective 12 μm filter; + = different from values for rabbit and human RBCs.

strating that endogenous NO was a determinant of pulmonary vascular resistance in the presence of these RBCs.[29] Thus, only the RBCs of species that release ATP in response to mechanical deformation (rabbits and humans) stimulated endogenous NO synthesis in the intact pulmonary circulation.[7,25,29]

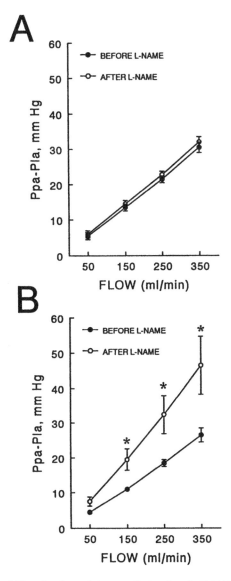

Figure 4. Effect of N$^{\omega}$-nitro-L-arginine methyl ester (L-NAME, 100 μM) on the relationship between flow rate and the pressure difference across the pulmonary circulation in isolated rabbit lungs perfused with physiological salt solution (PSS) to which dog RBCs (hematocrit 32% ± 2%, panel A) or human RBCs (hematocrit 17% ± 2%, panel B) were added. *Different from values in the absence of L-NAME.

The Mechanism of ATP Release from RBCs

Although the studies described above are consistent with the hypothesis that deformation-induced ATP release from RBCs is an important determinant of vascular resistance in the lung of rabbits and healthy humans, they do not address the mechanism by which ATP is released from these cells. ATP is a highly charged molecule and, as such, cannot pass easily through cell membranes. Thus, it would be anticipated that a signal-transduction pathway exists for the regulation of ATP release from RBCs in response to mechanical deformation. Recently, a family of membrane-associated proteins grouped together as the ATP binding cassette have been described.[30] A member of the family, the cystic fibrosis transmembrane conductance regulator (CFTR),[30,31] was suggested to be a transporter of ATP from the interior of cells to the external milieu. Although not all properties of the CFTR channel have been fully characterized, the activity of this channel has been shown to be inhibited by sulfonlyureas such as tolbutamide and glibenclamide[32] as well as by some nonsteroidal anti-inflammatory agents such as niflumic acid.[33] We reported that incubation of rabbit RBCs with glibenclamide or niflumic acid blocked the release of ATP in response to mechanical deformation.[34] Importantly, these inhibitors of CFTR had no effect on either RBC deformability or total ATP content of the RBCs.[34] Although studies with inhibitors of the activity of CFTR strongly implicate this channel as a component of the signal-transduction pathway for the release of ATP from the RBC, questions regarding the selectivity of the inhibitors must always be considered.

The finding that human RBCs, like those of rabbits, release ATP in response to mechanical deformation[29] presented a unique opportunity for the study of the contribution of CFTR to deformation-induced ATP release from human RBCs. Cystic fibrosis is a genetic disorder characterized clinically by a constellation of symptoms related, in large part, to chronic pulmonary disease.[35] In spite of the fact that CF patients may have different patterns of organ involvement, severity of disease, and genetic mutation, they share a common pathophysiological problem: the expression of CFTR activity is deficient and the activity of CFTR is markedly diminished or lost.[35]

We reported that, in contrast to heathy humans, RBCs of patients with CF did not release ATP in response to mechanical deformation (Figure 5 B).[34] In patients with CF, the failure of RBCs of patients with CF to release ATP could not be attributed to either altered RBC deformability (Figure 5 A) or reduced ATP content of the RBCs. To demonstrate that the lack of ATP release in response to deformation could not be related simply to the presence of chronic lung disease, RBCs from patients with the clinical diagnosis of chronic obstructive

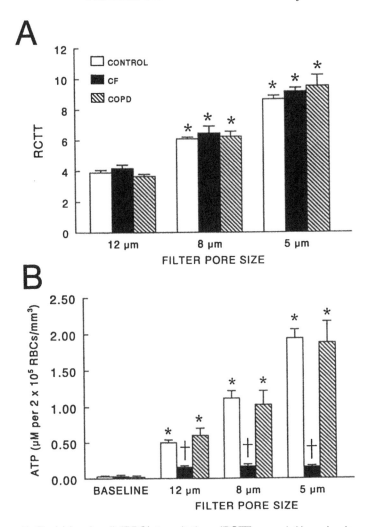

Figure 5. Red blood cell (RBC) transit time (RCTT, panel A) and adenosine triphosphate (ATP) release (concentration in filter effluent, panel B) in response to passage RBCs of healthy humans (open bars) or patients with cystic fibrosis (CF, solid bars) or chronic obstructive pulmonary disease (COPD, cross-hatched bars) through filters with decreasing average pore size. *Different from respective 12 μm filter (panel A) or baseline value (panel B); + = different from rabbit and human RBCs.

pulmonary disease were also studied. RBCs from the latter group released ATP in response to mechanical deformation and the response did not differ from that of healthy humans (Figure 5 A, B).[34]

Although these studies implicate CFTR as a component of the signal-transduction pathway for deformation-induced ATP release, they do not permit determination of the exact role of CFTR in the egress of ATP from the RBC. Thus, the possibility that CFTR functions as a conduit for ATP efflux cannot be excluded. However, the data are also consistent with the interpretation that CFTR activity is required for activation of another channel that functions as an ATP conduit. Resolution of this issue awaits further investigation.

The Failure of Deformation-Induced ATP Release from RBCs of Humans with Pulmonary Hypertension

Cystic fibrosis patients develop pulmonary hypertension.[35] However, the coexistence of severe airways disease, alveolar hypoxia, and pulmonary hypertension in these individuals makes investigation of the contribution of defective ATP release from RBCs to the development of pulmonary hypertension difficult. Severe airways disease and alveolar hypoxia are not, however, features of another human condition, namely, primary pulmonary hypertension (PPH). In patients with PPH, pulmonary vascular resistance is increased in the absence of known etiology,[36] i.e., the pathophysiological mechanisms responsible for the development and progression of PPH have not been defined. Interestingly, both PPH patients[37] and patients with CF[38] were reported to demonstrate decreased NO synthesis in the lungs when compared with those of healthy humans. The mechanism responsible for the failure of NO synthesis in the pulmonary circulation in these conditions was not determined. We hypothesized that the failure of deformation-induced ATP release from RBCs could be a common defect in patients with CF and PPH. This failure to release ATP into the vascular lumen would deprive the lung of an important stimulus for endogenous NO synthesis.

Previously, it was reported that RBCs of patients with PPH are distinct from those of healthy humans, i.e., the deformability of RBCs of patients with PPH was found to be decreased when compared to those of healthy humans.[39] Blood viscosity was increased in patients with PPH while plasma viscosity was normal, suggesting that decreased RBC deformability resulted in rheological changes of physiological significance.[39] Recently, we confirmed the observation that RBC deformability is decreased (increased RCTT) in patients with PPH (Figure 6 A). However, in addition to decreased deformability, these latter studies demonstrated that RBCs of patients with PPH failed to demonstrate increments in ATP release in response to increases in mechanical deformation (Figure 6 B). Although the inability of RBCs to release ATP in response to mechanical deformation was not related to a decrease in total ATP content of the cells, the effect of decreased RBC deformability on ATP release could not be de-

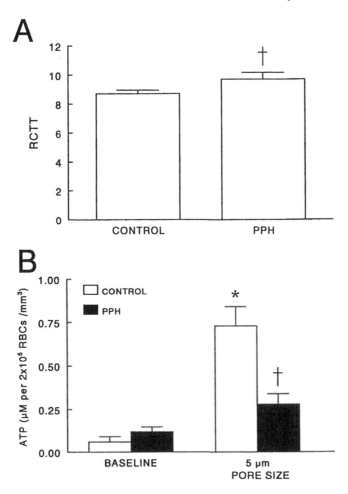

Figure 6. Red blood cell (RBC) transit time (RCTT, panel A) and ATP release (ATP concentration in filter effluent, panel B) in response to passage RBCs of healthy humans (CONTROL, open bars) and patients with primary pulmonary hypertension (PPH, solid bars) through filters with an average pore size of 5 μm. *Different from respective baseline value; + = different from CONTROL value.

termined. To address this important issue, additional experiments were performed in which ATP release from RBCs of healthy humans and patients with PPH was stimulated by a mechanism independent of deformation. Our studies in patients with CF suggested that CFTR was a component of a signal-transduction pathway for ATP release from rabbit and human RBCs. A major stimulus for the activation of CFTR is an increase in intracellular cAMP.[40] We hypothesized that incubation of RBCs with an active cAMP analog, adenosine 3'5'-cyclic monophosphorothioate, Sp-isomer (Sp-cAMP)[41] would result in ATP release. Indeed, in the presence of Sp-cAMP, ATP released from RBCs of healthy humans increased from a baseline value of 0.3 ± 0.1 to 1.1 ± 0.3 μM of ATP per 2 × 10⁵ RBCs/mm³ ($P<0.01$). In contrast, RBCs of patients with PPH demonstrated a baseline ATP release of 0.2 ± 0.1of ATP per 2 × 10⁵ RBCs/mm³ and this value did not increase upon incubation with Sp-cAMP. Although Sp-cAMP could have effects in addition to activation of CFTR, these findings demonstrate that, in contrast to RBCs of healthy humans, RBCs of patients with PPH fail to release ATP in response to a pharmacological stimulus. Importantly, this finding demonstrates that the failure of mechanical deformation to induce ATP release from RBCs of patients with PPH cannot be attributed solely to an effect on RBC deformability per se.

A Proposed Role for RBC-Derived ATP in the Regulation of Vascular Resistance

The finding that RBCs of rabbits and healthy humans are required for flow-induced NO synthesis in the pulmonary circulation, coupled with the findings that mechanical deformation of these RBCs results in ATP release which, in turn, can stimulate NO synthesis in the lung suggests a novel mechanism for the control of pulmonary vascular caliber (Figure 7). In this construct, as the RBC is increasingly deformed by in-

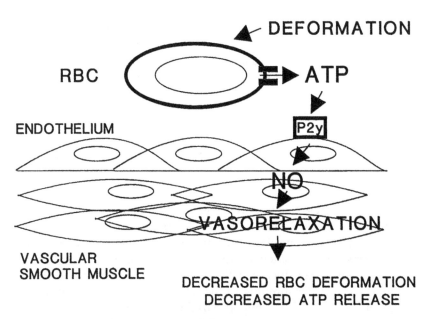

Figure 7. Proposed model of the contribution of red blood cell (RBC)-derived ATP to the control of vascular resistance.

crements in the velocity of blood flow through a vessel and/or by reductions in vascular caliber, it releases ATP, which stimulates endothelial synthesis of NO, resulting in relaxation of vascular smooth muscle and, thereby, an increase in vascular caliber. This vasodilation results in a decrease in pulmonary vascular resistance as well as a decrease in the stimulus for RBC deformation and ATP release. Thus, we propose that RBC-derived ATP contributes to the low resistance to blood flow present in the healthy lung. Failure of this mechanism for deformation-induced ATP release from RBCs could be expected to lead, ultimately, to the development of pulmonary hypertension.

References

1. Ignarro LJ, Buga G, Chaudhuri, G. EDRF generation and release from perfused bovine pulmonary artery and vein. *Eur J Pharmacol* 1988;149:79–88.
2. Ignarro LJ, Byrns RE, Buga GM, et al. Mechanisms of endothelium-dependent vascular smooth muscle relaxation elicited by bradykinin and VIP. *Am J Physiol* 1987;253:H1074–H1082.
3. Brashers VL, Peach MJ, Rose CE. Augmentation of hypoxic pulmonary vasoconstriction in the isolated perfused rat lung by in vitro antagonists of endothelium-dependent relaxation. *J Clin Invest* 1988;82:1495–1502.
4. Archer SL, Rist K, Nelson DP, et al. Comparison of the hemodynamic effects of nitric oxide and endothelium-dependent vasodilators in the lung. *J Appl Physiol* 1990;68:735–747.
5. Mazmanian GM, Baudet B, Brink C, et al. Methylene blue potentiates vascular reactivity in isolated rat lungs. *J Appl Physiol* 1989;66:1040–1045.
6. Sprague RS, Thiemermann C, Vane JR. Endogenous EDRF opposes hypoxic pulmonary vasoconstriction and supports blood flow to hypoxic alveoli in rabbits. *Proc Natl Acad Sci USA* 1992;89:8711–8715.
7. Sprague RS, Stephenson AH, Dimmit RA, et al. Effect of L-NAME on pressure-flow relationships in isolated rabbit lungs: Role of red blood cells. *Am J Physiol* 1995;269:H1941–H1948.
8. Wilson PS, Khimenko P, Moore TM, et al. Perfusate viscosity and hematocrit determine pulmonary vascular responsiveness to NO synthase inhibitors. *Am J Physiol* 1996;270:H1757–1765.
9. Uncles DR, Daugherty MO, Frank DU, et al. Nitric oxide modulation of pulmonary vascular resistance is red blood cell dependent in isolated rat lungs. *Anesth Analg* 1996;83:1212–1217.
10. Buga GM, Gold ME, Fukuto JM, et al. Shear stress-induced release of nitric oxide from endothelial cells grown on beads. *Hypertension* 1991;17:187–193.
11. Lamontagne D, Polh U, Busse R. Mechanical deformation of vessel wall and shear stress determine the basal release of endothelium-derived relaxing factor in the intact rabbit coronary vascular bed. *Circ Res* 1992;70:123–130.
12. Rubanyi GM, Romero JC, Vanhoutte PM: Flow-induced release of endothelium-derived relaxing factor. *Am J Physiol* 1986;250:H1145–H1149.
13. Hull SS Jr, Kaiser L, Jaffe MD, et al. Endothelium-dependent flow-induced dilation of canine femoral and saphenous arteries. *Blood Vessels* 1989;23:183–198.
14. Koller A, Sun D, Huang A, et al. Corelease of nitric oxide and prostaglandins

mediates flow-dependent dilation of rat gracilis muscle arterioles. *Am J Physiol* 1994;267:H326–H332.

15. McMurtry IF, Hookway MA, Roos S. Red blood cells play a crucial role in maintaining vascular reactivity to hypoxia in isolated rat lungs. *Chest* 1977;72(Suppl):253–256.

16. Bogle RG, Coade SB, Moncada S, et al. Bradykinin and ATP stimulate L-arginine uptake and nitric oxide release in vascular endothelial cells. *Biochem Biophys Res Commun* 1991;254:926–932.

17. Bergfeld GR, Forrester T. Release of ATP from human erythrocytes in response to a brief period of hypoxia and hypercapnea. *Cardiovasc Res* 1992;26:40–46.

18. Miseta A, Bogner P, Berenyi M, et al. Relationship between cellular ATP, potassium, sodium, and magnesium concentrations in mammalian and avian erythrocytes. *Biochem Biophys Acta* 1993;1175:133–139.

19. Houston DA, Burnstock G, Vanhoutte PM. Different P_2-purinergic receptor subtypes of endothelium and smooth muscle in canine blood vessels. *J Pharmacol Exp Ther* 1987;241:501–506.

20. Dull RO, Tarbell JM, Daves PF. Mechanism of flow-mediated signal transduction in endothelial cells: Kinetics of ATP surface concentrations. *J Vasc Res* 1992;29:410–419.

21. Ando J, Ohtsuka A, Korenaga R, et al. Effect of extracellular ATP level on flow-induced Ca^{++} response in cultured vascular endothelial cells. *Biochem Biophys Res Commun* 1991;179:1192–1199.

22. Korenaga R, Ando J, Tusboi H, et al. Laminar flow stimulates ATP- and shear stress-dependent nitric oxide production in cultured bovine endothelial cells. *Biochem Biophys Res Commun* 1994;198:213–219.

23. Hassessian H, Burnstock G. Interacting roles of nitric oxide and ATP in the pulmonary circulation of the rat. *Br J Pharmacol* 1995;114:846–850.

24. Strehler BL, McElroy WC. Assay of adenosine triphosphate. In Colowick SP, Kaplan NO, eds: *Methods in Enzymology, vol. 3.* New York: Academic Press; 1957.

25. Sprague RS, Ellsworth ML, Stephenson AH, Lonigro AJ. Increases in flow rate stimulate adenosine triphosphate release from red blood cells in isolated rabbit lungs. *Exp Clin Cardiol* 1998;3:73–77.

26. Ellsworth ML, Forrester T, Ellis CG, Dietrich HH. The erythrocyte as a regulator of vascular tone. *Am J Physiol* 1995;269:H2155–H2161.

27. Nishiwaki K, Nyhan DP, Rock P, et al. N^G-nitro-L-arginine and pulmonary vascular pressure-flow relationship in conscious dogs. *Am J Physiol* 1992;262:H1331–H1337.

28. Dormandy J, Flute P, Matrai A, et al. The new St. George's blood filtrometer. *Clin Hemorheol* 1985;5:975–983.

29. Sprague RS, Ellsworth ML, Stephenson AH, et al. ATP: The red blood cell link to NO and local control of the pulmonary circulation. *Am J Physiol* 1996;271:H2717–H2722.

30. Al-Awqati Q. Regulation of ion channels by ABC transporters that secrete ATP. *Science* 1995;269:805–806.

31. Reisin IL, Prat AG, Abraham EH, et al. The cystic fibrosis transmembrane conductance regulator is a dual ATP and chloride channel. *J Biol Chem* 1994;269:20584–20591.

32. Schultz BD, DeRoos ABG, Venglarik CJ, et al. Glibenclamide blockade of CFTR chloride channels. *Am J Physiol* 1996;271:L192–L200.

33. Cuthbert AW, Evans MJ, Colledge WH, et al. Kinin-stimulated chloride

secretion in mouse colon requires the participation of CFTR chloride channels. *Brazilian J Med Biol Res* 1994;27:1905–1910.

34. Sprague RS, Ellsworth ML, Stephenson AH, et al. Deformation-Induced ATP release from red blood cells requires cystic fibrosis transmembrane conductance regulator activity. *Am J Physiol* 1998;275:H1726–H1732.

35. Davis PB, Drumm M, Konstan MW. Cystic fibrosis. *Am J Respir Crit Care Med* 1996;154:1229–1256.

36. Rubin LJ. Pathology and pathophysiology of primary pulmonary hypertension. *Am J Cardiol* 1995;75:51A–54A.

37. Kaneko FT, Arroliga AC, Dweikl RA, et al. Biochemical reaction products of nitric oxide as quantitative markers of primary pulmonary hypertension. *Am J Respir Crit Care Med* 1998;158:917–923.

38. Lundberg JON, Nordvall SL, Weitzberg E, et al. Exhaled nitric oxide in pediatric asthma and cystic fibrosis. *Arch Dis Child* 1997;75:323–326.

39. Persson SU, Gustavasson CG, Larsson H, Persson S. Studies of blood rheology in patients with primary pulmonary hypertension. *Angiology* 1991; 42:836–842.

40. Hanrahan JW, Mathews CJ, Grygorczyk R, et al. Regulation of the CFTR chloride channel from humans and sharks. *J Exp Zoology* 1996;275:283–291.

41. Holen B, Gordon PB, Stromhaug PE, Seglen PO. Role of cAMP in the regulation of hepatotoxic autophagy. *Eur J Biochem* 1996;236:169–170.

Chapter 10

Malaria and the Microcirculation

May Ho, MD, Msc

Introduction

Malaria is a parasitic infection that is transmitted by the bite of a female anopheline mosquito. Over half of the human population is at risk for this infection, resulting in an estimated 300 to 500 million infections and up to 2 million deaths annually, particularly among children in sub-Saharan Africa.[1] There are 4 *Plasmodium* species that infect humans, namely, *P. falciparum, P. vivax, P. ovale,* and *P. malariae, P. falciparum* is the causative agent of the most severe form of malaria. The molecular basis of the pathophysiology of severe falciparum malaria that results primarily from the sequestration of infected erythrocytes in the microcirculation is reviewed in this chapter.[2]

Falciparum malaria is an acute febrile illness characterized by fever, chills, headache, myalgia, anemia, and splenomegaly. The infection responds promptly to antimalarial treatment. Untreated, less than 5% of patients will die in the acute attack. The majority will survive with almost no immunity against the next infection unless he or she has been exposed to years of repeated challenge. Not only is immunity to *P. falciparum* slow to develop, it is also lost quickly when the individual leaves the endemic area. Once acquired, immunity is maintained by the presence of a low-grade infection, a phenomenon referred to as concomitant immunity or premunition.[3]

Complications of falciparum malaria develop in about 1% of infected individuals, and are manifested as coma (cerebral malaria),

Grant support: Medical Research Council of Canada, Alberta Heritage Foundation for Medical Research and Wellcome – Mahidol University, Oxford Tropical Medicine Research Program funded by the Wellcome Trust, United Kingdom.

From: Weir EK, Reeve HL, Reeves JT (eds). *Interactions of Blood and the Pulmonary Circulation.* Armonk, NY: Futura Publishing Company, Inc.; ©2002.

metabolic acidosis, hypoglycemia, anemia, and in adults, renal failure and pulmonary edema.[4] The multiorgan disease carries a mortality of 15–30% despite intensive treatment. The most dramatic clinical manifestation is cerebral malaria, when patients present in coma that has developed suddenly following a seizure or more gradually over a period of hours through the stages of confusion, delirium, obtundation, and finally unarousable coma. Localizing neurological signs are rare, suggesting that the underlying pathology is a diffuse symmetrical encephalopathy. Permanent residual neurological sequelae, including cognitive impairment, are seen in less than 5% of adults, but can be detected in approximately 10% of children.

Acute pulmonary edema resulting from an increase in pulmonary capillary permeability as in other forms of acute respiratory distress syndrome is another severe but rare complication of falciparum malaria. It often occurs in association with renal impairment, typically at a time when the patient appears to be recovering from other manifestations of severe disease. Hypoalbuminemia is a contributing factor, as is overzealous fluid therapy in these patients who are very vulnerable to volume overload.

Acute renal failure is another major cause of death in adults with severe falciparum malaria. Renal impairment, and ultimately acute tubular necrosis, in severe falciparum malaria presumably results from a reduction in renal microvascular blood flow. In some patients, dehydration and hemoglobinuria contribute to the process.

Two major metabolic disturbances seen in severe falciparum malaria are hypoglycemia and metabolic acidosis. These 2 disorders commonly coexist. Hypoglycemia arises as a result of several processes. There is impairment of gluconeogenesis secondary to liver dysfunction, and increased glucose consumption by both the febrile host and parasites. Hypoglycemia may also be iatrogenic in that the antimalarial drug quinine can by itself stimulate insulin secretion. Pregnant women are particularly vulnerable to hyperinsulinemic hypoglycemia because of the accelerated ketogenic response to starvation and an exaggerated islet cell response to the secretory stimulus of quinine. The biochemical features of quinine-induced hypoglycemia are raised plasma insulin, lactate, and alanine levels in the presence of low concentrations of ketone bodies.

Lactic acidosis results from anaerobic glycolysis of the host and parasite, and reduced lactate clearance. The contribution of the host in the form of L (+) lactate is the more important factor. Elevated concentrations of lactate occur in both the arterial and the venous circulation as well as in the cerebrospinal fluid. The anion gap remains within normal limits initially, but arterial pH eventually falls to critical levels, requiring dialysis for effective correction.

Cytoadherence

When postmortem tissues from patients who died of severe falciparum malaria are examined, the most striking pathological feature is the intense sequestration of infected erythrocytes in the microvasculature of vital organs (Figure 1). The resulting microcirculatory obstruction leads to tissue hypoxia, metabolic disturbances, and multiorgan dysfunction as described above. The organ distribution of sequestration varies and tends to reflect the clinical features of the preceding clinical illness. For example, sequestration is the highest in the brain compared to that in other organs in patients who died of cerebral malaria.[5] Even within the brain, variation in the degree of sequestration is seen between cerebral and cerebellar vessels, and white and gray matter.[6] At the microvascular level, there is considerable heterogeneity among the individual vessels. The majority of vessels are packed with infected erythrocytes containing parasites that are fully developed, but there are others that contain the immature ring stages of the parasite.[7] This synchronous clustering suggests that once the erythrocytes have adhered, detachment does not occur. In the acute phase of severe falciparum malaria, there is

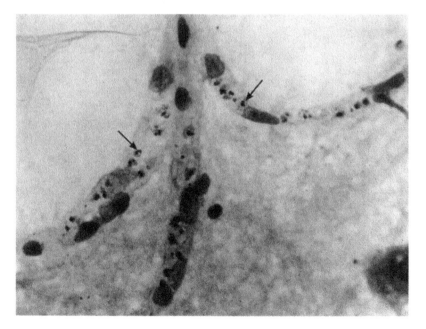

Figure 1. Cerebral venules packed with infected erythrocytes (arrows) in a fatal case of cerebral malaria. Reproduced from *The American Journal of Physiology* (*Cell Physiol* 45) 1999;C1231–C1242, by copyright permission of The American Physiological Society.

remarkably little extravascular pathology, and although occasional fibrin strands may be seen, platelets are also notable by their absence.

At the ultrastructural level, electron-dense, knob-like protrusions of the erythrocytic membrane are seen at the points of contact between the infected erythrocyte and the endothelial cells (Figure 2). These knobs are made up of parasite-encoded proteins that have been exported to the surface of the infected erythrocyte and inserted into the cytoskeleton. They are essential for firm adhesion to the endothelial cell under flow conditions by concentrating parasite ligands at specific sites,[8] thus serving a similar function as microvilli on the surface of leukocytes, where ligands for interaction with vascular endothelium are presented.[9]

The word *cytoadherence* was coined to describe the unique ability of *P. falciparum* to adhere to capillary and postcapillary venular endothelium during the second half of its 48-hour parasite life cycle. Although the transit of infected erythrocytes can be delayed in microvessels due to a loss of deformability,[10] it has been widely postulated that parasites actively adhere to microvascular endothelium in order to evade clearance by the spleen. The stage and host cell specificity of the adhesion

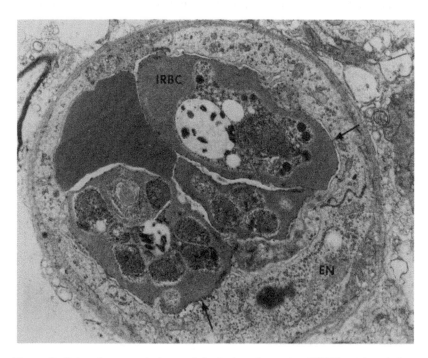

Figure 2. Cytoadherence between infected erythrocytes (IRBC) and endothelial cells (EN) showing knobs (arrows) at the points of attachment. Reproduced from *The American Journal of Physiology* (*Cell Physiol* 45) 1999;C1231–C1242, by copyright permission of The American Physiological Society.

process indicate that the adhesive interactions involve specific parasite ligands and endothelial receptors. Because of the implications for anti-adhesive therapy, there has been intense research on the adhesion molecules and parasite ligands involved in mediating cytoadherence.

Endothelial Receptors: Static Binding Studies

A number of endothelial receptors have been identified based on their ability to support the adhesion of laboratory-adapted or selected parasite lines and clones to cell lines and purified receptor proteins in static binding assays in vitro.[11] The molecules include thrombospondin, CD36, intercellular adhesion molecule-1 (ICAM-1), vascular cell adhesion molecule-1 (VCAM-1), E-selectin, platelet endothelial cell adhesion molecule-1 (PECAM-1), and $\alpha_v\beta_3$. However, these adhesive phenotypes cannot be directly extrapolated to malaria parasites causing clinical infections, since clinical parasite isolates are genetically and phenotypically heterogeneous. In addition, the adhesion phenotype of parasites is known to be influenced by long-term culture in vitro and by the selection and cloning process itself.

When infected erythrocytes taken directly from the peripheral blood of acutely infected patients were studied, greater than 90% of the isolates tested adhered to CD36, whereas about 10% adhered to ICAM-1. For isolates that adhered to both molecules, the degree of adhesion to CD36 was at least 10-fold higher than adhesion to ICAM-1. There was minimal or no adhesion to VCAM-1, E-selectin, or PECAM-1.

Adhesion molecule specificity has also been studied by immuno-histological examination of postmortem tissues. In these studies, the co-localization of sequestration with increased ICAM-1 expression and the relative paucity of CD36 staining in the brain have been taken as evidence that ICAM-1 is the principal receptor for cytoadherence in the cerebral circulation. This interpretation fails to take into account 2 very important features of adhesion molecule biology, namely: (1) that adhesion molecules expression can occur as a result of the ischemia associated with cytoadherence rather than as the initiating event, and (2) that the relative intensity of adhesion molecule expression by immunofluorescence bears no direct relationship to its functional role.

From a parasite population perspective, results from static binding assays suggest that about 30% of infected erythrocytes in a given parasite isolate adhered to CD36, whereas 2–3% were adherent to ICAM-1. The percentage of infected erythrocytes adherent to E-selectin and VCAM-1 was negligible. This means that greater than 60% of infected erythrocytes do not bind to any of the receptor molecules in vitro. These observations suggest that there might be as yet unidentified receptor molecules for infected erythrocytes. A more likely explanation is that infected erythrocytes may need to interact with more than one adhesion molecule for optimal adhesion. The interaction with some of the adhesion molecules such as E-selectin, P-selectin, and VCAM-1 may be revealed only under flow conditions. To ensure their own survival, infected erythrocytes will likely use a number of adhesion molecules to adhere to the vascular endothelium in vivo in order to evade clearance by the spleen.

Endothelial Receptors: Flow Chamber Studies

The hypothesis that infected erythrocytes may in fact interact with a number of adhesion molecules mimicking the cascade of adhesive events involved in leukocyte recruitment under flow conditions was tested by studying cytoadherence in a parallel plate flow chamber assay in vitro.[12,13] The interactions between infected erythrocytes and various cellular substrata at fluid shear stresses approximating those in the microvasculature were directly visualized. A suspension of infected erythrocytes was drawn through the flow chamber at varying rates with an infusion pump attached to the outlet. Attached infected erythrocytes and their motion could be clearly observed with phase contrast objectives and quantitated by analysis of videotaped images. Tethering referred to the initial contact between infected erythrocytes and the endothelial monolayer. A rolling cell was defined as one that displayed a typical end-on-end rolling motion at a velocity 10- to 20-fold lower than the centerline flow rate of red blood cells which exceeds 1000 μm/sec. An infected erythrocyte was considered adherent if it remained stationary for more than 10 seconds.

Using the flow chamber assay, infected erythrocytes from clinical parasite isolates were observed to interact with individual adhesion molecules in a stepwise process that involved tethering, rolling and firm adhesion.[12] Infected erythrocytes initially tethered and then rolled on CD36, ICAM-1, P-selectin, and VCAM-1, but not E-selectin. However, the strength of the rolling interaction with each receptor molecule varied, as reflected in differences in rolling velocity, and significant adhesion under shear was almost exclusively to CD36. Some infected erythrocytes bypassed the rolling event and were arrested on CD36 immediately after tethering. On C32 melanoma cells, which co-express CD36 and ICAM-1, inhibition of rolling by an anti-ICAM-1 antibody reduced subsequent adhesion of some isolates to CD36. Similarly, inhibition of rolling by an anti-P-selectin antibody reduced adhesion of infected erythrocytes to CD36 on activated platelets.[13]

The above studies were performed using transfectants, cell lines, and purified receptor proteins, which ensured that maximal numbers of adhesion molecules were provided as substrata. To determine if the same synergistic adhesive interactions occur on microvascular endothelial cells, where the distribution and expression of adhesion molecules are considerably less, we conducted studies using human dermal microvascular endothelial cells.[14] These are the only readily accessible cells that express or can be induced to express all the adhesion molecules (CD36, ICAM-1, P-selectin, and VCAM-1) that have so far been implicated in mediating cytoadherence under flow conditions. These adhesion molecules are of clinical significance because all of them are expressed or up-regulated on the microvasculature of brain, liver, kidney, and lung tissues from patients who died from severe falciparum malaria.[15]

Our results indicate that infected erythrocytes tethered, rolled, and adhered on both resting and cytokine-stimulated microvascular endothelial cells in a shear-dependent manner. Adhesion was largely via CD36. We have shown previously on CD36 transfectants that the molecule can in fact mediate all 3 phases of infected red blood cell (IRBC)-endothelial cell interactions, i.e., tethering, rolling, and adhesion. However, interaction with CD36 on microvascular endothelium, where the expression of the molecule was much lower than on the transfectants (mean fluorescent intensity at least a log lower), did not appear to be sufficient for the arrest of approximately two-thirds of the rolling infected erythrocytes. On the other hand, stimulation with TNF-α for 24 hours, which upregulated ICAM-1 and induced VCAM-1 expression, resulted in the adhesion of nearly 100% of the rolling infected erythrocytes without affecting rolling flux. The expression of these molecules appeared to increase the stickiness of microvascular endothelial cells, so that a greater percentage of rolling infected erythrocytes was arrested. Inhibition of the rolling component by receptor-specific antibodies resulted in significant reduction of subsequent adhesion to CD36. On the other hand, P-selectin expression induced by oncostatin-M increased the number of rolling as well as adherent cells, indicating an actual increase in the number of infected erythrocytes recruited to the endothelial surface. This finding firmly establishes a major role for P-selectin in mediating cytoadherence under flow conditions, which is consistent with the key role of selectins in the initial tethering and rolling of leukocytes on vascular endothelium.[16]

Endothelial Receptors: In Vivo Studies

Even the above experiments with microvascular endothelial cells have their limitations. The shear stress used in the flow chamber assay in vitro is at the lowest limit of the shear stress in the microvasculature in vivo.[16] The lack of a suitable animal model for cytoadherence has meant that the hypothesis that infected erythrocytes can actively adhere in the microcirculation to allow for propagation of the infection has never been tested directly in vivo. To this end, we recently made use of a well-established model of human skin grafted onto SCID mice[17] but extended the model to directly visualize the human microvasculature by epi-fluorescence intravital microscopy.[18] The skin graft retains the human microvascular bed of the superficial dermis, and the graft blood supply is restored by spontaneous anastomosis of the mouse and human microvessels at the base of the graft. By fluorescently labeling the microvessels in vivo with the lectin *Ulex europaeus*, which specifically recognizes human endothelial cells of vessels of all sizes, we were able to directly observe the adhesive interactions of rhodamine-labeled infected erythrocytes in the fields of observation.

In all animals examined, infected erythrocytes were observed to roll and/or adhere in postcapillary venules of the human skin graft (Figure 3). Surprisingly, infected erythrocytes also interacted with arterioles in some of the grafts examined. The interaction in arterioles was predominantly one of rolling, while adhesion of infected erythrocytes occurred mainly in postcapillary venules. Approximately two-thirds of the adherent infected erythrocytes rolled for various distances before becoming arrested, while the rest adhered immediately after tethering. In addition, occlusion of some capillaries by infected erythrocytes was observed after parasite injection. The administration of an anti-CD36 monoclonal antibody rapidly reduced rolling and adhesion of infected erythrocytes in postcapillary venules. More importantly, already adherent infected erythrocytes quickly detached, although no effect was seen on infected erythrocytes in the capillaries. The residual rolling of infected erythrocytes after anti-CD36 treatment was largely inhibited by anti-ICAM-1 treatment, resulting in further reduction in the number of adherent cells. Treatment of the SCID mice with anti-ICAM-1 alone also reduced rolling and adhesion, although the parasite isolates tested were not known to adhere to ICAM-1 under flow conditions in vitro.

These data in the human/SCID mouse chimera demonstrate for the first time that *Plasmodium falciparum*-infected erythrocytes undergo adhesive interactions similar to those of leukocytes under the unique physiological shear conditions and configurations of adhesion molecule expression present in a human microvasculature in vivo. As 2 very different cell systems, leukocytes and an intra-erythrocytic pathogen, appear to make use of the rolling to adhesion cascade, from an evolutionary standpoint it suggests that the stepwise mechanism is likely the optimal strategy for cellular recruitment under flow in blood vessels many times the cell diameter in vivo.

There are also some important differences between the adhesive

Figure 3. Interactions of infected erythrocytes and human endothelial cells in the human/SCID mouse model. Panels a–c illustrate the same vascular field within the human skin graft. To aid identification, the vascular walls are indicated by lines. Adherent or slowly moving (rolling) infected erythrocytes are visible as discrete circular objects, while non-interacting infected erythrocytes are observed as streaks in the centerline of blood flow. Uninfected erythrocytes are unlabeled. Panels a and b are separated by approximately 3 seconds. Arrows indicate infected erythrocytes undergoing rolling interactions with the endothelial surface of a postcapillary venule within the graft. Over the 3-second time course, the rolling infected erythrocytes have moved slowly along the vascular wall. At the same time, the patency of the microcirculation is apparent as rapidly moving, noninteracting infected erythrocytes are observed throughout this period. Panel c illustrates the same area of microvasculature following dual treatment with monoclonal antibodies against human CD36 and ICAM-1. Very few interacting infected erythrocytes are observed despite many cells continuing to pass through the graft microvasculature. Reproduced from *The Journal of Experimental Medicine* 2000;192;1205–1211, by copyright permission of The Rockefeller University Press.

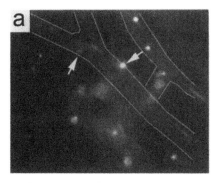

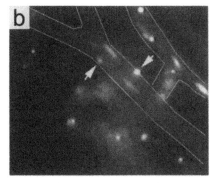

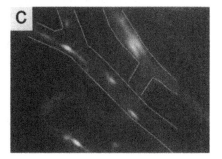

mechanisms used by leukocytes and infected erythrocytes. First, CD36, the scavenger receptor, was the dominant adhesive molecule for rolling and adhesion of infected erythrocytes. This molecule does not support interactions with leukocytes (unpublished observations). Second, ICAM-1 supported the rolling of erythrocytes, whereas leuckocytes adhere but do not roll on ICAM-1. Furthermore, ICAM-1 and CD36 acted synergistically in the recruitment of infected erythrocytes. These 2 molecules by themselves appeared to be sufficient to support rolling and adhesion of infected erythrocytes on noninflamed microvessels. However, it is well documented that TNF-α, IL-1β, IL-6, and IFN-γ are elevated during severe falciparum malaria,[19,20] and it is likely that these cytokines would induce the expression of adhesion molecules such as P-selectin and VCAM-1, which have been shown to enhance the adhesion of infected erythrocytes on human microvascular endothelial cells in vitro.

Third, rolling and active adhesion of infected erythrocytes occurred on both the arteriolar and the venular sides of the circulation, whereas leukocytes adhere predominantly in venules and not at all in uninflamed microvessels. This finding suggests that adherent infected erythrocytes can withstand very high shear rates. However, it should be stressed that the interaction of infected erythrocytes with arterioles was mainly of the rolling phenotype. Whether the adhesion seen in some arterioles reflects lower shear stress in the murine compared with human microcirculation remains to be determined.

Collectively, the in vitro and in vivo observations strongly support the hypothesis that (1) infected erythrocytes interact with multiple adhesion molecules on microvascular endothelium under physiological flow conditions, and that the different interactions are synergistic in promoting adhesion, (2) the degree of cytoadherence in vivo may very well depend on secondary interactions with adhesion molecules such as ICAM-1, VCAM-1, and P-selectin, which accompany and enhance CD36-mediated adhesion of infected erythrocytes, and (3) rolling interactions with other adhesion molecules may be a prerequisite for adhesion to CD36 for some although not all infected erythrocytes, mimicking the adhesive cascade that is involved in the recruitment of leukocytes to sites of inflammation (Figure 4). The human/SCID mouse chimera provides an excellent model to further elucidate the role of adhesion molecules in the pathogenesis of *P. falciparum* malaria, and to

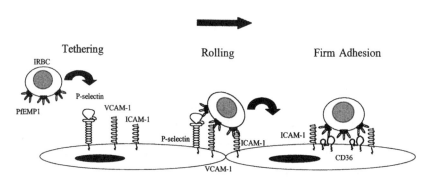

Postcapillary venule

Figure 4. Schematic diagram of the different phases of IRBC interaction with endothelial receptors observed under physiological flow conditions.

evaluate potential therapeutic interventions that would disrupt the adhesive interactions of infected erythrocytes with vascular endothelium.

Parasite Cytoadherent Ligands

Compared to the growing number of host receptors described for infected erythrocytes, relatively few ligands on the surface of the infected red blood cell (IRBC) have been identified. The best-studied cytoadherent ligand on IRBC is *P. falciparum* erythrocyte membrane protein 1 (PfEMP1) that is expressed on the surface of infected erythrocytes in the second half of the parasite life cycle.[11] It is a variant protein both in terms of antigenicity and molecular size. The protein is encoded by a large family of *var* genes, many of which are transcribed in the early stages of the parasite cycle. In parasite clones selected on a particular receptor, only one variant corresponding to the cytoadherent phenotype is expressed on the surface of infected erythrocytes when they adhere to endothelium, which suggests that a silencing mechanism at the transcriptional level becomes operational as the parasite matures.[21] PfEMP1 has been shown to interact with CD36, ICAM-1, thrombospondin, chondroitin-4-sulfate (CSA), and P-selectin (Ho et al., manuscript in preparation). In addition, the domains of PfEMP1 involved in interaction with CD36, ICAM-1, and CSA have been mapped.[22–24]

A second gene family, the cytoadherence-linked asexual gene (*clag9*), has been shown to be essential for cytoadherence. This gene was originally detected on chromosome 9, but recent data from sequencing of the *P. falciparum* genome has revealed that *clag9* is part of a multigene family with sequences present on a number of chromosomes throughout the parasite genome. The gene is transcribed in mature parasites, and translates into a 220 kDA protein that is distinct from PfEMP1. Both subtelomeric deletions at one of the ends of chromosome 9[25] and knocking out *clag9*[26] were associated with a loss of binding of infected erythrocytes to CD36. There is preliminary evidence that the *clag* protein may be expressed on the surface of infected erythrocytes, but its precise cellular location and function have not been defined. It has been postulated that the *clag9* protein may interact directly with CD36, or act as an accessory molecule for the binding of PfEMP1 to CD36, or it may be involved in the transport and correct folding of PfEMP1 on the red cell surface.

Cytoadherence and the Pathogenesis
of *P. falciparum* Malaria

Despite the exciting new molecular findings concerning ligands and receptors, and the demonstration that cytoadherence does indeed occur in a human microvasculature in vivo, many aspects of cytoadherence remain poorly understood. For example, we do not as yet know what determines the sites of sequestration in vivo. Parasites may display tropism for certain microvasculature, which may in turn reflect the expression of organ-specific receptors, and/or the unique architecture of the microcirculation in relation to infected erythrocytes. The adhesion of infected erythrocytes to chondroitin sulfate A[27] and hyaluronic acid[28] expressed on syncytiotrophoblasts in the human placenta clearly demonstrates the existence of organ-specific adhesion molecules for infected erythrocytes that may contribute to local pathology. The accumulation of mononuclear leukocytes in the pulmonary,[4] but not other, microcirculation in severe falciparum malaria serves as additional evidence for the differential recruitment of blood cells to different vital organs in this infection. These questions can be resolved only by closely examining the interactions between clinical parasite isolates and human tissues, and correlating the findings with well-documented clinical manifestations.

A more fundamental issue that has been hotly debated over the past 2 decades is the relative role of vascular obstruction, as described in this chapter, and the systemic and local release of inflammatory cytokines in the pathogenesis of severe falciparum malaria. These 2 mechanisms in fact do not need to be mutually exclusive, as it is well established that inflammatory cytokines can upregulate adhesion molecule expression and thus enhance cytoadherence. In addition, hypoxia as a result of sequestration can synergize with inflammatory cytokines to induce nitric oxide synthase, leading to an increase in nitric oxide production. Nitric oxide was originally postulated to have a pathological role in causing coma in cerebral malaria by disrupting local neurotransmission.[29] Elevated levels of iNOS and nitrosotyrosine have been demonstrated in various cellular locations from fatal cases of falciparum malaria. On the other hand, nitric oxide also appears to have a protective role in inhibiting the growth of *P. falciparum* in vitro.[30] More importantly, recent studies in our laboratory have shown that nitric oxide has an antiadhesive effect on cytoadherence to both resting and TNF-α-stimulated microvascular endothelial cells (Serirom and Ho, manuscript in preparation). These observations are consistent with a dichotomous function for nitric oxide in falciparum malaria, as in other areas of inflammation.[31]

Conclusion

In human *P. falciparum* malaria infection, infected erythrocytes either sequester or are removed from the circulation, primarily by the spleen. The balance between splenic clearance and sequestration, which allows the parasite to survive to initiate a new life cycle, is a major determinant of the rate of increase and magnitude of the infecting parasite burden. Within this paradigm, pathogenicity is proportional to the size of the sequestered parasite burden and the pattern of vital organ sequestration. We have come a long way in our understanding of the molecular mechanisms of cytoadherence under physiological flow conditions. The next challenge lies in translating the advances in our understanding of pathogenesis into improved treatment for the many millions who are affected by falciparum malaria.

Acknowledgment: I am grateful to Professor Nicholas J. White, Centre for Tropical Medicine, Nuffield Department of Clinical Medicine, University of Oxford, United Kingdom, for insightful discussions.

References

1. World Health Organization. Malaria. *WHO Fact Sheet* 1996;94:1–3.
2. MacPherson GG, Warrell MJ, White NJ, et al. Human cerebral malaria: A quantitative ultrastructural analysis of parasitized erythrocyte sequestration. *Am J Pathol* 1985;119:385–401.
3. Smith T, Felger I, Tanner M, et al. Premunition in *Plasmodium falciparum* infection: Insights from the epidemiology of multiple infections. *Trans R Soc Trop Med Hyg* 1999;93(Suppl 1):1–59–64.
4. White NJ, Ho M. The pathophysiology of malaria. *Adv Parasitol* 1992;31: 83–173.
5. Pongponratn E, Riganti M, Punpoowong B, et al. Microvascular sequestration of parasitized erythrocytes in human falciparum malaria: A pathological study. *Am J Trop Med Hyg* 1991;44:168–175.
6. Sein KK, Maeno Y, Thuc HV, et al. Differential sequestration of parasitized erythrocytes in the cerebrum and cerebellum in human cerebral malaria. *Am J Trop Med Hyg* 1993;48:504–511.
7. Silamut K, Phu NH, Whitty C, et al. A quantitative analysis of microvascular sequestration of malaria parasites in the human brain. *Am J Pathol* 1999;155:395–410.
8. Crabb BS, Cooke BM, Reeder JC, et al. Targeted gene disruption shows that knobs enable malaria-infected red cells to cytoadhere under physiological shear stress. *Cell* 1997;89:287–296.
9. Moore KP, Patel KD, Bruehl RE, et al. P-selectin glycoprotein ligand-1 mediates rolling of human neutrophils on P-selectin. *J Cell Biol* 1995;128: 661–671.
10. Cranston HA, Boylan CW, Carroll GL, et al. *Plasmodium falciparum* maturation abolishes physiologic red cell deformability. *Science* 1984;223:400–402.
11. Ho M, White NJ. Molecular mechanisms of cytoadherence in malaria. *Am J Physiol* 1999;276 (*Cell Physiol* 45):C1231–C1242.
12. Udomsangpetch R, Reinhardt PH, Schollaardt T, et al. Promiscuity of clinical *Plasmodium falciparum* isolates for multiple adhesion molecules under flow conditions. *J Immunol* 1997;158:4358–4364.
13. Ho M, Schollaardt T, Niu X, et al. Characterization of *Plasmodium falciparum*-infected erythrocytes and P-selectin interaction under flow conditions. *Blood* 1998;91:4803–4809.
14. Yipp BG, Anand S, Schollaardt T, et al. Synergism of multiple adhesion

molecules in mediating cytoadherence of *Plasmodium falciparum*-infected erythrocytes to microvascular endothelial cells under flow. *Blood* 2000;96: 2292–2298.

15. Turner GD, Morrison H, Jones M, et al. An immunochemical study of the pathology of fatal malaria: Evidence for widespread endothelial activation and a potential role for intercellular adhesion molecule-1 in cerebral sequestration. *Am J Pathol* 1994;145:1057–1069.

16. Lawrence MB, Springer TA. Leukocytes roll on a selectin at physiological flow rates: Distinction from and prerequisite for adhesion through integrins. *Cell* 1991;85:859–873.

17. Murray AG, Petzelbauer P, Hughes CCW, et al. Human T-cell-mediated destruction of allogeneic dermal microvessels in a severe combined immunodeficient mouse. *Proc Natl Acad Sci USA* 1994;91:9146–9150.

18. Ho M, Hickey MJ, Murray AG, et al. Visualization of *Plasmodium falciparum*-endothelium interactions: Mimicry of the leukocyte recruitment paradigm. *J Exp Med* 2000;192:1205–1211.

19. Kwiatkowski D, Hill AVS, Sambou I, et al. TNF concentration in fatal cerebral, non-fatal cerebral, and uncomplicated *Plasmodium falciparum* malaria. *Lancet* 1990;336:1201–1204.

20. Day NPJ, Hien TT, Schollaardt T, et al. The prognostic and pathophysiological role of pro- and anti-inflammatory cytokines in severe malaria. *J Infect Dis* 1999;180:1288–1297.

21. Scherf A, Hernandez-Rivas R, Buffet E, et al. Antigenic variation in malaria: In situ switching, relaxed and mutually exclusive transcription of *var* genes during intra-erythrocytic development of *Plasmodium falciparum*. *EMBO* 1998;17:5418–5426.

22. Baruch DI, Ma XC, Singh HB, et al. Identification of a region of PfEMP1 that mediates adherence of *Plasmodium falciparum*-infected erythrocytes to CD36: Conserved function with variant sequence. *Blood* 1997;90:3766–3775.

23. Smith JD, Craig AG, Kriek N, et al. Identification of a *Plasmodium falciparum* intercellular adhesion molecule-1 binding domain: A parasite adhesion trait implicated in cerebral malaria. *Proc Natl Acad Sci USA* 2000;97: 1766–1771.

24. Reeder JC, Cowman AF, Davern KM, et al. The adhesion of *Plasmodium falciparum*-infected erythrocytes to chondroitin sulfate A is mediated by PfEMP1. *Proc Natl Acad Sci USA* 1999;96:5198–5202.

25. Day KP, Karamalis F, Thompson J, et al. Genes necessary for expression of a virulence determinant and for transmission of *Plasmodium falciparum* are located on a 0.3 megabase region of chromosome 9. *Proc Natl Acad Sci USA* 1993;90:8292–8296.

26. Trenholme KR, Gardiner DL, Holt DC, et al. *clag9*: A cytoadherence gene in *Plasmodium falciparum* essential for binding of parasitized erythrocytes to CD36. *Proc Natl Acad Sci USA* 2000;97:4029–4033.

27. Fried M, Duffy PE. Adherence of *Plasmodium falciparum* to chondroitin sulfate A in the human placenta. *Science* 1996;272:1502–1504.

28. Beeson JG, Rogerson SJ, Cooke BM, et al. Adhesion of *Plasmodium falciparum*-infected erythrocytes to hyaluronic acid in placental malaria. *Nat Med* 2000;6:86–90.

29. Clark IA, Rockett KA, Cowden WB. Proposed link between cytokines, nitric oxide, and human cerebral malaria. *Parasitol Today* 1991;7:205–207.

30. Rockett AK, Awburn MM, Cowden WB, et al. Killing of *Plasmodium falciparum* in vitro by nitric oxide derivatives. *Infect Immun* 1991;59:3280–3283.

31. Kubes P. Inducible nitric oxide synthase: A little bit of good in all of us. *Gut* 2000;47:6–9.

Section III

Platelets

Chapter 11

The Role of Platelets in Pulmonary Hypertension

Andrew J. Peacock, MPhil, MD,
Paul Egermayer, MA, MB, ChB, and
G. Ian Town, MD

Introduction

The various syndromes of pulmonary hypertension were recently reclassified at the Evian International Symposium in 1998.[1] This classification divided pulmonary hypertension into pulmonary arterial hypertension, pulmonary venous hypertension, pulmonary hypertension due to thromboembolism and hypoxic lung disease, and pulmonary vasculitis. Pulmonary arterial hypertension may have multiple etiologies such as genetic predisposition, anorexigen use, HIV infection, and others but, rather surprisingly, a common histology and a common response to treatment, most notably intravenous prostacyclin.[2,3] This suggests there may be a common pathway that leads to pulmonary arterial hypertension.

Pulmonary hypertension occurs because of vasoconstriction of resistance pulmonary arterioles and also remodeling of the pulmonary vasculature. This raises the question of whether pulmonary vasoconstriction is a necessary prerequisite to the development of pulmonary vascular remodeling or can it occur independently. In particular, is there a common pathway leading to vasoconstriction and histological change not withstanding the etiologic stimulus? When considering the role of platelets in this process, it is worth considering whether platelets

Supported by Chest, Heart and Stroke (Scotland), British Lung Foundation, and National Services Division, Scotland.

From: Weir EK, Reeve HL, Reeves JT (eds). *Interactions of Blood and the Pulmonary Circulation*. Armonk, NY: Futura Publishing Company, Inc.; ©2002.

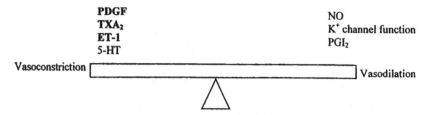

Figure 1. Vasoconstriction in "normal" (unremodeled) pulmonary artery. Hypoxia and various vasoactive compounds cause vasoconstriction, both by direct effects on pulmonary vascular smooth muscle and also indirectly via endothelial cell release of vasoconstrictors. Platelet-derived vasoactive factors could be involved either as primary initiators of vasoconstriction or acting in synergy with other vasoconstrictors such as hypoxia or other vasoactive compounds.

are a necessary component of this pathway and, if so, is platelet activation necessary for platelet involvement? If, as it appears, activation is necessary, then how can the products released by platelets cause vasoconstriction (Figure 1) or pulmonary vascular remodeling (Figure 2) but lead in either case to marked restriction of the pulmonary vascular bed (Figure 3)?

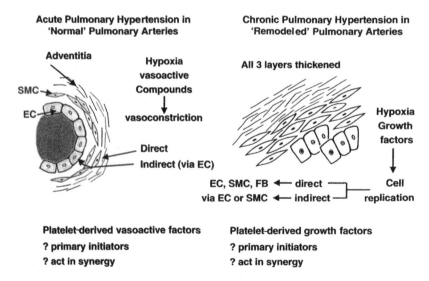

Figure 2. Mechanism of pulmonary artery remodeling. All 3 layers (adventitia, media, and intima) may become thickened in chronic pulmonary hypertension due to replication of pulmonary vascular cells. It is possible that hypoxia and growth factors work either directly on these cells or indirectly via the endothelial cells, or platelet-derived growth factors may act as primary initiators of cellular replication or act in synergy with other mitogens including hypoxia.

Pulmonary Hypertension

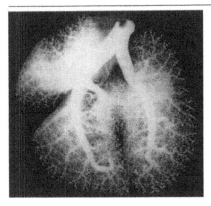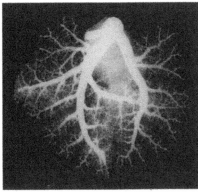

Figure 3. Rat pulmonary arteriogram. Left: normal. Right: widespread loss of pulmonary arterial branch filling after 28 days hyperoxia (which causes endothlelial cell injury). Reproduced with permission from Jones R, Zapol WM, Reid L. Oxygen toxicity and restructuring of pulmonary arteries: A morphometric study. *Am J Pathol* 1985;121:212–223.

Platelet Physiology

Platelets are small anuclear cells derived from megakaryocytes. Their principal activity is the control of hemostasis via the development of the mechanical plug in response to vascular trauma. It is known that, in the face of endothelial cell injury or other stimuli such as hypoxia, there is *activation* of platelets within seconds, and they then adhere to the site of vascular injury aided by endothelial cell release of von Willebrand factor (vWF) and factor VIII. Platelets then *aggregate* and contract at the site of injury and *release* contents from dense granules within the cytoplasm. (Figure 4). This process of *aggregation and release* is aided by the arachidonic acid derivative, thromboxane A_2 (TXA_2). It is clear, therefore, that for platelets to have a function, they must first be *activated* then *aggregated* and finally *release* their complex store of cytokines, mitogens, and other elements.

Platelets release many compounds capable of initiating and maintaining pulmonary hypertension, including vasoconstrictors known to be active in the pulmonary circulation and growth factors with known effects on cells comprising the pulmonary artery wall (Table 1). What is not clear is whether platelet activation and release are necessary components of all pathways to pulmonary hypertension in both acute and chronic situations.

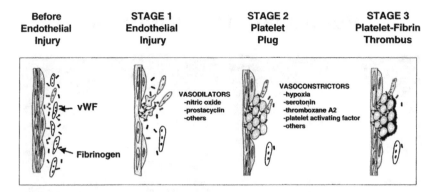

Figure 4. Diagram illustrating the stages in interaction of platelets with the walls of pulmonary arteries following endothelial injury. Stage 1: platelets adhere to the damaged endothelial wall by the mediation of von Willebrand factor. Stage 2: platelets form a plug over the injury and release vasoactive compounds. Stage 3: fibrin clot is formed to seal endothelial cell injury. Reprinted from Egermayer P, Town IG, Peacock AJ. The role of serotonin in the pathogenesis of acute and chronic pulmonary hypertension. *Thorax* 1999;54:161–168.

Mechanisms of Pulmonary Artery Vasoconstriction

The mechanism of pulmonary artery vasoconstriction is outside the scope of this chapter and has been dealt with in a number of reviews elsewhere,[4] but is likely to be due to an imbalance of vasodilators and vasoconstrictor factors as a consequence of endothelial cell injury, hypoxia, or other stimulus.

It is clear that at least 3 platelet-derived compounds (platelet-derived growth factor—PDGF; thromboxane—TXA_2; and serotonin—5-HT) are capable of causing pulmonary arterial vasoconstriction.

Mechanisms of Pulmonary Artery Remodeling

This subject is also dealt with elsewhere[2,3] but several platelet-derived compounds are believed important and each could be causal or a modulator of the initiating process or even a consequence of that process. It appears that there are at least 2 important predispositions to pulmonary vascular remodeling:

- Genetic.[5] It appears that there is a PPH gene present in both familial pulmonary hypertension and a significant number of cases of sporadic pulmonary hypertension. It codes for a receptor member of the TGF-β family, raising the question

Table 1

Major Products Released by Stimulated
Platelets that Participate in Inflammation

Lipids	Growth Factors (cont'd)
Thromboxane A2	Epidermal growth factor
Lipoxygenase products	Platelet-derived endothelial cell
12-Hydroxyeicosatetraenoic acid	growth factor
(12-HETE)	Transforming growth factor-β
12-hydroxyperoxy-eicosatetrae-	Adenine nucleotides
noic acid (12-HPETE)	ADP
Platelet-activating factor	ATP
Arachidonic acid	Complement proteins
Endoperoxides	Oxidants
Cationic proteins	Superoxide anion
Platelet factor 4	Hydrogen peroxide
β-Thromboglobulin	Hydroxyl radical
Permeability factor	Enzymes
Platelet basic protein	Chemotactic factor
β-Lysin	Heparinase
Vasoactive amines	Acid hydrolase
Histamine	Elastase
Serotonin	Collagenase
Growth factors	Anti-inflammatory products
Platelet-derived growth factor	Glutathione redox cycle
Interleukin-1	Adenosine
Hepatocyte growth factor	Catalase
	Superoxide dismutase—CuZn, Mn

Reprinted with permission from *Platelets*. Heffner JE, Repine JE. In Crystal RG, West JB, et al. *The Lung.* Lippincott: Philadelphia; 1997:947–959.

of the importance of this compound in the development of pulmonary vascular remodeling.

- Endothelial cell injury by toxins, drugs, ischemia/reperfusion, inflammation, and hemodynamic forces such as shear stress and pressure. Inflammatory mediators from "professional cells" such as lymphocytes, macrophages, and neutrophils combine with factors from "nonprofessional cells," for example, lung parenchymal cells and platelets,[3] to act via pathways where growth factors and cytokines are released. These include:
  1. TGF-β, which is localized to the smooth muscle cells of remodeled pulmonary arteries in pulmonary hypertension and known to stimulate PDGF and vascular endothelial growth factor (VEGF) synthesis.
  2. PDGF, which is found in macrophages in the lungs of pa-

tients with primary pulmonary hypertension and is known to increase VEGF production in the face of hypoxia.

3. VEGF, which is increased in the endothelial cells of patients with primary pulmonary hypertension and is increased by hypoxia via the HIF-1α transcription factor.

4. Platelet activation factor (PAF) is found in the cell membrane. It is known that PAF antagonists decrease pulmonary hypertension in both hypoxia and the monocrotaline lung model.

Activated platelets produce at least 3 of these mitogens, namely PDGF, VEGF, and 5-HT, which are capable of stimulating replication of endothelial cells, smooth muscle cells, and fibroblasts in the pulmonary vascular wall.

Possible Role of Platelets in the Genesis of Pulmonary Hypertension

It appears that platelet activation is necessary if platelets are to have a role (Figure 5). It is no coincidence that some platelet products have dual function, an example of "cell growth vasomotor coupling."[6]

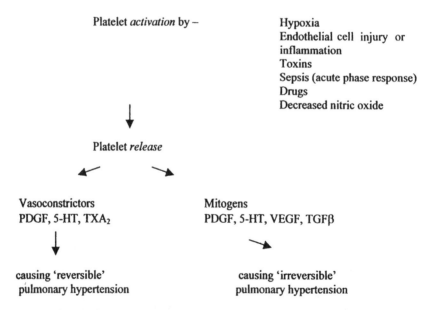

Platelet *activation* by –

Hypoxia
Endothelial cell injury or inflammation
Toxins
Sepsis (acute phase response)
Drugs
Decreased nitric oxide

Platelet *release*

Vasoconstrictors
PDGF, 5-HT, TXA$_2$

Mitogens
PDGF, 5-HT, VEGF, TGFβ

causing 'reversible' pulmonary hypertension

causing 'irreversible' pulmonary hypertension

Figure 5. Role of platelet activation in causing pulmonary hypertension. Platelet activation gives rise to the release of substances that can cause vasoconstriction and cellular proliferation.

Evidence for Role of Platelets in Pulmonary Arterial Hypertension

Most of the evidence for a role of platelets in pulmonary arterial hypertension comes from studies showing that platelet-derived compounds are capable of causing pulmonary hypertension and are found to be present in excessive amounts in some cases of pulmonary arterial hypertension.

Platelet Abnormalities in Pulmonary Arterial Hypertension

Increased aggregation and decreased survival of platelets is seen in most cases of pulmonary hypertension[7,8] but it is not clear whether this is the cause of the pulmonary hypertension or an effect of pulmonary hypertension. These changes are seen especially in portal hypertension, where they could be due to hypersplenism, adult respiratory distress syndrome (ARDS),[9] primary pulmonary hypertension,[10] and primary pulmonary hypertension of the newborn.[11] It is also known that immune mediated thrombocytopenia is associated with pulmonary arterial hypertension.[12] It appears that at least part of the reason for the reduction in platelet count in patients with pulmonary hypertension is because shear stress results in release of vWF from endothelial cells, increasing platelet adherence. But whether this is the sole cause of the loss of platelets or whether the platelets themselves promote adherence by a self-perpetuating process is unknown.

It is also known that platelet cell membrane disorders, e.g., antiphospholipid syndrome, are responsible for about 10% of cases of chronic thromboembolic pulmonary hypertension.[13,14]

Platelet Products and the Pulmonary Circulation

Thromboxane (TXA$_2$)

Thromboxane is synthesized from arachidonic acid following activation of platelets (it is also synthesized by endothelial cells, alveolar macrophages, and neutrophils). Thromboxane levels are known to be increased in ARDS associated with septic shock.[15] Hypoxia induces release of thromboxane A_2[16] and endotoxin infusion increases thromboxane levels in the plasma,[17-19] but the TXA_2 responsible for the pulmonary hypertension may not all derive from platelets because pulmonary hypertension can occur in the face of thrombocytopenia. However, if thrombocytopenia is induced prior to the endotoxin infusion, then pulmonary hypertension does not occur.[20]

Platelet-Derived Growth Factor (PDGF)

This is the most important mitogen for cell division in injured vessels[21] and it is known to stimulate the replication of endothelial cells, smooth muscle cells, and fibroblasts, including fibroblasts derived from pulmonary arteries.[22] Increased levels of PDGF can be seen in the bronchoalveolar lavage of patients with ARDS, a condition where both pulmonary arterial hypertension and lung fibrosis occur.[23]

Serotonin (5-HT)

Serotonin (5-HT), which is produced in the neuroendocrine cells of the gastrointestinal tract and lung and stored in the dense granules of platelets, has been widely implicated in the genesis and modulation of pulmonary arterial hypertension and is associated with conditions of pulmonary arterial hypertension in humans. It is known to have effects on the intact pulmonary circulation, isolated pulmonary vascular rings, and harvested pulmonary vascular cells both as a vasoconstrictor and a mitogen. Studies on 5-HT have provided the greatest evidence for a role of platelets in the development of acute and chronic pulmonary hypertension, but increased pulmonary neuroendocrine production of 5-HT may also be important. In this section we will summarize what is known.

Studies in Humans:

5-HT is known to be one of the most powerful vasoconstrictors in the pulmonary circulation,[24] but unlike other vasoactive compounds (except in hypoxia), it is a systemic vasodilator.[25]

Twenty-five percent of patients with *carcinoid syndrome* have pulmonary hypertension.[26] 5-HT is metabolized by the liver and possibly it is because of this that only 25% develop pulmonary hypertension. Patients with carcinoid syndrome also get valvular lesions, usually of the tricuspid valve.[27,28] Interestingly, these valvular lesions have also been seen in patients who have used anorexigens. These drugs are known to have serotonergic properties,[29] suggesting that 5-HT is the culprit in the valvular abnormality.

Patients with *adult respiratory distress syndrome* are known to have 5-HT levels up to 4 times higher than normal, particularly in the face of gram-negative sepsis.[30,31] Pulmonary hemodynamics may improve after ketanserin, a 5-HT receptor antagonist.[32–34] Ketanserin does not affect the early rise in pulmonary artery pressure after endotoxin but does diminish the late rise.[35] 5-HT is associated with acute vasoconstriction, but the mitogenic properties may also be responsible for pulmonary vascular remodeling.[36]

Pulmonary embolism causes pulmonary hypertension by obstruction of pulmonary arteries, but there may also be a vasospastic element due in part to 5-HT release from platelets aggregated at the site of thrombus.[37,38] Evidence for this comes from several sources:

a. there is a decrease in platelets in the circulation of patients suffering from pulmonary thromboembolism[39]
b. embolization with beads rather than clot does not cause as great a rise in pulmonary artery pressure[25,40]
c. ketanserin, the 5-HT receptor antagonist, decreases postembolic pulmonary hypertension in dogs[41,42]
d. if animals are rendered thrombocytopenic prior to embolization, then pulmonary hypertension is less severe.[43]

A role for 5-HT in *primary pulmonary hypertension* was originally suggested by Herve, who found that a patient with platelet storage disorder who had also developed primary pulmonary hypertension was found to have high plasma 5-HT levels and the pulmonary hypertension improved using ketanserin.[44] Herve then went on to show in 16 patients with primary pulmonary hypertension that the patients had decreased platelet levels of 5-HT but increased plasma levels of 5-HT when compared with controls.[10] These abnormalities remained after heart/lung transplant, suggesting they were a primary initiating phenomenon rather than a consequence of the disease. Subsequent studies have suggested that 80% of patients with primary pulmonary hypertension have increased plasma 5-HT levels, which may be up to 20 times normal (more than is seen in the carcinoid syndrome) (Herve, personal communication). The cause of the increase in 5-HT levels is not known because the 5-HT transporter (5-HTT) responsible for the active transport of 5-HT and 5-HT metabolism are both normal. There is additional evidence for a role of 5-HT in primary pulmonary hypertension in studies of patients who have developed pulmonary hypertension in association with the anorexigens fenfluramine and dexfenfluramine. These drugs have been shown to increase the risk of PPH in women who use them[45] and are known to affect 5-HT metabolism.[46] They cause pulmonary hypertension in dogs, probably via a serotonergic mechanism.[47] The effect of the anorexigen is thought to be associated with an increase in plasma 5-HT as a consequence of the inhibition of the 5-HT transporter,[48] raising the specter that other drugs that also affect the 5-HT transporter, such as the popular antidepressants paroxetine and fluoxetine, may also cause pulmonary hypertension.

Chronic hypoxic lung disease is the most common cause of pulmonary hypertension in the western world, but the pulmonary hypertension is usually mild and there is controversy about whether there is additional mortality/morbidity of the disease contributed by the abnormalities in the pulmonary circulation. It is known that hypoxia decreases platelet survival and increases aggregation of platelets and that the patients with chronic obstructive pulmonary disease have increased activation of platelets.[49] Hypoxia is known to increase the transcription of the 5-HT transporter gene,[50] probably by its hypoxia response element stimulated by the transcription factor HIF-1.

Studies in Animals:

Monocrotaline is commonly used to induce experimental pulmonary hypertension in animals. It appears to cause pulmonary hypertension by inducing endothelial cell injury, which in turn causes platelet accumulation in the lung and an increase in plasma 5-HT. This results in an increase in pulmonary artery pressure and pulmonary artery remodeling, which can be reversed by 5-HT blockade or by drugs that cause a decrease in 5-HT synthesis[51,52] but not by TXA_2 inhibition.[53]

The *fawn hooded rat* is a strain of rat that has a hereditary bleeding tendency due to a defect in platelet aggregation. This is an animal model of platelet storage pool disease. These rats develop pulmonary hypertension when exposed to an additional stimulus such as mild hypoxia. Sato et al.[54] have shown that the rats develop much greater pulmonary hypertension and pulmonary vascular remodeling than Sprague-Dawley rats for the same degree of hypoxia. Furthermore, pulmonary artery smooth muscle cells from these rats proliferate more rapidly in response to standard mitogens.[55]

Mechanisms of Action 5-HT

5-HT is a known vasoconstrictor and appears to cause this effect via $5\text{-}HT_1$ receptors, at least in bovine pulmonary arteries and pulmonary arteries from the chronic hypoxic rat.[56] It is also a mitogen, and work in our own laboratory on isolated pulmonary artery fibroblasts from chronic hypoxic rats has shown that it acts via the $5\text{-}HT_{2A}$ receptor (Welsh, personal communication). What is unclear is whether 5-HT acts principally via cell surface receptors or whether, following its active transport into the cell by the transport system 5-HT transporter, it acts in the cytosol. It may be that 5-HT transporter is merely a mechanism for removing active hormones from the circulation (Figure 6), but it seems that cytosolic 5-HT (via the 5-HT transporter) may have a role, because 5-HT causes a dose response increase in pulmonary artery smooth muscle cell replication that can be blocked by the 5-HT transporter inhibitors paroxetine and fluoxetine but not by ketanserin, the 5-HT receptor antagonist.[50] Further, a mouse knockout model of 5-HT transporter deficiency that does not take up 5-HT synthesized in the gut into liver, lung, or platelets, does not develop remodeling in the pulmonary vasculature in response to hypoxia (Adnot, personal communication).

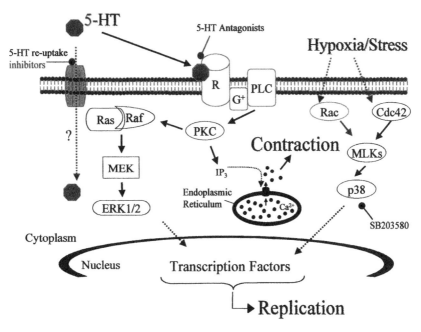

Figure 6. Diagram of possible mechanisms by which 5-HT could influence cellular function. 5-HT is thought to act principally on a g-protein-linked receptor which in turn activates protein kinase-C and then leads either to stimulation of the MAP-kinase pathways to increase transcription or, via the phosphoinositide pathway, results in cytosolic release of calcium with reduction. It is to be noted that hypoxia and other forms of stress appear to act via a separate stress-activated MAP-kinase pathway. 5-HT is also transported into the cytosol and it may have an activity within a cytosol as yet undetermined. R = receptor; G = g protein; PLC = phosolipase C; P38 = stress kinase pathway; PKC = protein kinase C; IP3 = inosotide triphosphate.

Conclusion

There is considerable evidence in animals and humans supporting the role of platelets in the initiation and development of pulmonary hypertension, both by vasoconstriction and by pulmonary vascular remodeling. The bulk of the evidence centers on platelet function in terms of 5-HT release. 5-HT is both a powerful pulmonary vasoconstrictor and a mitogen for pulmonary vascular cells. At present, it is unclear whether platelet activation and subsequent release of vasoactive mitogens such as 5-HT are necessary in all forms of pulmonary hypertension or only in those associated with endothelial injury such as adult respiratory distress syndrome and sepsis. It is also unclear whether 5-HT has different roles at the cell surface (at specific 5-HT repectors) versus the cytosol, where its concentration depends on the activity of the active transport system 5-HT transporter. The transcription of the 5-HTT gene is known to depend on hypoxia and other stimuli. It is tempting to speculate that vasospastic and some mitogenic effects of 5-HT are due to cell surface receptor activation, whereas the action in the cytosol causes similar effects but via different mechanisms and in response to different stimuli.

References

1. Rich S, ed. Primary pulmonary hypertension: Executive summary from the World Symposium. *Primary Pulmonary Hypertension:* World Health Organization, 1998.
2. Fishman AP, Fishman MC, Freeman BA, et al. Mechanisms of proliferative and obliterative vascular diseases. *Am J Respir Crit Care Med* 1998;158: 670–674.
3. Voelkel NF, Tuder RM. Cellular and molecular mechanisms in the pathogenesis of severe pulmonary hypertension. *Eur Respir J* 1995;8:2129–2138.
4. Peacock AJ. Primary pulmonary hypertension. *Thorax* 1999;54:1107–1118.
5. Thomson JR, Machado RD, Pauciulo MW, et al. Sporadic primary pulmonary hypertension is associated with germline mutations of the gene encoding BMPR-II, a receptor member of the TGF-β family. *J Med Genet* 2000;37:741–745.
6. Scott PH, Peacock AJ. Cell signaling in pulmonary vascular cells: Do not shoot the messenger! *Thorax* 1996;8:864–866.
7. Nakonechnicov S, Gabbasov Z, Chazova I, et al. Platelet aggregation in patients with primary pulmonary hypertension. *Blood Coagul Fibrinol* 1996;7:225–227.
8. Chouat A, Weitzenblum E, Higgenbottam T. The role of thrombosis in severe pulmonary hypertension. *Eur Respir J* 1996;9:356–363.
9. Bone R, Francis P, Pierce A. Intravascular coagulations associated with the adult respiratory distress syndrome. *Am J Med* 1976;61:585–589.
10. Herve P, Launay JM, Scrobohaci ML, et al. Increased plasma serotonin in primary pulmonary hypertension. *Am J Med* 1995;99:249–254.
11. Segall ML, Goetzman BW, Schick JB. Thrombocytopenia and pulmonary hypertension in the perinatal aspiration syndromes. *J Pediatr* 1980;96:727–730.

12. Jubelirer SJ. Primary pulmonary hypertension: Its association with microangiopathic hemolytic anemia and thrombocytopenia. *Arch Intern Med* 1991;151:1221–1223.

13. Hillderdal G. The lung physician and the antiphospholipid syndrome. *Eur Resp J* 1997;10:511–512.

14. Arnout J. The pathogenesis of the antiphospholipid syndrome: A hypothesis based on parallelisms with heparin-induced thrombocytopenia. *Thromb Haemost* 1996;75:536–541.

15. Reines H, Cook J, Halashka P, et al. Plasma thromboxane concentrations are raised in patients dying with septic shock. *Lancet* 1982;1:174–175.

16. Castle V, Coates G, Mitchell L, et al. The effect of hypoxia on platelet survival and site of sequestration in the newborn rabbit. *Thromb Haemost* 1988;59:45–48.

17. Hales C, Sonne L, Peterson M, et al. Role of thromboxane and prostacyclin in pulmonary vasomotor changes after endotoxin in dogs. *J Clin Invest* 1981;68:497–505.

18. Kubo K, Kobayoshi T. Effects of OKY-046, a selective thromboxane synthetase inhibitor, on endotoxin-induced lung injury in unanesthetized sheep. *Am Rev Respir Dis* 1985;132:494–499.

19. Snapper J, Hutchinson A, Ogletree M, et al. Effects of cyclooxygenase inhibitors on the alterations in lung mechanics caused by endotoxemia in the unanesthetized sheep. *J Clin Invest* 1983;72:63–76.

20. Bredenberg C, Taylor G, Webb W. The effect of thrombocytopenia on the pulmonary and systemic hemodynamics of canine endotoxin shock. *Surgery* 1980;87:59–68.

21. Deuel T, Huang J. Platelet-derived growth factor: Structure, function, and roles in normal and transformed cells. *J Clin Invest* 1984;74:669–676.

22. Peacock AJ, Dawes KE, Shock A, et al. Endothelin-1 and endothelin-3 induce chemotaxis and replication of pulmonary artery fibroblasts. *Am J Respir Cell Mol Biol* 1992;7:492–499.

23. Thorson S, Madtes D, Shimokado K, et al. Fibroblast replication is stimulated by bronchoalveolar lavage fluids from patients with adult respiratory distress syndrome. *Am Rev Respir Dis* 1985;131:A139 (abstract).

24. Heffner JE, Sahn SA, Repine JE. The role of platelets in the adult respiratory distress syndrome: Culprits or bystanders? *Am Rev Respir Dis* 1987; 135:482–492.

25. Comroe JH, van Lingen B, Stroud RC. Reflex and direct cardiopulmonary effects of 5-OH tryptamine (serotonin): Their possible role in pulmonary embolism and coronary thrombosis. *Am J Physiol* 1953;173:379–386.

26. Tornebrandt K, Eskilsson J, Nobin A. Heart involvement in metastatic carcinoid disease. *Clin Cardiol* 1986;9:13–19.

27. Jacobsen MB, Nitter-Hauge S, Bryde PE, et al. Cardiac manifestations of mid-gut carcinoid disease. *Eur Heart J* 1995;16:263–268.

28. Robiolo PA, Rigolin VH, Wilson JS, et al. Carcinoid heart disease: Correlation of high serotonin levels with valvular abnormalities detected by cardiac catheterization and echocardiography. *Circulation* 1995;92:790–795.

29. Connolly HM, Crary JL, McGoon MD, et al. Valvular heart disease associated with fenfluramine-phentermine. *N Engl J Med* 1997;337:581–588.

30. Hechtman H, Huval W, Mathieson M, et al. Prostaglandin and thromboxane mediation of cardiopulmonary failure. *Surg Clin North Am* 1983; 63:263–283.

31. Sibbald W, Peters S, Lindsay RM. Serotonin and pulmonary hypertension in human septic ARDS. *Crit Care Med* 1980;8:490–494.

32. Vincent JL, Degaute JP, Domb M, et al. Ketanserin, a serotonin antagonist: Administration in patients with acute respiratory failure. *Chest* 1984;85: 510–513.
33. Kasajima K, Ozdemir A, Webb WR, et al. Role of serotonin and serotonin antagonist on pulmonary haemodynamics and microcirculation in hemorrhagic shock. *J Thorac Cardiovasc Surg* 1974;67:908–914.
34. Huval W, Lelcuk S, Shepro D, et al. Role of serotonin in patients with acute respiratory failure. *Ann Surg* 1984;200:166–172.
35. Demling R, Wong C, Fox R, et al. Relationship of increased lung serotonin levels to endotoxin-induced pulmonary hypertension in sheep: Effect of a serotonin antagonist. *Am Rev Respir Dis* 1985;132:1257–1261.
36. Tomashefski JF, Davies P, Boggis C, et al. The pulmonary vascular lesions of the adult respiratory distress syndrome. *Am J Pathol* 1983;112:112–126.
37. Smith G, Smith AN. The role of serotonin in experimental pulmonary embolism. *Surg Gynecol Obstet* 1995;101:691–699.
38. Gurewich V, Cohen ML, Thomas DP. Humoral factors in massive pulmonary embolism: An experimental study. *Am Heart J* 1968;76:784–791.
39. Monreal M, Lafoz E, Casals A, et al. Platelet count and venous thromboembolism: A useful test for suspected pulmonary embolism. *Chest* 1991;100:1493–1496.
40. Williams GD, Westbrook KC, Campbell GS. Reflex pulmonary hypertension and systemic hypotension after microsphere pulmonary embolism: A myth. *Am J Surg* 1969;118:925–930.
41. Huval WV, Mathieson MA, Stemp LI, et al. Therapeutic benefits of 5-hydroxytryptamine inhibition following pulmonary embolism. *Ann Surg* 1983;197:220–225.
42. Huet Y, Brun-Buisson C, Lemaire F, et al. Cardiopulmonary effects of ketanserin infusion in human pulmonary embolism. *Am Rev Respir Dis* 1987;135:114–117.
43. Mlczoch J, Tucker A, Weir EK, et al. Platelet-mediated hypertension and hypoxia during pulmonary microembolism: Reduction by platelet inhibition. *Chest* 1978;74:648–653.
44. Herve P, Drouet L, Dosquet C, et al. Primary pulmonary hypertension in a patient with a familial pool disease: Role of serotonin. *Am J Med* 1990;89 (1):117–120.
45. Abenhaim L, Moride Y, Brenot F, et al. Appetite suppressant drugs and the risk of primary pulmonary hypertension. *N Engl J Med* 1996;335:609–616.
46. Fristrom S, Airaksinen MM, Halmekoski J. Release of platelet 5-hydroxytryptamine by some anorexic and other sympathomimetics and their acetyl derivatives. *Acta Pharmacol Toxicol* 1977;41:218–224.
47. Naeije R, Maggiorini M, Delcroix M, et al. Effects of chronic dexfenfluramine treatment on pulmonary hemodynamics in dogs. *Am J Respir Crit Care Med* 1996;154(5):1347–1350.
48. Weir EK, Reeve HL, Johnson G, et al. A role for potassium channels in smooth muscle cells and platelets in the etiology of primary pulmonary hypertension. *Chest* 1998;114(Suppl):200S–204S.
49. Rostagno C, Prisco D, Boddie M, et al. Evidence for local platelet activation in pulmonary vessels in patients with pulmonary hypertension secondary to chronic obstructive pulmonary disease. *Eur Respir J* 1991;4:147–151.
50. Eddahibi S, Fabre V, Boni C, et al. Induction of serotonin transporter by hypoxia in pulmonary vascular smooth muscle cells: Relationship with the mitogenic action of serotonin. *Circ Res* 1999;84:329–336.

51. Kay JM, Keane PM, Suyama KL. Pulmonary hypertension induced in rats by monocrotaline and chronic hypoxia is reduced by p-chlorophenylalanine. *Respiration* 1985;47:48–56.

52. Kanai Y, Hori S, Tanaka T, et al. Role of 5-hydroxytryptamine in the progression of monocrotaline-induced pulmonary hypertension in rats. *Cardiovasc Res* 1993;27:1619–1623.

53. Langleben D, Carvalho AC, Reid LM. The platelet inhibitor, dazmegrel, does not reduce monocrotaline-induced pulmonary hypertension. *Am Rev Respir Dis* 1986;133:789–791.

54. Sato K, Webb S, Tucker A, et al. Factors influencing the idiopathic development of pulmonary hypertension in the fawn hooded rat. *Am Rev Respir Dis* 1992;145(Pt 1):793–797.

55. Janakidevi K, Tiruppathi C, del Vecchio PJ, et al. Growth characteristics of pulmonary artery smooth muscle cells from fawn-hooded rats. *Am J Physiol* 1995;268:L465–470.

56. MacLean MR, Clayton RA, Hillis SW, et al. $5-HT_1$-receptor-mediated vasoconstriction in bovine isolated pulmonary arteries: Influences of vascular endothelin and tone. *Pulm Pharm* 1994;7:65–72.

Chapter 12

Emerging Concepts of the Mechanisms of Platelet Secretion

Guy L. Reed, MD

Platelet Secretion and Vascular Disease

The occlusion of a blood vessel by a thrombus is the critical pathological event in pulmonary embolism, myocardial infarction, stroke, and other vascular diseases. Thrombi that do not occlude the vessels also contribute to vascular remodeling in diseases such as pulmonary hypertension and arteriosclerosis.[1-4] Platelets trigger thrombus formation and initiate cellular processes that cause vascular remodeling. There is evidence of increased platelet activation and secretion, as well as decreased platelet survival in patients and animals with pulmonary and arteriosclerotic vascular diseases.[5-7] Platelets are specialized secretory cells that contain 3 types of large intracellular vesicles or granules: alpha, dense, and lysosomal.[8] Platelets are activated by ligands that signal the presence of vascular injury or dysfunction.[9,10] After cellular activation, platelets secrete the contents of their intracellular granules and aggregate with each other. Platelet secretion (Figure 1) releases key effector molecules that (1) amplify thrombus formation (e.g., coagulation factor V), (2) activate platelets and other cells (e.g., ADP), (3) promote the adhesion of leukocytes (e.g., P-selectin), and (4) activate a genetic program of remodeling in the cells of the blood vessel wall (e.g., platelet-derived growth factor, serotonin).

This work was supported in part by NIH grant HL-64057.

From: Weir EK, Reeve HL, Reeves JT (eds). *Interactions of Blood and the Pulmonary Circulation*. Armonk, NY: Futura Publishing Company, Inc.; ©2002.

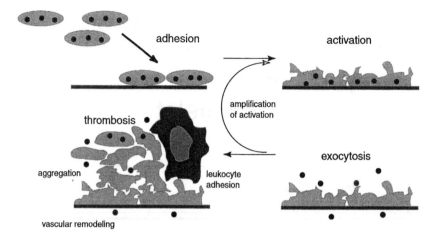

Figure 1. Platelet activation and secretion. Platelets adhere at sites of vascular injury. Platelets are activated by several agents such as thrombin, ADP, collagen, PAF, epinephrine, thromboxane A2, serotonin, etc. After activation platelets release or exocytose the contents of their intracellular granules; secreted agents such as ADP amplify platelet activation. Released factor Va accelerates thrombin generation, which further amplifies platelet activation. Thrombin promotes platelet aggregation and generates fibrin, the protein matrix of the thrombus. Secreted P-selectin promotes leukocyte adhesion. The exocytosis of growth modulators such as platelet-derived growth factor, TGF-β, serotonin, etc., activate a program of vascular remodeling.

Platelet Granule Development and Disorders

Platelets are anuclear cells that bud from megakaryocytes through a highly regulated process of segmentation. At the time of segmentation, platelets contain a fully developed and complex membrane system.[11] There are large intracellular granules, a surface-connected canalicular system, and a dense tubular system. The granules contain proteins synthesized by the megakaryocyte or taken up by endocytosis because there is no significant protein synthesis in platelets. Disorders of platelet secretion result in impaired hemostasis.[12] These disorders are rare, and the most frequent abnormalities described are the secretory pool disorders (SPD).[9,12–16] Humans with diminished or absent alpha granules have alpha SPD and those with decreased or missing dense granules have dense SPD. Alpha SPD is associated with a mild bleeding abnormality, while dense SPD can be associated with severe hemorrhage. The ontogeny of the platelet granules is not understood, but both the alpha and dense granules appear to arise from endogenous synthesis in the megakaryocytes and from fusion with endocytic and perhaps other vesicles. There is increasing evidence that the dense granules derive in part from lysosomes. Genetic diseases that are associated with dense granule SPD and albinism such as Hermansky-Pudlak and Chédiak-Higashi syndrome also display abnormalities of melanosomes and lysosomes. These disorders lead to abnormal lysosomal lipofuscin ceroid deposition or large cellular inclusion bodies that can cause pulmonary fibrosis, neurological abnormalities, as well as a number of other problems.[17] Three genes have recently been identified as being responsible for these defects: *HPS1, ADTB3A, LYST/Beige*.[18-21] *ADTB3A* codes for a protein subunit (β3a) of the AP-3 complex, which is involved in protein trafficking. The LYST protein may be involved in vesicle fusion or fission and the HPS1 protein has no known function at present. The molecular causes of dense SPD that are not associated with melanosomal abnormalities are unknown. These diseases may be heterogeneous with phenotypes ranging from mild to severe reductions in dense granule number.[22,23] There have been occasional reports of pulmonary hypertension developing in patients with dense SPD, presumably from inability of platelets to store serotonin in the granules.[1] The fact that these patients are frequently normal except for their bleeding tendency suggests that the molecular defect is limited to the production, maintenance, or packaging of dense granules.

Unfortunately, at present, the molecular defects responsible for alpha SPD are unknown and there are no good animal models for this disease. Similar to isolated dense SPD, alpha SPD appears to result from a lesion that affects only the packaging or maintenance of these particular cellular organelles because the endothelial Weibel-Palade body, which resembles the alpha granule, appears unaffected in these patients.[24] Finally, in addition to the SPDs, there are isolated reports of patients with normal platelet granules that have signaling disorders that lead to diminished secretion and aggregation in response to different platelet-activating agents.[12,16]

Molecular Machinery for Exocytosis in Platelets

Until recently, the molecular machinery for platelet secretion was unknown. In a search for molecules that may be important for mediating the secretory or exocytotic process, platelet Sec1 protein (PSP) was cloned.[25] PSP is a homologue of Sec1, a protein originally identified as required for secretion in yeast. It was found that platelets also contain specific SNARE proteins.[25,26] The SNARE proteins have been identified as playing a critical role in exocytosis in other specialized secretory cells such as neurons. These independent findings suggested that platelets use a molecular machinery for exocytosis, which has important similarities to the machinery used by neurons or other secretory cells.

In fact, there are important similarities in the physiology of exocytosis in platelets and other secretory cells such as neurons. Both platelets and neurons have vesicles that contain small excitatory molecules and protein effector molecules. Still, platelet granules tend to be significantly larger and more complex (up to 500 nm in diameter). In both cells, secretion is triggered by specific signals. In platelets, secretion is triggered by intracellular signaling that occurs after the interaction of a membrane receptor with an intracellular ligand.[27,28] Typically these ligands activate phospholipase C to produce diacylglycerol and inositol 1,4,5-trisphosphate (IP_3). Diacylglycerol in turn activates protein kinase C, while IP_3 increases intracellular Ca^{2+} levels. Ca^{2+} alone is sufficient to trigger secretion but activated protein kinase C interacts synergistically to lower the Ca^{2+} levels required for secretion. In neurons, propagation of action potentials down the axon increases intracellular Ca^{2+} and induces exocytosis; the role of kinases and other molecules in this process remains unclear.[29] One of the most remarkable differences between neurons and platelets is in the kinetics of exocytosis. As little as 200 μs is required for neuronal secretion, while platelets require up to 25,000-fold longer (5 s).

Studies of exocytosis in neuronal cells, yeast, flies, and worms have defined molecules that are required for vesicle exocytosis.[29–31] Regulated secretion requires certain "SNARE protein"-related molecules (Table 1). These molecules include the quintessential SNARE proteins: vesicle-associated membrane protein (VAMP or synaptobrevin), SNAP-25 (or its related molecules SNAP-23, SNAP-29), and syntaxin. All 3 of these molecules are membrane-bound proteins that form a tight, stable trimolecular complex (SNARE complex). This complex is required for the late stages of fusion between secretory vesicles and the plasmalemma. This complex can also be dissociated by the combined action of alpha (or beta or gamma) SNAP and the ATPase, N-ethylmaleimide-sensitive factor or NSF. At the present time, it is not clear at what stage in the secretory process alpha-SNAP/NSF interacts with the SNARE complex to dissociate it. However, NSF activity has been found to be required for many secretory processes.

In neurons, the neuronal Sec1-related protein (nSec1 or Munc18a) interacts with syntaxin 1 with high affinity.[32] The binding of nSec1 to syntaxin 1 blocks the interaction of syntaxin 1 with SNAP-25 and VAMP, thereby preventing SNARE complex formation. Overexpression of the Sec1 homologue Rop has been shown to inhibit secretion, indicating that Sec1 has an inhibitory effect on exocytosis, through its binding interactions with syntaxin.[33] At the same time, Sec1, Rop, and their homologues are required for secretion.[34,35] Thus, in addition to their inhibitory effects, the Sec1 proteins appear to be involved in interactions with other molecules that are required for exocytosis. A number of other molecules have been implicated in secretion in neurons such as the Rab proteins, Munc13, Doc2, etc. However, their role in other secretory cells such as platelets is just being defined.[29–31]

Table 1

Platelet Secretory Molecules[25,29-31,38,39,42,47,51-55]

Gene Family	Homologues		Molecular Interactions	Role in Neuronal Exocytosis	Role in Exocytosis of	
	Platelets	Neurons			Alpha Granules	Dense Granules
Syntaxin	Syntaxin 2,4	Syntaxin 1	SNARE complex	Required	Required**	Required
SNAP-23/25	SNAP-23	SNAP-25	SNARE complex	Required	Required	Required
VAMP	VAMP 1,2,3	VAMP 3	SNARE complex	Required	Required	Required
NSF	NSF	Same	SNARE complex dissociation	Required	Required	Required
SNAP (α,β,γ)	α,γ	α,β,γ	Cofactor for NSF	Required	Required	Required
Sec1	PSP	Nsec1	Binds syntaxins	Required	Probable***	Probable
Rab	3b,6,8,11,31	3a, and others	Indirect interaction with SNAREs?	Rab 3a may inhibit exocytosis	?	?
Munc-13	?*	Munc-13–1	Syntaxin	Required for triggered synaptic vesicle fusion	?	?
Doc2	?		Syntaxin, Sec1	Probable	?	?
Synaptotagmin	?	Synapto. 1	Syntaxin	Required for Ca2+-depend. exocytosis	?	?

?*There is not clear evidence for the presence of these molecules in platelets.

**Required—there is strong evidence for the role of this secretory molecule in this process.

***Probable— there is suggestive published or unpublished data to support a role for this molecule in secretion.

Platelet Secretion Proceeds Through a SNARE-Dependent Process

The finding that platelets contain PSP, the SNARE proteins, and NSF suggested that platelet secretion proceeded through a SNARE-dependent mechanism. The initial evidence for this came from studies of peptide inhibitors of NSF ATPase activity induced by interactions with alpha SNAP.[36] Peptides that inhibited NSF activity in vitro also inhibited exocytosis of alpha and dense granules in permeabilized platelets. Scrambling the sequence of these peptides eliminated their inhibitory effects, and peptides without inhibitory effects in vitro also had no activity in platelet secretion. Moreover, antibodies that inhibited NSF activity in vitro also significantly attenuated secretion. These inhibitory effects were overcome by incubation with recombinant NSF and control antibodies had no inhibitory effect. Other studies have also confirmed that NSF activity is required for secretion of both granules.[37,38]

Inhibitors of the SNARE protein function have also established that platelet secretion occurs through a SNARE-dependent mechanism. For example, antibodies against syntaxin 4, VAMP, and SNAP-23 strongly inhibit alpha granule secretion in streptolysin O-permeabilized platelets.[38,39] Other studies have suggested that syntaxin 2 may also play a role in alpha granule secretion, which provides the first example of 2 forms of syntaxin being required for exocytosis of 1 type of vesicle.[38] Studies with antibodies introduced into permeabilized cells indicate that dense granule secretion requires syntaxin 2 and SNAP-23.[37]

PSP forms a complex with syntaxin 4 in platelets. In vitro, the binding of PSP to syntaxin 4 inhibits syntaxin 4 from forming a SNARE complex with SNAP-25 or VAMP.[25] Because SNARE complex formation is required for exocytosis, PSP-syntaxin 4 interactions are likely to have an inhibitory effect on secretion. In support of this notion, antibodies against PSP appear to enhance secretion in permeabilized platelets.[40] Although interactions between the Sec1 proteins and syntaxins have not been previously shown in vivo, the PSP-syntaxin 4 interaction can be demonstrated in platelets by immunoprecipitation with monoclonal antibodies.[41]

Signaling Events That Link Platelet Activation to Exocytosis

Unregulated platelet secretion could lead to fatal thrombotic occlusion or render platelets unable to respond effectively to extreme vascular injuries. Platelet secretion occurs only after cells are activated by the interaction of a membrane receptor with its cognate ligand such as thrombin, ADP, etc. This activation signal is transmitted by second messengers such as Ca^{2+} and protein kinase C to effect secretion. A major unanswered question in the field of exocytosis is how these second messengers signal to the secretory machinery to cause exocytosis. Protein kinase C plays an important role in eliciting secretion. Recent studies have shown that PSP is phosphorylated when cells are activated to secrete by thrombin.[25] This phosphorylation is blocked by inhibitors of protein kinase C with an attendant decrease in secretion.[25,42] In vitro PSP is a direct protein kinase C substrate and is phosphorylated with a stoichiometry of 0.9 mole phosphate per mole of protein.[25] Phosphorylation of PSP prevents it from binding with syntaxin 4, thus relieving PSP's inhibitory effects on SNARE complex formation.

Syntaxins, by virtue of their interactions with the SNARE proteins, the Sec1 proteins, and a number of other molecules, also play a critical role in modulating secretion. As such, the function of syntaxin 4 may be regulated by intracellular signaling events that link cell activation to secretion. Indeed, syntaxin 4 is phosphorylated when cells are activated by thrombin, through a protein kinase C-dependent mechanism.[42] Like PSP, syntaxin 4 is a direct protein kinase C substrate, and monomeric syntaxin is phosphorylated with a stoichiometry of up to 0.8 mole of phosphate per mole of syntaxin.[42] Interestingly, phosphorylation of syntaxin 4 in vitro inhibits its interactions with SNAP-23. A similar pattern is seen in intact platelets. Immunoprecipitation studies show that platelet activation by thrombin or protein kinase C activators (phorbol ester) decreases syntaxin 4—SNAP-23 interactions in platelets. Phosphatase inhibitors further diminish syntaxin 4—SNAP-23 binding, arguing that phosphorylation events diminish SNARE complex formation. However, when platelets are activated to secrete in the presence of protein kinase C inhibitors, syntaxin 4—SNAP-23 interactions return to baseline.[42] Thus platelet activation signals that lead to secretion appear to enhance SNARE complex dissociation through a protein kinase C-dependent mechanism.

A critical question for understanding this mechanism is whether protein kinase C is acting preferentially on monomeric syntaxin 4 or syntaxin 4 in the SNARE complex. The interaction of syntaxin 1 with other SNARE proteins in a SNARE complex significantly alters the conformation of syntaxin and it may change syntaxin's properties as a substrate for protein kinase C or other kinases.[43–45] Recent in vitro studies have suggested that formation of the SNARE complex significantly alters the phosphorylation of syntaxin 4 by protein kinase C, increasing it by up to 300%. The effects of these phosphorylation events on SNARE complex disassembly and the sites of phosphorylation are currently being identified.

A Working Model for Platelet Exocytosis

These studies suggest a model for platelet exocytosis (Figure 2). This is a hypothetical model because certain key insights into exocytosis are missing in platelets and in other types of cells. Platelet exocytosis is homologous to regulated secretion in neurons and other cells but it contains a platelet-selective machinery that is uniquely coupled to signaling events triggered by cell activation. Platelets contain syntaxin 4, VAMP, SNAP-23, and PSP as well as other secretory molecules (Figure 2B). Platelets also contain a number of different Rab molecules but there is at present relatively little information about their potential function in exocytosis.[46,47]

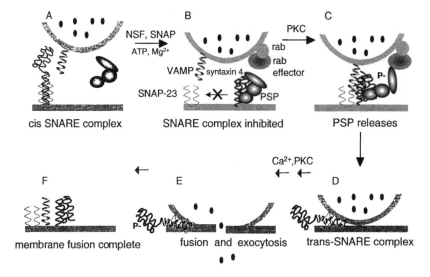

Figure 2. Working model for platelet secretion. Platelets contain syntaxin 4, VAMP, SNAP-23, PSP, as well as other secretory molecules. Platelets also contain Rab proteins and Rab-interacting molecules. Although there is genetic evidence in other cells that the Rab proteins interact with the Sec1 proteins, there is at present no direct evidence for their involvement in platelet exocytosis.[9] SNAP-triggered NSF activity plays a key role in platelet exocytosis, perhaps through dissociation of pre-engaged SNARE proteins on the same membrane (cis-SNARE complexes) (A). Alternatively, NSF activity may play a critical role in dissociating the SNARE complex during the final process of fusion and exocytosis (F). Once syntaxin 4 is disengaged from the SNARE complex, PSP binding to syntaxin 4 prevents SNARE complex formation (B). Phosphorylation of PSP prevents it from binding to syntaxin 4 and relieves PSP's inhibitory effects on SNARE protein interactions (C). The release of PSP permits trans-SNARE complex formation (D). Increases in intracellular Ca^{2+}, mediated through an unidentified Ca^{2+} sensor protein(s) leads to membrane fusion and exocytosis (E). Preferential phosphorylation of syntaxin 4 in the SNARE complex may also have a role, which is yet to be defined, in fusion and exocytosis (E), and/or the eventual dissociation of the SNARE complex (F).

The Rab proteins have been genetically linked to the secretory machinery in yeast and Rab3A has been shown to play an inhibitory role in neuronal secretion.[48–58] SNAP-triggered NSF activity plays a key role in platelet exocytosis. This suggests that in resting platelets (prior to cell activation), the SNARE proteins could be engaged in cis-SNARE complexes (Figure 2A), which prevent the formation of the trans-SNARE complexes (Figure 2D) necessary for exocytosis. Alternatively, NSF activity could be required for the final dissociation of SNARE complexes, which appears to occur in platelets that have been activated to secrete (Figure 2F).[39,42] PSP binding to syntaxin 4 prevents SNARE complex formation (Figure 2B). Phosphorylation of PSP relieves its inhibitory effects on SNARE protein interactions (Figure 2C) and permits SNARE complex formation (Figure 2D). Increased intracellular Ca^{2+}, acting through as yet unidentified molecules, drives membrane fusion and exocytosis (Figure 2E). Preferential phosphorylation of syntaxin 4 in the SNARE complex may have a role (which is yet to be defined) in the process of fusion and exocytosis, and/or the eventual dissociation of the SNARE complex (Figure 2F).

Summary and Future Directions

Platelets are specialized secretory cells that release a number of biologically active molecules at the site of vascular injury. These secreted molecules play key roles in thrombosis and vascular remodeling processes. Studies of patients with platelet secretory disorders suggest that some of the molecular processes of granule development and granule packaging are unique to this cell type. At the same time, platelets utilize some of the same molecules for dense granule formation that are required for the generation of other membrane-bound organelles in other cells. The molecular machinery required for the final stages of platelet exocytosis is homologous to the SNARE proteins used for secretion in other cell types. However, the signaling mechanisms that couple platelet exocytosis to the process of cell activation by extracellular agonists appears to be platelet-selective. Although critical aspects of the exocytotic process remain poorly understood, insights into the mechanisms underlying platelet secretion may lead to the generation of agents to improve hemostasis and/or to inhibit thrombosis and vascular remodeling.

Acknowledgments: The author gratefully acknowledges many stimulating discussions with Drs. Janos Polgar, Sul-Hee Chung, Michael Fitzgerald, and with Aiilyan Houng.

References

1. Herve P, Launay JM, Scrobohaci ML, et al. Increased plasma serotonin in primary pulmonary hypertension. *Am J Med* 1995;99:249–254.

2. Ashmore RC, Rodman DM, Sato K, Webb SA, et al. Paradoxical constriction to platelets by arteries from rats with pulmonary hypertension. *Am J Physiol* 1991;260:H1929–1934.

3. Nenci GG. Platelets, hypoxemia and pulmonary hypertension. *Adv Exp Med Biol* 1984;164:325–333.

4. Mlczoch J, Tucker A, Weir EK, Reeves JT, et al. Platelet-mediated pulmonary hypertension and hypoxia during pulmonary microembolism: Reduction by platelet inhibition. *Chest* 1978;74:648–653.

5. Hassell KL. Altered hemostasis in pulmonary hypertension. *Blood Coagul Fibrinolysis* 1998;9:107–117.

6. Smith FB, Lowe GD, Fowkes FG, et al. Smoking, haemostatic factors and lipid peroxides in a population case control study of peripheral arterial disease. *Atherosclerosis* 1993;102:155–162.

7. Blann AD, Lip GY, Beevers DG, McCollum CN. Soluble P-selectin in atherosclerosis: A comparison with endothelial cell and platelet markers. *Thromb Haemost* 1997;77:1077–1080.

8. White JG. Anatomy and structural organization of the platelet. In Colman RW, Hirsch J, Marder VJ, Salzman EW, eds: *Hemostasis and Thrombosis: Basic Principles and Clinical Practice, 3rd ed.* Philadephia: Lippincott; 1994:538.

9. Reed GL, Fitzgerald ML, Polgar J. Molecular mechanisms of platelet exocytosis: The Secret Life of Thrombocytes. *Blood.* In press.

10. Gordon JL, ed. *Platelets in Biology and Pathology.* New York: North Holland Publishing; 1976.

11. Cramer EM, Norol F, Guichard J, et al. Ultrastructure of platelet formation by human megakaryocytes cultured with the Mpl ligand. *Blood* 1997;89:2336–2346.

12. Weiss HJ. Inherited abnormalities of platelet granules and signal transduction. In Colman RW, Hirsh J, Marder VJ, et al., eds: *Hemostasis and Thrombosis.* Philadelphia: J.P. Lippincott Company; 1994:524–545.

13. Gerrard JM, Phillips DR, Rao GH, et al. Biochemical studies of two patients with the gray platelet syndrome: Selective deficiency of platelet alpha granules. *J Clin Invest* 1980;66:102–109.

14. Fuse I. Disorders of platelet function. *Crit Rev Oncol Hematol* 1996;22:1–25.

15. Smith MP, Cramer EM, Savidge GF. Megakaryocytes and platelets in alpha-granule disorders. *Baillieres Clin Haematol* 1997;10:125–148.

16. Rao AK. Congenital disorders of platelet function: Disorders of signal transduction and secretion. *Am J Med Sci* 1998;316:69–76.

17. Dell'Angelica EC, Mullins C, Caplan S, Bonifacino JS. Lysosome-related organelles. *Faseb J* 2000;14:1265–1278.

18. Oh J, Bailin T, Fukai K, et al. Positional cloning of a gene for Hermansky-Pudlak syndrome, a disorder of cytoplasmic organelles. *Nat Genet* 1996;14:300–306.

19. Dell'Angelica EC, Shotelersuk V, Aguilar RC, et al. Altered trafficking of lysosomal proteins in Hermansky-Pudlak syndrome due to mutations in the beta 3A subunit of the AP-3 adaptor. *Mol Cell* 1999;3:11–21.

20. Barbosa MD, Nguyen QA, Tchernev VT, et al. Identification of the homologous beige and Chdiak-Higashi syndrome genes. *Nature* 1996;382:262–265.

21. Nagle DL, Karim MA, Woolf EA, et al. Identification and mutation analysis of the complete gene for Chediak- Higashi syndrome. *Nat Genet* 1996;14:307–311.

22. McNicol A, Israels SJ, Robertson C, Gerrard JM. The empty sack syn-

drome: A platelet storage pool deficiency associated with empty dense granules. *Br J Haematol* 1994;86:574–582.
23. Weiss HJ, Witte LD, Kaplan KL, et al. Heterogeneity in storage pool deficiency: Studies on granule-bound substances in 18 patients including variants deficient in alpha- granules, platelet factor 4, beta-thromboglobulin, and platelet-derived growth factor. *Blood* 1979;54:1296–1319.
24. Gebrane-Younes J, Cramer EM, Orcel L, Caen JP. Gray platelet syndrome: Dissociation between abnormal sorting in megakaryocyte alpha-granules and normal sorting in Weibel-Palade bodies of endothelial cells. *J Clin Invest* 1993;92:3023–3028.
25. Reed GL, Houng AK, Fitzgerald ML. Human platelets contain SNARE proteins and a Sec1p homologue that interacts with syntaxin 4 and is phosphorylated after thrombin activation: Implications for platelet secretion. *Blood* 1999;93:2617–2626.
26. Lemons PP, Chen D, Bernstein AM, et al. Regulated secretion in platelets: Identification of elements of the platelet exocytosis machinery. *Blood* 1997;90:1490–1500.
27. Brass LF, Manning DR, Cichowski K, Abrams CS. Signaling through G proteins in platelets: To the integrins and beyond. *Thrombosis Haemostasis* 1997;78:581–589.
28. Barnes MJ, Knight CG, Farndale RW. The collagen-platelet interaction. *Curr Opin Hematol* 1998;5:314–320.
29. Calakos N, Scheller RH. Synaptic vesicle biogenesis, docking, and fusion: A molecular description. *Physiolog Rev* 1996;76:1–29.
30. Sollner T, Bennett MK, Whiteheart SW, et al. A protein assembly-disassembly pathway in vitro that may correspond to sequential steps of synaptic vesicle docking, activation, and fusion. *Cell* 1993;75:409–418.
31. Jahn R, Sudhof TC. Membrane fusion and exocytosis. *Ann Rev Biochem* 1999;68:863–911.
32. Hata Y, Slaughter CA, Sudhof TC. Synaptic vesicle fusion complex contains unc-18 homologue bound to syntaxin. *Nature* 1993;366:347–351.
33. Schulze KL, Littleton JT, Salzberg A, et al. Rop, a Drosophila homolog of yeast Sec1 and vertebrate n-Sec1/Munc-18 proteins, is a negative regulator of neurotransmitter release in vivo. *Neuron* 1994;13:1099–1108.
34. Wu MN, Fergestad T, Lloyd TE, et al. Syntaxin 1A interacts with multiple exocytic proteins to regulate neurotransmitter release in vivo. *Neuron* 1999;23:593–605.
35. Novick P, Field C, Schekman R. Identification of 23 complementation groups required for post-translational events in the yeast secretory pathway. *Cell* 1980;21:205–215.
36. Polgar J, Reed GL. A critical role for N-ethylmaleimide-sensitive fusion protein (NSF) in platelet granule secretion. *Blood* 1999;94:1313–1318.
37. Chen D, Bernstein AM, Lemons PP, Whiteheart SW. Molecular mechanisms of platelet exocytosis: Role of SNAP-23 and syntaxin 2 in dense core granule release. *Blood* 2000;95:921–929.
38. Lemons PP, Chen D, Whiteheart SW. Molecular mechanisms of platelet exocytosis: Requirements for alpha-granule release. *Biochem Biophys Res Commun* 2000;267:875–880.
39. Flaumenhaft R, Croce K, Chen E, et al. Proteins of the exocytotic core complex mediate platelet alpha-granule secretion: Roles of vesicle-associated membrane protein, SNAP-23, and syntaxin 4. *J Biol Chem* 1999;274:2492–2501.

40. Polgar J, Reed GL. Unpublished observations.1999.
41. Houng AK, Reed GL. Unpublished observations. 2000.
42. Chung SH, Polgar J, Reed GL. Protein kinase C phosphorylation of syntaxin 4 in thrombin-activated human platelets. *J Biol Chem* 2000;275:25286–25291.
43. Fasshauer D, Bruns D, Shen B, et al. A structural change occurs upon binding of syntaxin to SNAP-25. *J Biol Chem* 1997;272:4582–4590.
44. Fasshauer D, Otto H, Eliason WK, et al. Structural changes are associated with soluble N-ethylmaleimide-sensitive fusion protein attachment protein receptor complex formation. *J Biol Chem* 1997;272:28036–28041.
45. Sutton RB, Fasshauer D, Jahn R, Brunger AT. Crystal structure of a SNARE complex involved in synaptic exocytosis at 2.4 A resolution. *Nature* 1998;395:347–353.
46. Fitzgerald ML, Reed GL. Rab6 is phosphorylated in thrombin-activated platelets by a protein kinase C-dependent mechanism: Effects on GTP/GDP binding and cellular distribution. *Biochem J* 1999;342:353–360.
47. Karniguian A, Zahraoui A, Tavitian A. Identification of small GTP-binding rab proteins in human platelets: Thrombin-induced phosphorylation of rab3B, rab6, and rab8 proteins. *Proc Natl Acad Sci USA* 1993;90:7647–7651.
48. Geppert M, Goda Y, Stevens CF, Sudhof TC. The small GTP-binding protein Rab3A regulates a late step in synaptic vesicle fusion. *Nature* 1997;387: 810–814.
49. Sogaard M, Tani K, Ye RR, et al. A rab protein is required for the assembly of SNARE complexes in the docking of transport vesicles. *Cell* 1994;78 :937–948.
50. Lian JP, Stone S, Jiang Y, et al. Ypt1p implicated in v-SNARE activation. *Nature* 1994;372:698–701.
51. Richards-Smith B, Novak EK, Jang EK, et al. Analyses of proteins involved in vesicular trafficking in platelets of mouse models of Hermansky-Pudlak syndrome. *Mol Genet Metab* 1999;68:14–23.
52. Bernstein AM, Whiteheart SW. Identification of a cellubrevin/vesicle-associated membrane protein 3 homologue in human platelets. *Blood* 1999;93:571–579.
53. Whiteheart SW, Griff IC, Brunner M, et al. SNAP family of NSF attachment proteins includes a brain-specific isoform. *Nature* 1993;362:353–355.
54. Geppert M, Goda Y, Hammer RE, et al. Synaptotagmin I: A major Ca^{2+} sensor for transmitter release at a central synapse. *Cell* 1994;79:717–727.
55. Augustin I, Rosenmund C, Sudhof TC, et al. Munc13–1 is essential for fusion competence of glutamatergic synaptic vesicles. *Nature* 1999;400:457–461.
56. Raccuglia G. Gray platelet syndrome: A variety of qualitative platelet disorder. *Am J Med* 1971;51:818–828.
57. Rosa JP, George JN, Bainton DF, et al. Gray platelet syndrome: Demonstration of alpha granule membranes that can fuse with the cell surface. *J Clin Invest* 1987;80:1138–1146.
58. Breton-Gorius J, Vainchenker W, Nurden A, et al. Defective alpha-granule production in megakaryocytes from gray platelet syndrome: Ultrastructural studies of bone marrow cells and megakaryocytes growing in culture from blood precursors. *Am J Pathol* 1981;102:10–19.

Chapter 13

Platelet Activation:
Communication with Integrin Cytoplasmic Domains

Leslie V. Parise, PhD

Introduction

Platelets circulate freely in the vasculature but are poised to adhere rapidly to damaged sites in order to maintain hemostasis. Platelets are initially stimulated by a variety of agonists, including abnormally exposed extracellular matrix molecules such as collagen or von Willebrand factor (vWF) or adherent plasma proteins such as fibrinogen. In addition, soluble platelet agonists are generated or released at sites of injury including thrombin, epinephrine, thrombospondin, adenosine diphosphate (ADP), thromboxane A_2, and serotonin. Many of these soluble agonists are generated, activated, or released from the platelets themselves, and/or may be provided by neighboring cells. These agonists act together to activate adjacent platelets, ultimately causing multiple changes in platelets, including platelet shape change, cytoskeletal assembly, granule secretion, $\alpha IIb\beta 3$ activation, platelet aggregation, and clot retraction. One of the most important events in this regard is the activation of the major platelet integrin $\alpha IIb\beta 3$. Activation of this integrin is defined as a conversion of $\alpha IIb\beta 3$ from a resting to an active conformation, such that it acquires the ability to bind large soluble ligands such as fibrinogen or vWF. The impingement of intracellular signals on $\alpha IIb\beta 3$ that causes this conversion is often referred to as "inside-out signaling." Fibrinogen, which bridges platelets together under low shear conditions, and vWF, which bridges platelets together under high shear

Support provided by: 2-P01-HL45100, 5-P01-HL06350, 1-R01-HL58939.

From: Weir EK, Reeve HL, Reeves JT (eds). *Interactions of Blood and the Pulmonary Circulation*. Armonk, NY: Futura Publishing Company, Inc.; ©2002.

conditions, have multiple platelet binding sites that promote platelet aggregate formation. When ligands such as fibrinogen or vWF bind to αIIbβ3, additional specific signaling events are initiated intracellularly, in a process termed "outside-in integrin signaling." These outside-in signals appear to be crucial for maximal platelet aggregation and clot retraction.[1] The resultant platelet plug formation and subsequent retraction require the synchronization of cell signaling and cell adhesive events. A detailed understanding of these events is vital to obtaining precise therapeutic targets in the platelet, beyond those that currently exist. These targets are necessary for ultimately controlling the contribution of platelets to aggregate formation on ruptured atherosclerotic plaques, and thus to myocardial infarction, stroke, and a variety of additional thrombotic disorders. In this chapter is a discussion of signaling pathways leading to the activation of αIIbβ3, with special attention to the integrin cytoplasmic domains, and proteins that may bind to these domains to regulate platelet function.

Platelet Agonists and Their Receptors

One of the most potent platelet agonists known is the proteolytic enzyme, thrombin. Thrombin circulates as a zymogen and is activated by coagulation factors Va and Xa, which assemble on exposed phosphatidylserine on the surface of activated platelets and other cells. Thrombin activates human platelets by binding to and cleaving the protease-activated receptors PAR-1 and PAR-4, which are 7-transmembrane G-protein-coupled receptors on platelets and other cells.[2,3] Murine platelets utilize a slightly different combination of receptors, PAR-3 and PAR-4.[4,5] Thrombin cleaves the N-terminus of these receptors, releasing a 41-amino-acid cleavage product. Removal of the N-terminus exposes the so-called "tethered ligand," which is believed to bind back on itself to activate the cellular receptor to which it is attached.[2]

A different type of platelet agonist is thrombospondin (TSP), which, unlike thrombin, is not an enzyme, but is instead a large adhesive protein present in the subendothelial matrix and platelet α-granules. Minimal TSP is found free in circulation, unless platelets become activated and release their granular contents. TSP induces platelet activation through its interaction with a 5-transmembrane spanning receptor termed CD47 integrin-associated protein (IAP).[6,7] IAP received its name due to its ability to co-isolate with several integrins including αIIbβ3,[6] αvβ3,[8] and α2β1.[9] While it was originally proposed that IAP activates integrins via a direct interaction, more recent evidence suggests that this activation is indirect and G-protein-mediated. Thus, IAP appears to associate directly with the large G-protein,

Gαi, making this receptor unique, since to date the only other membrane spanning receptors known to couple to large G-proteins are the 7-transmembrane-spanning family. TSP-induced signaling through Gαi is evident by the finding that pertussus toxin, a Gαi inhibitor, blocks IAP-mediated αIIbβ3 activation.[10]

An additional large adhesive protein that is also a platelet agonist is collagen. Several collagen-binding sites exist on the platelet but only two, glycoprotein VI and the α2β1 integrin, appear necessary for collagen-induced platelet activation. Glycoprotein VI was recently cloned and sequenced.[11,12] This receptor contains Ig-like domains and appears to span the membrane once. It is physically coupled to another membrane protein, the Fc receptor γ chain,[13] a component that is necessary for transmission of collagen signals. In addition to GPVI, the α2β1 integrin is necessary for collagen signaling[14]; patients who lack either GPVI[15] or α2β1[16] expression do not aggregate in response to collagen. It is currently controversial as to whether the α2β1 integrin merely acts as a necessary attachment site for collagen, while the simultaneous binding of collagen to GPVI actually transmits signals into the platelet as some recent evidence suggests,[17] or whether the α2β1 integrin also participates directly in the signaling process as it does in other cells.[18] One of the most immediate signaling events post-collagen binding is the phosphorylation of the FcR γ chain on tyrosine residues within the ITAM or immune-receptor tyrosine-based activation motif by the tyrosine kinase Fyn or Lyn.[19] Phosphorylation of this motif creates an SH2 binding site that is recognized by this domain in the tyrosine kinase, Syk. Syk is then recruited, phosphorylated, and activated.[20] Activation of Syk appears critical to the collagen activation process, as pharmacological inhibition of Syk[14] or lack of Syk in knockout mice results in loss of collagen-stimulated platelet aggregation. Some evidence suggests that the next kinase activated in this cascade is Bruton's tyrosine kinase (BTK). Platelets from individuals lacking this kinase exhibit a decrease in phospholipase (PL)Cγ2 activation and collagen-induced platelet aggregation, in addition to a B-cell deficiency.[21] Thus, PLCγ2 activation appears to occur downstream of BTK, leading to phosphoinositide turnover. A very simplified view of the phosphoinositide cycle is that activation of PLCγ2, via the collagen pathway or PLC downstream of 7-transmembrane-spanning G-protein coupled receptors, hydrolyzes membrane-associated phosphatidylinositol biphosphate (PIP_2), generating inositol trisphosphate (IP_3) and diacylglycerol (DAG). DAG contributes to the activation of protein kinase C (PKC), and IP_3 causes a receptor-mediated release of intracellular Ca^{2+}. Both events, especially the activation of PKC, appear to play a major role in platelet activation. However, beyond these steps, the events that lead to activation of the fibrinogen-binding function of αIIbβ3 are less well understood.

Small G-Proteins

Small G-proteins may play a role in subsequent steps of platelet activation. H-Ras is activated in platelets downstream of PKC.[22] Whether H-Ras contributes to platelet activation is unclear, however, since separate evidence in a CHO cell system suggests that H-Ras transmits inhibitory signals to at least one integrin construct.[23] However, recent evi-

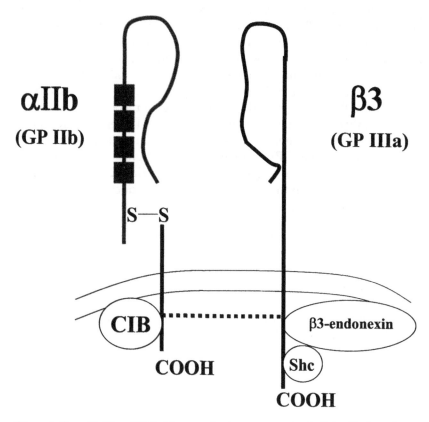

Figure 1. The αIIbβ3 or GPIIb-IIIa complex is a noncovalently linked heterodimer that spans the platelet membrane. The αIIbβ3 integrin exists in an inactive conformation on resting platelets that prevents it from binding large soluble ligands such as fibrinogen or von Willebrand factor. The integrin cytoplasmic domains appear to play an important role in maintaining the resting conformation and in allowing a change to the active conformation to occur. The resting state may be maintained in part by interactions between the αIIb and β3 cytoplasmic domains.[31,32] Molecules that bind to the integrin cytoplasmic domains, such as CIB to αIIb[40,44] or β3 endonexin to β3[35] may play a role in stabilizing or destabilizing the integrin cytoplasmic domains or may bind once the integrin is activated, as in the case of Shc.[38] The actual role of any of these molecules in directly modulating αIIbβ3 function in platelets remains to be determined.

dence suggests that two other small G-proteins, R-Ras and Rap1b, do play a role in activation of some integrins in some cell types. Thus, a constitutively active construct of R-Ras was shown to potentially activate the αIIbβ3 integrin in a CHO cell system.[24] In a separate study, R-Ras was shown to stimulate α2β1-mediated cell migration that was specifically dependent on the presence of the α2 integrin cytoplasmic domain.[25]

Rap1 is an abundant small G-protein in platelets that is activated in two distinct phases in thrombin-stimulated platelets. It is first activated downstream of the PLC-mediated increase in intracellular Ca^{2+} mentioned above, and second, downstream of PCK activation.[26] Rap1 appears to be involved in the activation of integrins LFA-1 (αLβ1)[27] and VLA-4 (α4β1).[28] Whether Rap1 plays a role in activating αIIbβ3 on platelets is currently unknown, but is an intriguing possibility.

Integrin Cytoplasmic Domains

It is apparent that the relatively short integrin cytoplasmic domains contribute to the activation of αIIbβ3.[29,30] A direct binding of these cytoplasmic domains to one another was detected in vitro by fluorescence quenching, terbium luminescence, circular dichroism, and mass spectrometry[31] (Figure 1). Hughes et al. provided evidence that a salt bridge exists between the integrin α and β cytoplasmic domains and that mutation of amino acids involved in this potential interaction resulted in an active conformation of the integrin.[32] It is therefore possible that the natural activation mechanism of the platelet also involves disruption of this salt bridge, perhaps through proteins that bind to integrin cytoplasmic domains (Figure 1).

Cytoplasmic Domain-Binding Proteins

Evidence for the existence of regulatory proteins that bind to integrin cytoplasmic domains is provided by studies in which overexpression of the β3 or β1 integrin cytoplasmic domain in CHO cells inhibited the activated state of an expressed integrin.[30] The mechanism of this inhibition was proposed to be a competition by the overexpressed cytoplasmic domain for molecules that normally bind to the integrin that are necessary for integrin activation.

In addition to these types of studies, proteins have been identified that bind directly to the integrin cytoplasmic domains. A few of the numerous candidate integrin-binding proteins are discussed here. Most of the proteins identified to date bind to the β-cytoplasmic domains. One of these proteins is talin,[33,34] which may also bind by a separate site to the α-cytoplasmic domain.[33] Overexpression of the talin head domain in CHO cells causes a shift of αIIbβ3 to a high affinity state.[34]

β3-endonexin was identified in a yeast 2-hybrid screen as a novel β3 cytoplasmic domain protein. When overexpressed in CHO cells with recombinant αIIbβ3, β3 endonexin causes the integrin to assume an active conformation.[35] Whether β3 endonexin has the same effect on αIIbβ3 in platelets is currently unknown, but places β3 endonexin, along with talin, as a promising candidate activator of αIIbβ3 in vivo (Figure 1).

Two muscle proteins have been identified as binding to the β3 integrin cytoplasmic domain. One such protein, skelemin, is known to regulate the organization of myosin filaments, and binds to the membrane proximal portion of the β3 cytoplasmic domain.[36] The other protein, myosin,[37] binds to the tyrosine phosphorylated β3 cytoplasmic domain. Because tyrosine phosphorylated β3 preferentially associates with the cytoskeleton, it is hypothesized that myosin, or in the above study, skelimin, provides this link to the cytoskeleton.

In addition to myosin, another protein that binds to tyrosine phosphorylated β3 integrin is the adapter molecule Shc[38] (Figure 1). Tyrosine phosphorylation of the β3 integrin cytoplasmic domain occurs during platelet activation, and this phosphorylation and subsequent recruitment of adapter proteins such as Shc appear to be crucial to the full aggregation response of platelets; mice expressing the β3 integrin, with two tyrosines converted to phenylalanines, such that tyrosine phosphorylation cannot occur in vivo, display an impaired aggregation response induced by a number of agonists,[1] and aggregation-induced Shc phosphorylation does not occur in these platelets.[38] Although the subsequent pathways stimulated by integrin-associated Shc in platelets are unknown, phosphorylated Shc in other cells, via Grb2 binding, activates the Ras pathway.

Less is known about the exact role of the αIIb cytoplasmic domain and molecules that bind to it. Proteins identified as binding to the a cytoplasmic domain include calreticulin[39] and CIB.[40] Calreticulin binds to the GFFKR sequence common to many integrins including αIIb. The role of calreticulin, if any, in αIIbβ3 activation and platelet function is unknown but can be surmised from studies in other cells. Calreticulin binds transiently to some integrins during cell attachment and spreading, when that integrin is specifically engaged in the adhesive process.[41] In embryonic stem cells lacking calreticulin, integrin-mediated adhesion is severely impaired, but is rescued by introduction of recombinant calreticulin into these cells.[42] Moreover, the transient increase in cytosolic calcium that normally occurs upon integrin engagement is impaired in cells lacking calreticulin. Thus, calreticulin may couple integrin engagement to calcium transients.

A potential intracellular regulatory molecule termed CIB for "calcium and integrin binding protein" was discovered to bind to the cytoplasmic domain of αIIb in the yeast 2-hybrid system.[40] This 22-kDa molecule is homologous to calcineurin B, the regulatory subunit for a serine/threonine phosphatase called calcineurin, and calmodulin, a ubiquitous regulatory molecule. Like these molecules, CIB contains several EF-hand, Ca^{2+} binding domains. CIB is most homologous (64%), however, to a protein termed KIP2 (kinase interacting protein 2), a relatively unstudied protein of unknown function.[43] CIB is found not only in platelets but also appears from Northern blots to be widely distributed in various organs and tissues.[44] Studies to measure the binding of recombinant CIB to the synthetic αIIb peptide by either of two biophysical techniques, isothermal titration calorimetry or intrinsic protein fluorescence, indicate that the αIIb peptide binds to CIB in a Ca^{2+}-dependent manner with a Kd of $\sim$0.7μM, by an interaction that is most likely hydrophobic.[44] A separate study indicates that CIB binds preferentially to the activated conformation of αIIbβ3.[45] CIB appears to have a number of binding partners other than the αIIb integrin, including several serine/threonine kinases such as DNA-dependent protein kinase,[46] FNK and SNK,[47] the apoptotic enzyme caspase 2,[48] and the Alzheimer's-related protein, presenilin 2.[49] Which of these potential binding partners are in platelets is unknown and whether CIB actually regulates integrin function is unknown, but it appears that CIB has the potential, like calmodulin, to regulate enzyme function and/or serve as a docking molecule at the cytoplasmic domain of the αIIb integrin (Figure 1).

Conclusions and Future Directions

Although numerous molecules have been identified that either modulate integrin function or bind directly to integrins, the mechanism by which signals are transduced to the integrin and thereby converted to a change in conformation and function of the integrin remains to be delineated. The terminally differentiated, anucleate platelet is not yet directly amenable to molecular approaches that allow for overexpression of wild type or mutated molecules of interest, or knockout of protein expression. While ingenious models of αIIbβ3 integrin activation have been devised in other cell systems, these models have limitations in that they most probably lack portions of the relevant activation machinery present in platelets. Despite these limitations, several very specific conditions have been identified in CHO cells, as discussed above, that allow αIIbβ3 activation. Nonetheless, the only current means of reliably altering specific protein expression in platelets is through the more laborious transgenic and knockout mouse technology. For this reason, the recent advances in technology to recover, culture, and induce maturation of the platelet precursors, megakaryoctes, which can be genetically manipulated, is a promising model for more rapid study of platelet signaling pathways.[50] Further development of these types of systems will facilitate a more precise understanding of how multiple molecules and signaling pathways cooperate to regulate integrin function.

References

1. Law DA, DeGuzmann FR, Heiser P, et al. The integrin cytoplasmic motif, ICY, is required for outside-in alphaII bbeta3 signaling and normal platelet function. *Nature* 1999;401:808–811.
2. Vu TK, Hung DT, Wheaton VI, Coughlin SR. Molecular cloning of a functional thrombin receptor reveals a novel proteolytic mechanism of receptor activation. *Cell* 1991;64:1057–1068.
3. Hung DT, Vu TK, Wheaton VI, et al. Cloned platelet thrombin receptor is necessary for thrombin-induced platelet activation. *J Clin Invest* 1992;89: 1350–1353.
4. Ishihara H, Connolly AJ, Zeng D, et al. Protease-activated receptor 3 is a second thrombin receptor in humans. *Nature* 1997;386:502–506.
5. Ishihara H, Zeng D, Connolly AJ, et al. Antibodies to protease-activated receptor 3 inhibit activation of mouse platelets by thrombin. *Blood* 1998;91: 4152–4157.
6. Chung J, Gao AG, Frazier WA. Thrombspondin acts via integrin-associated protein to activate the platelet integrin alphaIIb beta3. *J Biol Chem* 1997;272:14740–14746.
7. Dorahy DJ, Thorne RF, Fecondo JV, Burns GF. Stimulation of platelet activation and aggregation by a carboxyl-terminal peptide from thrombospondin binding to the integrin-associated protein receptor. *J Biol Chem* 1997;272:1323–1330.
8. Lindberg FP, Gresham HD, Schwarz E, Brown EJ. Molecular cloning of integrin-associated protein: An immunoglobulin family member with multiple membrane-spanning domains implicated in alpha v beta 3-dependent ligand binding. *J Cell Biol* 1993;123:485–496.
9. Wang XQ, Frazier WA. The thrombospondin receptor CD47 (IAP) modulates and associates with alpha2 beta1 integrin in vascular smooth muscle cells. *Mol Biol Cell* 1998;9:865–874.
10. Frazier WA, Gao AG, Dimitry J, et al. The thrombospondin receptor integrin-associated protein (CD47) functionally couples to heterotrimeric Gi. *J Biol Chem* 1999;274:8554–8560.
11. Clemetson JM, Polgar J, Magnenat E, et al. The platelet collagen receptor glycoprotein VI is a member of the immunoglobulin superfamily closely related to Fc alphaR and the natural killer receptors. *J Biol Chem* 1999;274: 29019–29024.
12. Miura Y, Ohnuma M, Jung SM, Moroi M. Cloning and expression of the platelet-specific collagen receptor glycoprotein VI. *Thromb Res* 2000;98: 301–309.
13. Poole A, Gibbins JM, Turner M, et al. The Fc receptor gamma-chain and

the tyrosine kinase Syk are essential for activation of mouse platelets by collagen. *Embo J* 1997;16:2333–2341.

14. Keely PJ, Parise LV. The alpha2 beta1 integrin is a necessary co-receptor for collagen-induced activation of Syk and the subsequent phosphorylation of phospholipase C gamma2 in platelets. *J Biol Chem* 1996;271:26668–26676.

15. Moroi M, Jung SM, Okuma M, Shinmyozu K. A patient with platelets deficient in glycoprotein VI that lack both collagen-induced aggregation and adhesion. *J Clin Invest* 1989;84:1440–1445.

16. Nieuwenhuis HK, Akkerman JWN, Houdijk WPM, Sixma JJ. Human blood platelets showing no response to collagen fail to express surface glycoprotein Ia. *Nature* 1985;318:470–472.

17. Hers I, Berlanga O, Tiekstra MJ, et al. Evidence against a direct role of the integrin alpha2 beta1 in collagen- induced tyrosine phosphorylation in human platelets. *Eur J Biochem* 2000;267:2088–2097.

18. Ivaska J, Reunanen H, Westermarck J, et al. Integrin alpha2beta1 mediates isoform-specific activation of p38 and upregulation of collagen gene transcription by a mechanism involving the alpha2 cytoplasmic tail. *J Cell Biol* 1999;147:401–416.

19. Briddon SJ, Watson SP. Evidence for the involvement of p59fyn and p53/56lyn in collagen receptor signaling in human platelets. *Biochem J* 1999;338:203–209.

20. Tsuji M, Ezumi Y, Arai M, Takayama H. A novel association of Fc receptor gamma-chain with glycoprotein VI and their co-expression as a collagen receptor in human platelets. *J Biol Chem* 1997;272:23528–23531.

21. Quek LS, Bolen J, Watson SP. A role for Bruton's tyrosine kinase (Btk) in platelet activation by collagen. *Curr Biol* 1998;8:1137–1140.

22. Shock DD, He K, Wencel-Drake JD, Parise LV. Ras activation in platelets after stimulation of the thrombin receptor, thromboxane A2 receptor or protein kinase C. *Biochem J* 1997;321:525–530.

23. Hughes PE, Renshaw MW, Pfaff M, et al. Suppression of integrin activation: A novel function of a Ras/Raf-initiated MAP kinase pathway. *Cell* 1997;88:521–530.

24. Zhang Z, Vuori K, Wang H, et al. Integrin activation by R-ras. *Cell* 1996;85:61–69.

25. Keely PJ, Rusyn EV, Cox AD, Parise LV. R-Ras signals through specific integrin alpha cytoplasmic domains to promote migration and invasion of breast epithelial cells. *J Cell Biol* 1999;145:1077–1088.

26. Franke B, van Triest M, de Bruijn KM, et al. Sequential regulation of the small GTPase Rap1 in human platelets. *Mol Cell Biol* 2000;20:779–785.

27. Katagiri K, Hattori M, Minato N, et al. Rap1 is a potent activation signal for leukocyte function-associated antigen 1 distinct from protein kinase C and phosphatidylinositol-3-OH kinase. *Mol Cell Biol* 2000;20:1956–1969.

28. Reedquist KA, Ross E, Koop EA, et al. The small GTPase, Rap1, mediates CD31-induced integrin adhesion. *J Cell Biol* 2000;148:1151–1158.

29. O' Toole TE, Mandelman D, Forsyth J, et al. Modulation of the affinity of integrin alpha IIb beta 3 (GPIIb-IIIa) by the cytoplasmic domain of alpha IIb. *Science* 1991;254:845–847.

30. Chen YP, Te OT, Shipley T, et al. "Inside-out" signal transduction inhibited by isolated integrin cytoplasmic domains. *J Biol Chem* 1994;269:18307–18310.

31. Haas TA, Plow EF. The cytoplasmic domain of alphaIIb beta3: A ternary complex of the integrin alpha and beta subunits and a divalent cation. *J Biol Chem* 1996;271:6017–6026.

32. Hughes PE, Diaz-Gonzalez F, Leong L, et al. Breaking the integrin hinge: A defined structural constraint regulates integrin signaling. *J Biol Chem* 1996;271:6571–6574.
33. Knezevic I, Leisner TM, Lam SCT. Direct binding of the platelet integrin alphaIIbbeta3 (GPIIb-IIIa) to talin: Evidence that interaction is mediated through the cytoplasmic domains of both alphaIIb and beta3. *J Biol Chem* 1996;271:16416–16421.
34. Calderwood DA, Zent R, Grant R, et al. The talin head domain binds to integrin {beta} subunit cytoplasmic tails and regulates integrin activation. *J Biol Chem* 1999;274:28071–28074.
35. Kashiwagi H, Schwartz MA, Eigenthaler M, et al. Affinity modulation of platelet integrin alphaIIbbeta3 by beta3-endonexin, a selective binding partner of the beta3 integrin cytoplasmic tail. *J Cell Biol* 1997;137:1433–1443.
36. Reddy KB, Gascard P, Price MG, et al. Identification of an interaction between the m-band protein skelemin and beta-integrin subunits: Colocalization of a skelemin-like protein with beta1- and beta3-integrins in nonmuscle cells. *J Biol Chem* 1998;273:35039–35047.
37. Jenkins AL, Nannizzi-Alaimo L, Silver D, et al. Tyrosine phosphorylation of the beta3 cytoplasmic domain mediates integrin-cytoskeletal interactions. *J Biol Chem* 1998;273:13878–13885.
38. Cowan KJ, Law DA, Phillips DR. SHC identified as the primary protein associated with the beta 3 diphosphorylated cytoplasmic tail peptide of alphaIIb beta3 (GPIIbIIIa) in human platelets. *J Biol Chem* 2000;275:36423–36429.
39. Rojiani MV, Finlay BB, Gray V, Dedhar S. In vitro interaction of a polypeptide homologous to human Ro/SS-A antigen (calreticulin) with a highly conserved amino acid sequence in the cytoplasmic domain of integrin alpha subunits. *Biochemistry* 1991;30:9859–9866.
40. Naik UP, Patel PM, Parise LV. Identification of a novel calcium-binding protein that interacts with the integrin alphaIIb cytoplasmic domain. *J Biol Chem* 1997;272:4651–4654.
41. Coppolino MG, Dedhar S. Ligand-specific, transient interaction between integrins and calreticulin during cell adhesion to extracellular matrix proteins is dependent upon phosphorylation/dephosphorylation events. *Biochem J* 1999;340(Pt 1):41–50.
42. Coppolino MG, Woodside MJ, Demaurex N, et al. Calreticulin is essential for integrin-mediated calcium signaling and cell adhesion. *Nature* 1997;386:843–847.
43. Seki N, Hattori A, Hayashi A, et al. Structure, expression profile and chromosomal location of an isolog of DNA-PKcs interacting protein (KIP) gene. *Biochim Biophys Acta* 1999;1444:143–147.
44. Shock DD, Naik UP, Brittain JE, et al. Calcium-dependent properties of CIB binding to the integrin alphaIIb cytoplasmic domain and translocation to the platelet cytoskeleton. *Biochem J* 1999;342:729–735.
45. Vallar L, Melchior C, Plancon S, et al. Divalent cations differentially regulate integrin alphaIIb cytoplasmic tail binding to beta3 and to calcium- and integrin-binding protein. *J Biol Chem* 1999;274:17257–17266.
46. Wu X, Lieber MR. Interaction between DNA-dependent protein kinase and a novel protein, KIP. *Mutat Res* 1997;385:13–20.
47. Kauselmann G, Weiler M, Wulff P, et al. The polo-like protein kinases Fnk and Snk associate with a Ca(2+)- and integrin-binding protein and are regulated dynamically with synaptic plasticity. *EMBO J* 1999;18:5528–5539.

48. Ito A, Uehara T, Nomura Y. Isolation of Ich-1S (caspase-2S)-binding protein that partially inhibits caspase activity. *FEBS Lett* 2000;470:360–364.
49. Stabler SM, Ostrowski LL, Janicki SM, Monteiro MJ. A myristoylated calcium-binding protein that preferentially interacts with the Alzheimer's disease presenilin 2 protein. *J Cell Biol* 1999;145:1277–1292.
50. Shiraga M, Ritchie A, Aidoudi S, et al. Primary megakaryocytes reveal a role for transcription factor NF-E2 in integrin alpha IIb beta 3 signaling. *J Cell Biol* 1999;147:1419–1430.

Chapter 14

Control of Platelet Reactivity by Endothelial Ecto-ADPase/CD39:
Significance for Occlusive Vascular Diseases

Aaron J. Marcus, MD, M. Johan Broekman, PhD, Joan H.F. Drosopoulos, PhD, Naziba Islam, MS, Richard B. Gayle, III, PhD, David J. Pinsky, MD, and Charles R. Maliszewski, PhD

Introduction

Cell-cell interactions and cell-vessel wall interactions are critical components of the hemostatic process. Several of these interactions occur via "transcellular metabolism," that is, reciprocal or collaborative metabolism of signaling molecules by different cell types. This is particularly relevant with regard to endothelial cells and circulating cells in the blood, especially platelets. Endothelial cells (ECs) in proximity to platelets downregulate their reactivity via at least 3 different metabolic pathways. The first involves a cell-associated, aspirin-insensitive nucleotidase, ecto-ADPase/CD39.[1] The second involves short-lived fluid-phase signals–eicosanoids such as thromboxane (TXA_2), prostacyclin (PGI_2), and PGD_2.[2] The third is the nitric oxide (NO) system, also a fluid-phase autacoid, which inhibits platelet reactivity.[3] When we prevented the actions of TXA_2 and PGI_2 (by aspirin treatment), and NO (by inclusion of the NO-scavenger oxyhemoglobin), platelet inhibition by EC appeared to be due solely to metabolism of ADP emerging in the releasate

Supported in part by a Merit Review grant from the Department of Veterans Affairs, and by National Institutes of Health grants HL 47073 and HL 46403.

From: Weir EK, Reeve HL, Reeves JT (eds). *Interactions of Blood and the Pulmonary Circulation.* Armonk, NY: Futura Publishing Company, Inc.; ©2002.

following agonist-induced platelet activation. Moreover, metabolism of ADP by endothelial ADPase results in loss of platelet activation, release, recruitment, and aggregation.[1] We consider the platelet inhibition by CD39 unique because there is no other consequent blockade of platelet function per se; the mere deletion of ADP from the releasate is solely responsible for abolition of platelet recruitment.

Identification of CD39 as the
Endothelial Cell Ecto-ADPase

It was initially presumed that the ability of ECs to inhibit platelet reactivity was due to eicosanoids and/or NO. However, aspirin-treated ECs are able to reverse platelet aggregation in a manner reminiscent of apyrase-mediated inhibition of platelet reactivity to ADP (data not shown). To test whether ECs were able to metabolize ADP in the milieu, we incubated aspirin-treated human umbilical vein ECs (HUVECs) with radio-labeled ADP. Under these conditions, no PGI_2 is formed, and any NO generated was blocked by addition of purified oxyhemoglobin. ADP and its metabolites were separated and identified by radio-thin layer chromatography (TLC) (Figure 1). AMP accumulates transiently and is further metabolized to adenosine and then deaminated to inosine (Figure 1). Importantly, cell-free supernates from incubations of HUVECs with ^{14}C-ADP did not induce aggregation in platelet-rich plasma (PRP) because the ADP had been metabolized, while the same concentration of ^{14}C-ADP incubated in the absence of HUVECs did lead to platelet aggregation.[1]

Thus, the molecule responsible for the inhibitory activity cited above was an ADPase. We have identified HUVEC ADPase as a membrane-associated ecto-nucleotidase of the E-type.[4] Characteristics of this enzyme include Ca/Mg dependence, ineffectiveness of specific inhibitors of P-, F-, and V-type ATPases, and the capacity to metabolize both ATP and ADP, but not AMP. Thus, the HUVEC enzyme is an apyrase (ATP diphosphohydrolase), ATPDase, EC3.6.1.5.[4] Recently, a new nomenclature has been proposed to unify usage in this rapidly evolving field.[5] According to this nomenclature, HUVEC ecto-ADPase/ CD39 is human E-NTPDase-1.

In 1996, a soluble apyrase was purified from potato tubers, and its cDNA cloned.[6] Sequence analysis revealed 25% amino acid identity and 48% amino acid homology with human CD39.[6] CD39 had been cloned as a cell-surface glycoprotein,[7] expressed on activated B cells, NK cells, and subsets of T cells as well as some HUVEC preparations.[8] Nucleotidases with homology to CD39 and potato apyrase have now been found to be expressed throughout nature, in species as varied as

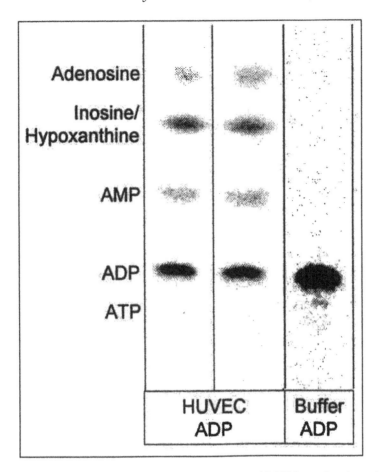

Figure 1. Metabolism of ADP by endothelial cells. HUVEC are incubated (5 minutes) with 50 μM [14C]-ADP. ADP metabolites are separated by radio-TLC. The activity of 5'nucleotidase, as well as adenosine deaminase, is inferred from the rapid appearance of adenosine and inosine in these scans. Detection and quantitation is performed with an InstantImager® (Packard Instrument Co., Meriden, CT).

the garden pea, *C. elegans*, and toxoplasma.[6] At least 4 regions within these molecules have extraordinary homology, and are designated apyrase conserved regions (ACR).[6]

We concluded that the HUVEC ADPase is identical to CD39[9] based on several observations. More than 95% of the ADPase activity from an ADPase preparation purified from HUVEC membranes was immuno-precipitated with any of several anti-human CD39 antibodies. Confocal microscopy and indirect immunofluorescence studies localized CD39 to the HUVEC cell surface. When COS cells were transfected with a vector containing the cDNA for either human or murine CD39, both CD39 and ecto-ADPase activity were expressed on the COS cell surface. PCR analyses using either authentic human CD39 cDNA or cDNA synthesized from HUVEC mRNA resulted in products of identical size for each of 4 different CD39-specific primer pairs. Sequencing the PCR products confirmed their identity. The PCR products encompassed 75% of the coding region of CD39, including the original 4 ACR (apyrase domain, Figure 2). In addition, Northern analyses demonstrated that HUVECs and MP-1 cells (from which CD39 was originally cloned) contained the same sized messages for CD39. Protein purification studies of ecto-ATPDases from different cell sources have been reported from other laboratories as well.[10,11]

For studies of the biological activity of CD39, we transfected COS cells with plasmids containing human or murine CD39 cDNA, or with an "empty" vector. The cells were then evaluated in our platelet aggregation assay system.[1] Only COS cells expressing CD39 blocked ADP-induced platelet aggregation.[9] These transfectants metabolized ADP to AMP within 3 minutes, which correlates with the time frame of events leading to formation of a hemostatic platelet plug or thrombus. Platelet adhesion to injured subendothelium leads to immediate release of ADP and recruitment of additional platelets to form an occlusive thrombus in less than 4 minutes. This chronology parallels the time course we observed for platelet inhibition by CD39-expressing cells and was also commensurate with their respective ADPase activities (Figure 3). The data emphasized the importance of CD39 as a thromboregulator and represented

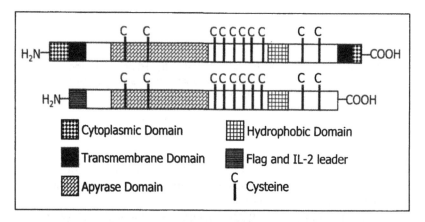

Figure 2. Domain structure of ecto-ADPase/CD39. Two transmembrane regions are located near the amino and carboxy termini; a hydrophobic sequence is centrally located. The putative apyrase conserved region (ACR) is shown on the left side as apyrase domain, adjacent to the N-terminal portion. Cysteine residues are marked as C. An engineered form of soluble CD39, containing a Flag tag and IL-2 secretion leader, and lacking the 2 transmembrane regions, is presented below for comparison.

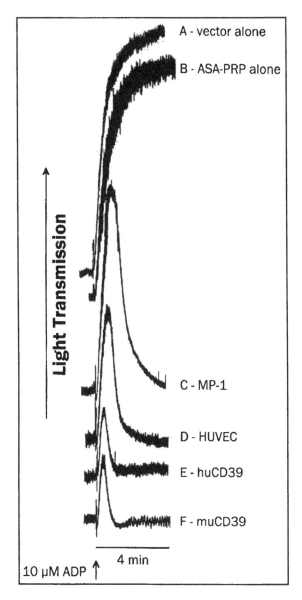

Figure 3. Blockade and reversal of platelet aggregation to ADP by intact HUVEC, MP-1 cells (an activated B-cell-line[7]), and COS cells transfected with full-length human or murine CD39. PRP from a donor who had ingested aspirin was stimulated with 10 μM ADP (A) in the presence of COS cells transfected with "empty" vector; (B) in the absence of any additions; and in the presence of (C) MP-1 cells, (D) HUVECs, and COS cells transfected with (E) human CD39 or (F) murine CD39. Expression of CD39 led to metabolism of the ADP component of the platelet releasate and acquisition of platelet inhibitory activity due to blockade of platelet recruitment.

the first direct demonstration of a physiological function for CD39 as an ADPase: blockade of platelet responsiveness to the prothrombotic agonist ADP via its metabolism to AMP. This phenomenon might represent evolution of an endothelial mechanism targeted toward metabolism of prothrombotic platelet-derived nucleotides, thereby controlling excessive platelet accumulation, as well as maintaining blood fluidity.

Recombinant Soluble Ecto-ADPase/CD39 (solCD39)

The biological properties of CD39 suggest a novel strategy for therapeutic intervention. Whereas aspirin treatment inhibits the prothrombotic action of thromboxane, it also prevents formation of the antithrombotic eicosanoid, prostacyclin, thereby limiting aspirin's effectiveness. Aspirin is a nondiscriminatory acetylating agent, as we demonstrated in 1970,[12] with undesirable side effects. CD39 is unaffected by aspirin and inhibits platelet reactivity even when eicosanoid formation and NO production are blocked. Since ADPase/CD39 is an effective physiological and constitutively expressed endothelial cell inhibitor of platelet reactivity, we postulated that a soluble form of the human enzyme could represent a promising new antithrombotic modality to be evaluated in vivo and ex vivo.

Soluble CD39, retaining nucleotidase activities, would constitute a novel antithrombotic agent that could be administered to thrombosis-prone patients who have a low threshold for platelet activation. Therefore, we generated a recombinant, soluble form of human CD39, based on the structure of CD39 (Figure 2). The 2 transmembrane regions near the amino and carboxyl termini of CD39 serve to anchor the native protein in the cell membrane. Modeling studies, antibody epitope analyses, and sequence homology have established that the portion of the molecule between the transmembrane regions is external to the cell.[7] The extracellular region contains the ACR characteristic of apyrase family members. This is in concordance with the notion that the external portion of CD39 is critical for its ecto-ADPase activity.[5,6,13]

To generate soluble CD39 (solCD39), we isolated the extracellular domain, encoding 439 amino acids, using oligonucleotide cassettes and PCR, and placed it in a mammalian expression vector.[14] Addition of the IL-2 leader sequence ensured secretion of the recombinant molecule. Following transfection with this solCD39-encoding plasmid, COS cells generated levels of ATPase and ADPase activity in their conditioned medium that increased linearly for a 5-day period, an initial indication of the stability of the recombinant protein. SolCD39 was isolated from conditioned medium derived from transiently transfected COS cells via immunoaffinity column chromatography using an anti-CD39 monoclonal antibody. This procedure yielded a single ~66 kDa protein with both ATPase and ADPase activities, suggesting that the molecule was properly glycosylated by COS cells. Incubation of the purified protein with N-glycanase to remove N-linked oligosaccharides yielded a band with the predicted molecular weight 52 kDa.[14]

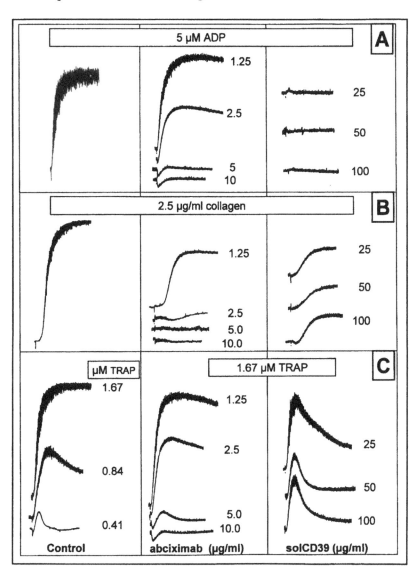

Figure 4. Inhibition and reversal of platelet aggregation. PRP from a donor who had ingested aspirin was stimulated with 5 μM ADP, 2.5 μg/mL collagen (Chrono-Log), or TRAP6 as indicated. In vitro platelet responses to these agonists were strongly inhibited by both abciximab and solCD39.

Purified solCD39 blocked ADP-induced platelet aggregation in vitro and also inhibited collagen-induced platelet reactivity.[14] Aggregation induced by the thrombin receptor activation peptide (TRAP) was strongly blocked by CD39 (Figure 4). Thus, we infer that collagen and TRAP depend more on released ADP for recruitment and aggregation than previously appreciated.

We then developed a CHO cell-based solCD39 expression system, capable of growing in serum-free medium, to increase protein production and to facilitate protein purification. Conditioned medium from this system contains 20-fold more ATPase and ADPase activity than that from COS cells.[14] Following administration of the latter solCD39 preparation to mice, enzyme activity was measurable for an extended period of time. The elimination phase half-life was ~2 days.[14]

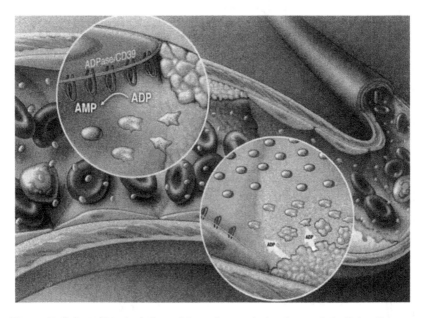

Figure 5. Schematic depiction of thromboregulation by endothelial cell ecto-ADPase/CD39. Platelet activation on or proximal to a site of vascular injury induces release of ADP from platelet dense granules (inset lower right). Released ADP activates and thereby recruits additional platelets that have arrived in the local microenvironment of the evolving thrombus. Activation and recruitment of platelets in proximity to endothelial cells is inhibited by metabolism of released ADP to AMP by endothelial cell ecto-ADPase/CD39. CD39 does not act on the platelet per se, but on the platelet releasate. These platelets then return to an unstimulated state, thereby limiting thrombus formation (inset upper left). Ecto-ADPase/CD39 has been identified and functionally characterized as a physiological, constitutively expressed thromboregulator.

Summary

A novel, soluble form of recombinant human ecto-ADPase, solCD39, demonstrates potential for a new class of antithrombotic agents acting via metabolism of ADP in an activated platelet releasate. SolCD39 blocked and reversed platelet activation, preventing recruitment of additional platelets into a growing thrombus. In this manner, solCD39, as a single therapeutic modality, may attenuate both the extent of occlusion as well as the vascular wall injury associated with cardiac and cerebrovascular events such as stroke, myocardial infarction, angioplasty, and stenting (Figure 5). Alternatively, since solCD39 acts independently of currently available antithrombotic approaches, a combination of solCD39 with the currently available therapeutic modalities, such as heparin, aspirin, and GPIIb/IIIa antagonists, may yield improved clinical results.

References

1. Marcus AJ, Safier LB, Hajjar KA, et al. Inhibition of platelet function by an aspirin-insensitive endothelial cell ADPase: Thromboregulation by endothelial cells. *J Clin Invest* 1991;88:1690–1696.
2. Marcus AJ, Weksler BB, Jaffe EA, et al. Synthesis of prostacyclin from platelet-derived endoperoxides by cultured human endothelial cells. *J Clin Invest* 1980;66:979–986.
3. Broekman MJ, Eiroa AM, Marcus AJ. Inhibition of human platelet reactivity by endothelium-derived relaxing factor from human umbilical vein endothelial cells in suspension: Blockade of aggregation and secretion by an aspirin-insensitive mechanism. *Blood* 1991;78:1033–1040.
4. Plesner L. Ecto-ATPases: Identities and functions. *Int Rev Cytol* 1995;158: 141–214.
5. Zimmermann H, Beaudoin AR, Bollen M, et al. Proposed nomenclature for two novel nucleotide hydrolyzing enzyme families expressed on the cell surface. In Vanduffel L, Lemmens R, eds: *Ecto-ATPases and Related Ectonucleotidases: Proceedings of the Second International Workshop on Ecto-ATPases and Related Ectonucleotidases.* Maastricht, The Netherlands: Shaker Publishing; 2000:1–8.
6. Handa M, Guidotti G. Purification and cloning of a soluble ATP-diphosphohydrolase (apyrase) from potato tubers (*Solanum tuberosum*). *Biochem Biophys Res Commun* 1996;218(3):916–923.
7. Maliszewski CR, Delespesse GJ, Schoenborn MA, et al. The CD39 lymphoid cell activation antigen: Molecular cloning and structural characterization. *J Immunol* 1994;153(8):3574–3583.
8. Kansas GS, Wood GS, Tedder TF. Expression, distribution, and biochemistry of human CD39: Role in activation-associated homotypic adhesion of lymphocytes. *J Immunol* 1991;146(7):2235–2244.
9. Marcus AJ, Broekman MJ, Drosopoulos JHF, et al. The endothelial cell ecto-ADPase responsible for inhibition of platelet function is CD39. *J Clin Invest* 1997;99(6):1351–1360.
10. Kaczmarek E, Koziak K, Sévigny J, et al. Identification and characteriza-

tion of CD39 vascular ATP diphosphohydrolase. *J Biol Chem* 1996;271(51): 33116–33122.

11. Christoforidis S, Papamarcaki T, Galaris D, et al. Purification and properties of human placental ATP diphosphohydrolase. *Eur J Biochem* 1995;234 (1):66–74.

12. Al-Mondhiry H, Marcus AJ, Spaet TH. On the mechanism of platelet function inhibition by acetylsalicylic acid. *Proc Soc Exp Biol Med* 1970;133:632–636.

13. Schulte EJ, Sévigny J, Kaczmarek E, et al. Structural elements and limited proteolysis of CD39 influence ATP diphosphohydrolase activity. *Biochemistry* 1999;38(8):2248–2258.

14. Gayle RB, III, Maliszewski CR, Gimpel SD, et al. Inhibition of platelet function by recombinant soluble ecto-ADPase/CD39. *J Clin Invest* 1998; 101(9):1851–1859.

Section IV

Leukocytes

Chapter 15

Neutrophil Degranulation:
Mechanisms of Regulation and Dysregulation in Interactions with Endothelial Cells

Tadaatsu Imaizumi, MD, Matthew K. Topham, MD, Thomas M. McIntyre, PhD, Stephen M. Prescott, MD, and Guy A. Zimmerman, MD

Leukocyte Degranulation: An Activation Response That Is Regulated in Physiological Inflammation and Dysregulated in Inflammatory Vascular Injury

Polymorphonuclear leukocytes (PMNs, neutrophils) and eosinophils are also known as "granulocytes" because they contain abundant cytoplasmic granules.[1,2] These granules are storage compartments for antimicrobial enzymes and peptides, hydrolases, proteases, and other enzymes that have a wide variety of substrates, surface receptors, β_1 and β_2 integrins, and NADPH oxidase and other intracellular enzymes and signaling kinases.[1-3] Upon appropriate stimulation, granular constituents are released into phagolysosomes where they participate in killing of ingested bacteria and degradation of engulfed particles.[1,4] In response to cellular activation, leukocyte granules and storage vesicles

Tadaatsu Imaizumi and Matthew K. Topham contributed equally to the work cited in this review and to preparation of the manuscript.

Work cited in this manuscript was supported by an NIH Special Center of Research in ARDS (P50 HL50153), NIH R01 HL44525, and an Asthma Research Center funded by the American Lung Association.

From: Weir EK, Reeve HL, Reeves JT (eds). *Interactions of Blood and the Pulmonary Circulation.* Armonk, NY: Futura Publishing Company, Inc.; ©2002.

can also be translocated to the cell surface and their molecular contents retained on the plasma membrane or locally released (Figure 1).[1-3] In this chapter, we focus on degranulation events that modify the surface phenotype and the local milieu by causing surface translocation and/or extracellular release of molecules that are resident in granular compartments. Granular exocytosis generally requires activation of the leukocyte except in conditions in which lysis of the cells causes wholesale release of intracellular components.

Factors that induce granulocyte activation and consequent degranulation include lipid mediators such as platelet-activating factor (PAF) and leukotriene B_4 (LTB_4), chemokines of the C-X-C class, bacterial peptides that are mimicked by N-formyl-methionyl-leucyl-phenylalanine (fMLP), and certain cytokines and complement factors.[4,5] There is a range of potencies for these degranulating factors. Each of these signaling molecules interacts with a plasma membrane receptor on the granulocyte and, under the appropriate conditions, can trigger cellular degranulation within minutes. Thus, degranulation is a mechanism that allows the granulocyte to rapidly change intracellular compartments, its surface phenotype, and its local extracellular milieu without requiring expression of new gene products. Leukocyte degranulation is a physiological response that is required for normal host defense against invading microbes and for wound

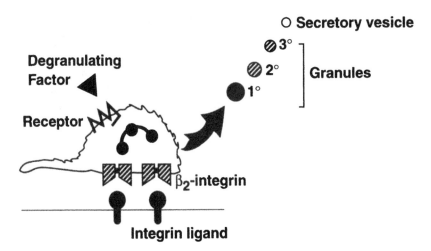

Figure 1. Neutrophil degranulation is induced by signaling molecules that activate the leukocytes via cell surface receptors. These signaling molecules, which can be thought of as degranulating factors, also induce other activation responses of PMNs, including polarization and adhesiveness mediated by β_2 integrins on the neutrophil plasma membrane. Exocytosis of primary (1°, azurophilic), secondary (2°, specific), and tertiary (3°, gelatinase-rich) granules and secretory vesicles occurs in a quantal and hierarchical fashion. See text for details.

repair.[5] Evidence for this includes the rare but informative congenital conditions known as neutrophil-specific granule deficiency and Chédiak-Higashi syndrome, in which impaired leukocyte degranulation contributes to delayed acute inflammation and increased susceptibility to infection.[1,6] In contrast, inappropriate or unregulated release of neutrophil and eosinophil granular constituents also contributes to inflammatory vascular and tissue injury in a variety of experimental and clinical conditions[7,8] (also see below). Thus, characterizing the factors that regulate degranulation of leukocytes is important in understanding both homeostatic and pathological inflammation.

PMNs, which this chapter will focus on, contain several types of granules that are heterogeneous in size and content and that are formed and loaded with enzymes and other constituents at specific times during maturation of the leukocytes in the marrow.[1-4] These include peroxidase-positive azurophilic or "primary" granules, secondary or "specific" granules, "tertiary" granules that are peroxidase-negative, and a population of secretory vesicles that are also peroxidase-negative.[1-3] Tertiary granules are enriched in gelatinase B (matrix metalloproteinase 9; MMP9) and are often called "gelatinase granules," although secondary granules also contain gelatinase.[1-3] Exocytosis of these granular compartments by activated PMNs is quantal in the sense that it varies with the magnitude of stimulation of the PMN and is also hierarchical, with secretory vesicles most rapidly mobilized followed by tertiary, specific, and primary granules, in that order[1] (Figure 1). This hierarchy of degranulation occurs both in vitro and in vivo.[1,3,9,10]

Activation-dependent degranulation of PMNs involves interaction of signaling factors with G-protein-coupled receptors or other classes of receptors on the plasma membrane of the leukocyte and a series of highly regulated intracellular signal transduction events. An increase in intracellular Ca^{2+} is critical; activation of phospholipases A_2, C, and D, protein kinase C, and phosphoinositide 3-kinase, phosphorylation events dependent on tyrosine kinases, and participation of Rho small GTP-binding proteins are also involved in neutrophil degranulation.[3] Engagement of surface integrins on PMNs can alter some of these events, increasing the magnitude of the degranulation response (see below). Fusion of primary, specific, and tertiary granules with the neutrophil plasma membrane involves intracellular proteins that facilitate docking of the granule membranes with the surface phospholipid bilayer and several protein-protein interactions. These proteins include members of the snare and annexin families.[3] The exocytotic process occurs in a fashion similar to that in other secretory cells such as platelets and neurons[11] but with cell-specific variations on the themes. Modification of the PMN cytoskeleton with cytochalasins[3,4] or by generation of endogenous ceramide enhances basal and stimulus-induced degranulation of PMNs.

Treatment of neutrophils with cytochalasins to enhance the release of markers of degranulation, such as elastase for primary granules and lactoferrin for specific granules,[2,3,5] is commonly done in in vitro assays.[4]

In contrast to the regulated quantal and hierarchical degranulation of PMNs in response to receptor-mediated activation by signaling factors, total release of neutrophil granular contents by cellular lysis sometimes occurs in inflammatory exudates.[4] Eosinophils also undergo cytolytic release of granular enzymes and proteins in asthma and other syndromes of immune inflammation.[8] Thus, this unregulated mechanism of degranulation may be particularly important in pathological inflammatory tissue injury. However, receptor-mediated neutrophil degranulation can also become dysregulated or unregulated. These events can occur if signaling factors that interact with cell surface receptors and trigger granular exocytosis are inappropriately generated (biochemical dysregulation) in response to pathological stimuli, if degranulating factors persist too long (temporal dysregulation), or if they activate the leukocytes while they are circulating or at sites distant from the inflamed or injured locus (spatial dysregulation). Therefore, cell lysis is not required for pathological vascular and tissue injury mediated by leukocyte granular release.

PMN Degranulation Is Modified by Engagement of Integrins and by Adhesive Interactions

Engagement of members of β_2 integrins on the surfaces of PMNs delivers outside-in signals that induce or regulate activation responses,[12,13] including degranulation. Crosslinking of β_2 integrins with an antibody, used as an experimental surrogate for engagement by ligand, induces elastase secretion and translocation of additional β_2 integrin heterodimers to the cell surface.[14] As noted above, elastase is a marker that detects exocytosis of primary (azurophilic) granules. Translocation of β_2 integrins to the cell surface indicates exocytosis of one or more of the other granular compartments, since each is an intracellular reservoir for $\alpha_M\beta_2$ integrin (MAC-1, CD11b/CD18).[1-3] Thus, β_2 integrins are markers of exocytosis of some granular compartments and also transmit outside-in signals that modify the degranulation response, in addition to their well-described functions as adhesion molecules. β_2 integrin-dependent neutrophil spreading triggers secretion of lactoferrin, a marker of the secondary or specific granules.[15] Blocking antibodies against integrin $\alpha_M\beta_2$ inhibit TNF_α-induced secretion of lactoferrin by adherent neutrophils.[16] Similarly, engagement of $\alpha_M\beta_2$ integrin by immobilized fibrinogen, an established ligand for this heterodimer,[12] induces release of lactoferrin when PMNs are stimulated with TNF_α.[17] The mechanism likely involves triggering of intracellular calcium transients by $\alpha_M\beta_2$ engagement.[12,16] Small increases in cytosolic free calcium mobilize secretory vesicles, although there is also a Ca^{2+}-independent mechanism for secretory vesicle release, whereas larger increases can trigger degranulation from other compartments.[3] Additional critical signaling events in β_2 integrin-mediated degranulation include activation of Src family kinases.[17] These observations indicate that β_2 integrin-dependent adhesion modifies degranulation of neutrophils when they adhere to matrix structures and also suggest that a similar mechanism operates when PMNs use β_2 integrins to bind to ICAM family members or other ligands in cell-cell interactions.[12,13,18,19] Engagement of β_2 integrins by immobilized ligands can be used in place of treatment of PMNs with cytochalasins as a more physiologically relevant assay of degranulation.[5,7] Engagement of β_2 integrins on eosinophils also enhances exocytosis by these granulocytes.[20,21]

Adhesive interactions mediated by other factors besides β_2 integrins can modify degranulation. Tethering of PMNs by P-selectin on the surfaces of stimulated human endothelial cells facilitates juxtacrine priming of the leukocytes by PAF, which is also displayed on the endothelial surface[22,23] (see below). Thus, adhesive interactions at cell surfaces can bring neutrophils into contact with membrane-anchored signaling factors that alter degranulation responses. In a second mechanism, PMNs roll on inflamed endothelial cells using L-selectin under certain conditions.[24,25] Engagement of L-selectin can trigger translocation of $\alpha_M\beta_2$ to the neutrophil surface,[26,27] which, as noted above, indicates exocytosis of secretory vesicles and/or tertiary and specific granules. In contrast, engagement of another neutrophil surface molecule, ICAM-3, does not cause degranulation even though it induces cytoskeletal reorganization,[28] indicating that additional intracellular events are involved (see above).

Adhesiveness and degranulation of neutrophils are interrelated in complex ways. Factors translocated to the surface from PMN granular compartments can secondarily enhance adhesive interactions. For example, surface lactoferrin augments neutrophil adhesiveness.[29,30] Enrichment of the PMN plasma membrane with copies of $\alpha_M\beta_2$ integrin that are stored in specific and tertiary granules and secretory vesicles has been outlined above; these heterodimers are then available for additional adhesive interactions. As a third example, urokinase plasminogen activator receptor (UPAR) is stored in secretory vesicles and secondary and tertiary granules in PMNs and is translocated to the surface in response to cellular activation.[1–3,31] UPAR mediates adhesion to vitronectin and modification of $\alpha_M\beta_2$ functions in addition to regulating surface proteolysis, and may be critical for leukocyte mobility under specific conditions.[32,33]

Human Endothelial Cells Modulate Neutrophil Degranulation

Adhesion of PMNs and their interactions with surfaces dramatically influence their degranulation responses (see above).[4,5] Furthermore, as outlined above, molecular adhesive and signaling events have the potential to alter degranulation during cell-cell interactions. Until recently, however, the mechanisms by which endothelial cells modify degranulation responses were unknown, even though PMNs adhere to the endothelial surface as the first step in their migration out of the blood and into the extravascular milieu in inflammation. There is now evidence that human endothelial cells can selectively regulate PMN degranulation.[3,5,7] The effect on granular secretion, and the molecular mechanisms involved, depend on whether the endothelial cells are in the resting state or have been activated by inflammatory or thrombotic stimuli, the nature of the endothelial agonist, and other factors. Endothelial signaling molecules inhibit, prime, or trigger granular secretion, establishing paradigms for regulated and selective degranulation in physiological inflammation and dysregulated exocytosis under pathological conditions.

Resting Human Endothelial Cells Inhibit Neutrophil Degranulation

Resting unstimulated human endothelial cells studied in culture were reported to inhibit release of primary and secondary granular markers from activated PMNs when the response was compared to that of PMNs incubated on acellular surfaces.[34] The mechanism was thought to involve antiadhesive factors that are constitutively present on the endothelial plasma membrane and/or are spontaneously released. More recently, we also found that resting endothelial cells inhibit exocytosis from primary and secondary granular compartments when PMNs are activated by fMLP, and that an inhibitory activity is associated with endothelial membrane preparations[5] (M. Topham et al., unpublished experiments). These experiments indicate that in the absence of an inflammatory stimulus, endothelial cells retard release of granular enzymes from PMN primary and secondary granules, an effect that may protect the endothelium from neutrophil-mediated injury (see below). Because of the pattern of sequential exocytosis of neutrophil storage vesicles and granules, however, translocation of β_2 integrins, UPAR, and other surface molecules from the more easily released compartments may still occur under these conditions[1-3] (also see above). Such selective degranulation would potentially favor emigration of the PMNs through intercellular junctions and across the subendothelial matrix without causing vascular injury.

Stimulated, inflamed endothelial cells can also generate factors that modulate PMN activation and, therefore, have the potential to inhibit degranulation. These include prostacyclin and nitric oxide.[35] Concurrent synthesis of inhibitory factors in temporal sequence with signaling molecules that trigger PMN degranulation (see below) provides a mechanism to edit and regulate PMN exocytosis at the endothelial surface in homeostatic inflammation.[22] Endothelial cells may locally modulate the activity of gelatinase and other enzymes released by exocytosis,[36] providing another mechanism for fine control.

Stimulated Endothelial Cells Prime PMNs for Enhanced Degranulation

In contrast to the inhibitory effect of resting endothelial cells, human endothelial cells stimulated with thrombin or leukotriene C_4 enhance degranulation responses of PMNs that are activated with fMLP.[37] In these experiments, lactoferrin was assayed as a marker of specific granule translocation and elastase as a primary granule marker. There was no granular release from these compartments when neutrophils were incubated with thrombin-stimulated endothelial monolayers in the absence of fMLP, indicating that the endothelial signaling molecule primes the PMNs for enhanced exocytosis but does not trigger it alone. The priming factor was rapidly induced in the endothelial cells—within minutes after stimulation—and was not released into solution but instead remained associated with the endothelial plasma membrane. Priming also occurred when the PMNs were activated with leukotriene B_4 rather than fMLP. The mechanism of priming involves juxtacrine signaling of the PMNs by PAF, which is rapidly synthesized by endothelial cells stimulated by thrombin or LTC_4 and is displayed on the endothelial surface together with P-selectin (Figure 2). P-selectin is rapidly translocated from intracellular storage granules to the endothelial surface in concert with PAF synthesis. Endothelial cell-associated PAF then binds to its receptor on the PMN and induces cellular activation and inside-out signaling of β_2 integrins,[38,39] a complex process that makes the integrin heterodimers competent to recognize ligands on the endothelial cells.[13] Thus, PAF triggers neutrophil adhesiveness that strengthens binding of the leukocytes to the endothelial surface in coordination with P-selectin.[22,40] In addition, PAF also acts as a juxtacrine priming signal for degranulation.[37] In contrast, P-selectin acts as a tether that facilitates the interaction of PAF with its receptor, but does not prime the neutrophil when it binds to its counterligand on the leukocyte, PSGL-1, even though PSGL-1 can transmit outside-in signals.[39,41] This was demonstrated using blocking experiments, selective display of PAF or P-selectin in model membranes, and other strategies.[37]

PAF is an excellent priming agent when it interacts with its receptor on neutrophils.[42,43] The mechanism of priming by PAF involves its ability to trigger intracellular calcium transients, which it does both in purified form and when displayed on the surfaces of stimulated endothelial cells.[37,42] As noted above, intracellular Ca^{2+} is a critical regulator of PMN degranulation.[3] Vercellotti et al.[44] also found that PAF synthesized by stimulated endothelial cells primes neutrophils for secretion of the primary granular marker elastase. More recently, PAF has been shown to potently prime neutrophils for translocation and retention of elastase on the leukocyte surface membrane, a location at which it is protected from inhibition by antiproteases.[45] In addition to its priming actions, PAF is a relatively potent direct stimulus for release of gelatinase, likely from tertiary granules.[46] By inference, this indicates that it is also an agonist for exocytosis of secretory vesicles (see above).[1-3] This again demonstrates the hierarchical exocytosis of particular populations of neutrophil granules and vesicles in response to specific stimuli.

The model outlined above and illustrated in Figure 2 provides a paradigm for rapid spatially targeted adhesion of PMNs to stimulated endothelial cells in acute inflammation.[22,40] The model also provides a paradigm for regulation of neutrophil degranulation responses as a result of this cell-cell interaction. Signaling by the PAF and P-selectin juxtacrine system does not trigger global release of primary or secondary granule enzymes, which might be injurious to the endothelium, but selectively translocates tertiary granules and secretory vesicles and primes the leukocytes in a spatially localized fashion for enhanced degranula-

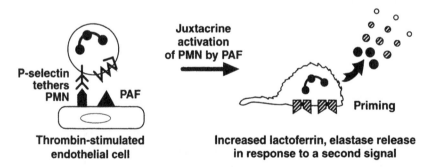

Figure 2. Neutrophils adherent to human endothelial cells stimulated by thrombin are primed for enhanced degranulation. The mechanism involves tethering by P-selectin and juxtacrine priming by PAF. When the neutrophils are stimulated by a second signaling molecule (fMLP, LTB_4), there is enhanced release of the primary granule marker elastase and of lactoferrin, a secondary granule marker. See text and reference 37 for details.

tion when they receive an additional stimulus. In vivo, this can occur when they encounter bacteria or debris for phagocytosis at extravascular sites and/or receive additional activating signals during transmigration. This paradigm may extend to interactions of PMNs with activated platelets, which also display P-selectin and PAF and use them to tether and signal PMNs in a juxtacrine fashion.[47,48]

Human Endothelial Cells Stimulated with Cytokines or Bacterial Lipopolysaccharide (LPS) Express Degranulating Factors

A different pattern of exocytosis of primary and secondary granular markers is seen when neutrophils are incubated with human endothelial monolayers that have been stimulated with interleukin-1 (IL-1), tumor necrosis factor α (TNF$_\alpha$), or bacterial lipopolysaccharide (LPS, endotoxin), which are agonists for endothelial activation in physiological and pathological inflammation[5,7] (Figure 3). There is a time-dependent release of elastase and lactoferrin that also depends on the time of stimulation of the endothelial cells and the concentration of the cytokine or LPS.[5] Under these conditions, no exogenous agonist is required to induce the PMN degranulation, in contrast to the priming of PMNs by thrombin-stimulated endothelial cells (see above and Figure 2), indicating that cytokine- or LPS-stimulated endothelial cells express

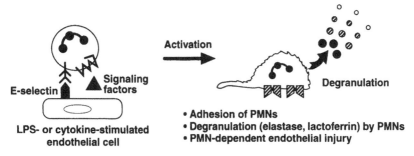

Activation

E-selectin ▲ Signaling factors

Degranulation

• Adhesion of PMNs
• Degranulation (elastase, lactoferrin) by PMNs
• PMN-dependent endothelial injury

LPS- or cytokine-stimulated endothelial cell

Figure 3. LPS- and cytokine-stimulated endothelial cells express signaling molecules that induce neutrophil degranulation. Expression of degranulating factors under these conditions requires new transcription of mRNA, as does expression of E-selectin and other proinflammatory proteins. The magnitude of release of degranulating activity, and therefore the degree of neutrophil degranulation, depends on the intensity of stimulation of the endothelial cells.[5,7] Thus, regulated degranulation induced by endothelial signaling molecules in a fashion that favors transmigration of PMNs can occur in physiological inflammation, but dysregulated signaling and degranulation may be triggered by activated or injured endothelial cells in pathological inflammatory injury. See text for details.

signaling molecules that directly trigger neutrophil degranulation (Figure 3). LPS was the most potent agonist for inducing synthesis of degranulating factors (DGFs) by endothelial monolayers.[7] Vascular injury mediated by elastase and other components of neutrophil granules occurs in vivo and may be a key pathogenetic mechanism in endotoxemia and sepsis syndromes and their complications, such as acute respiratory distress syndrome (ARDS) (see below). Thus, this in vitro model (Figure 3) has in vivo correlates.

A part of the degranulating activity synthesized by LPS- or cytokine-stimulated endothelial cells is released into solution,[5,7] indicating the generation of soluble degranulating factors with the potential to mediate neutrophil exocytosis and PMN-mediated vascular injury at distant sites. Synthesis of the degranulating activity is blocked by inhibiting transcription in the stimulated endothelial cells, indicating that genes coding for degranulating factors are induced in parallel with the genes for E-selectin and other inflammatory molecules (Figure 3) under these conditions.[5] The induction of transcripts coding for DGFs was confirmed by other experimental strategies, including heterologous translation of messenger RNAs in *Xenopus laevis* oocytes[7] (T. Imaizumi et al., unpublished experiments).

Identification of degranulating factors synthesized by cytokine- or LPS-stimulated endothelial cells has demonstrated a complex system of signaling molecules and is not yet complete. In cytokine- or LPS-stimulated human endothelial cells and cell lines, interleukin-8 (IL-8) is an immediate candidate DGF (Figure 4). The gene for IL-8 is induced in endothelial cells under these conditions, the protein is synthesized and secreted (Figure 4), and purified and recombinant IL-8 have degranulating activity.[7] However, complementary experimental approaches involving receptor desensitization, analysis of the degranulating activity generated by heterologous translation of transcripts in the *Xenopus* oocyte system, and purification and analysis of proteins from conditioned medium collected from LPS-stimulated endothelial cells demonstrated that additional degranulating factors are synthesized.[7]

A second candidate factor, epithelial neutrophil-activating peptide-78 (ENA-78), was identified using a degenerate polymerase chain reaction (PCR) strategy.[49] ENA-78, which is a member of the C-X-C family of chemokines, had previously been thought to be synthesized exclusively in epithelial cells but is now known to be expressed by primary human endothelial cells in response to LPS and several cytokines.[49,50] Both the transcript and the protein are induced in LPS-stimulated endothelial monolayers, the protein is secreted in concentrations sufficient to activate PMNs, and the protein is present in in situ endothelial cells in inflamed and injured human lung[49] (Figure 4). Furthermore, ENA-78 is a weak inducer of exocytosis of neutrophil primary and secondary granules and

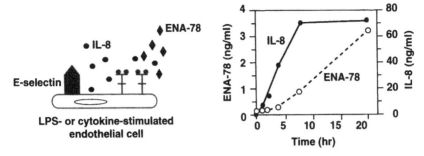

Figure 4. ENA-78 and IL-8 are synthesized and released by LPS- or cytokine-stimulated endothelial cells. ENA-78 and IL-8 are C-X-C chemokines that have degranulating activity. However, other degranulating factors are also synthesized by inflamed or injured endothelial cells. See text and references 5, 7, and 49 for details.

may also have priming activity when it binds to C-X-C receptor type II[49,51] (T. Imaizumi et al., unpublished experiments). However, the degranulating activity synthesized by cytokine- or LPS-stimulated endothelial cells could not be accounted for by ENA-78 alone or in combination with IL-8; furthermore, additional experiments using expression cloning and other approaches demonstrate that degranulating factors besides IL-8 and ENA-78 are induced in LPS-stimulated endothelial cells (T. Imaizumi et al., unpublished experiments). Functional experiments demonstrate that signaling molecules synthesized by stimulated endothelial cells can induce neutrophil activation responses in a combinatorial fashion[49] (T. Imaizumi et al., unpublished experiments), indicating that additive or synergistic actions of these signaling factors may be important in neutrophil activation and dysregulation in inflammatory injury syndromes. Further identification of these factors and characterization of their patterns of synthesis in stimulated and injured endothelial cells will yield additional insights into the mechanisms and consequences of leukocyte degranulation in endothelial interactions with PMNs. Importantly, the synthesis and secretion of degranulating factors is not stereotyped, but varies with the time of stimulation of the endothelial cells, the agonist, and other variables. This is true even for IL-8 and ENA-78 (Figure 4 and unpublished experiments), which are related gene products with similar promoter organization and structures of the mature proteins.[49]

Neutrophil Degranulation Contributes to Syndromes of Acute and Chronic Vascular Injury

As noted above, regulated neutrophil exocytosis is a physiological response that is important in defensive inflammatory responses and in tissue remodeling and repair. However, release of enzymes and other mediators by degranulating PMNs also contributes to cellular injury if it is inappropriately induced or occurs in an unregulated fashion.

Pathologic or dysregulated synthesis of neutrophil degranulating factors by endothelial cells is a likely mechanism of vascular and tissue damage in human syndromes. Several lines of evidence support this idea. In vitro experiments indicate that neutrophil granular enzymes cause endothelial monolayer disruption and cellular injury, and contribute an

Table 1

Evidence for Neutrophil Degranulation in Adult Respiratory Distress Syndrome (ARDS)

Stage of Syndrome	Marker(s)	Reference
Acute ARDS	Elastase	Lee et al., N Engl J Med 1981;304:192–196
Acute/subacute ARDS	Elastase	Cochrane et al., J Clin Invest 1983;71:754–761
At risk/acute/subacute ARDS	Glucosaminidase	Fowler et al., Am J Pathol 1984:116:427–435 Fowler et al., Am Rev Respir Dis 1987;136:1225–1235
Acute ARDS	Elastase	Idell et al., Am Rev Respir Dis 1985;132:1098–1105
Acute ARDS	Elastase, myeloperoxidase, collagenase	Weiland et al., Am Rev Respir Dis 1986;133:218–225
At risk/acute ARDS	Elastase, lactoferrin	Rocker et al., Lancet 1989;1:120–123
At risk/acute/subacute ARDS	Elastase	Suter et al., Am Rev Respir Dis 1992;145:1016–1022
At risk/acute/subacute ARDS	Gelatinase B (MMP-9)	Ricou et al., Am J Respir Crit Care Med 1996;154:346–352
At risk/acute ARDS	Elastase	Donnelly et al., Am J Respir Crit Care Med 1995;151:1428–1433
Acute/subacute ARDS	Gelatinase B (MMP-9)	Delclaux et al., Am J Physiol (Lung Cell Mol Physiol) 1997:16;L442–451

oxygen radical-independent mechanism of vascular damage.[7,52,53] Neutrophil proteases and oxygen radicals are, however, synergistic in mediating endothelial damage.[54] Elastase is a key granular enzyme in neutrophil-mediated endothelial injury in vitro[55] and can act in a protected fashion at the neutrophil cell surface.[45] In in vivo experiments, release of neutrophil elastase is involved in increased microvascular permeability in injury models.[7,56] There is, in addition, evidence for degranulation-induced endothelial and tissue injury in clinical studies of human diseases. As an example, all studies of samples from patients with ARDS that have looked for evidence of PMN degranulation have found it (Table 1), although none has identified the relevant degranulating factor(s). In addition, PMN degranulation has also been correlated with development of multiple organ failure and patient outcome after sepsis and trauma.[57] There is also experimental and/or clinical evidence that unregulated neutrophil accumulation and degranulation are facets of chronic inflammatory injury states as diverse as abdominal aortic aneurysm formation,[58] vasculitis,[59] destructive arthritic syndromes,[60] and many others. Further characterization of mechanisms of endothelial regulation of granular exocytosis may provide new strategies to modify these disorders and paradigms for other cell-cell interactions that can induce neutrophil degranulation.

Acknowledgments: The authors thank Edward Gill, MD, Holly Carveth, MD, Kurt Albertine, PhD, and other co-investigators and collaborators in studies cited in this review. We also thank technical associates who contributed to the work and Michelle Bills and Diana Lim, who prepared the manuscript and figures, respectively.

References

1. Borregaard N, Cowland JB. Granules of the human neutrophilic polymorphonuclear leukocyte. *Blood* 1997;89:3503–3521.
2. Bainton DF. Developmental biology of neutrophils and eosinophils. In Gallin JI, Snyderman R, eds: *Inflammation: Basic Principles and Clinical Correlates, 3rd ed.* Philadelphia: Lippincott Williams & Wilkins; 1999:13–34.
3. Berton G. Degranulation. In Gallin JI, Snyderman R, eds: *Inflammation: Basic Principles and Clinical Correlates, 3rd ed.* Philadelphia: Lippincott Williams & Wilkins; 1999:703–719.
4. Henson P, Henson J, Fittschen C, et al. Degranulation and secretion by phagocytic cells. In Gallin J, Goldstein I, Snyderman R, eds: *Inflammation: Basic Principles and Clinical Correlates, 2nd ed.* New York: Raven Press; 1992:511–540.
5. Topham MK, Carveth HJ, McIntyre TM, et al. Human endothelial cells regulate polymorphonuclear leukocyte degranulation. *Faseb J* 1998;12:733–746.
6. Holland SM, Gallin JI. Disorders of phagocytic cells. In Gallin JI, Snyderman R, eds: *Inflammation: Basic Principles and Clinical Correlates, 3rd ed.* Philadelphia: Lippincott Williams & Wilkins; 1999:895–914.
7. Gill EA, Imaizumi T, Carveth H, et al. Bacterial lipopolysaccharide induces

endothelial cells to synthesize a degranulating factor for neutrophils. *Faseb J* 1998;12:673–684.

8. Erjefalt JS, Persson CG. New aspects of degranulation and fates of airway mucosal eosinophils. *Am J Respir Crit Care Med* 2000;161:2074–2085.

9. Sengelov H, Kjeldsen L, Borregaard N. Control of exocytosis in early neutrophil activation. *J Immunol* 1993;150:1535–1543.

10. Sengelov H, Follin P, Kjeldsen L, et al. Mobilization of granules and secretory vesicles during in vivo exudation of human neutrophils. *J Immunol* 1995;154:4157–4165.

11. Guo W, Sacher M, Barrowman J, et al. Protein complexes in transport vesicle targeting. *Trends Cell Biol* 2000;10:251–255.

12. Kishimoto TK, Baldwin ET, Anderson DC. The role of beta 2 integrins in inflammation. In Gallin JI, Snyderman R, eds: *Inflammation: Basic Principles and Clinical Correlates, 3rd ed.* Philadelphia: Lippincott Williams and Wilkins; 1999:537–570.

13. Harris ES, McIntyre TM, Prescott SM, et al. The leukocyte integrins. *J Biol Chem* 2000;275:23409–23412.

14. Walzog B, Seifert R, Zakrzewicz A, et al. Cross-linking of CD18 in human neutrophils induces an increase of intracellular free Ca^{2+}, exocytosis of azurophilic granules, quantitative up-regulation of CD18, shedding of L-selectin, and actin polymerization. *J Leukoc Biol* 1994;56:625–635.

15. Suchard SJ, Boxer LA. Exocytosis of a subpopulation of specific granules coincides with H_2O_2 production in adherent human neutrophils. *J Immunol* 1994;152:290–300.

16. Richter J, Ng-Sikorski J, Olsson I, et al. Tumor necrosis factor-induced degranulation in adherent human neutrophils is dependent on CD11b/CD18-integrin-triggered oscillations of cytosolic free Ca^{2+}. *Proc Natl Acad Sci USA* 1990;87:9472–9476.

17. Mocsai A, Ligeti E, Lowell CA, et al. Adhesion-dependent degranulation of neutrophils requires the Src family kinases Fgr and Hck. *J Immunol* 1999;162:1120–1126.

18. Schleiffenbaum B, Moser R, Patarroyo M, et al. The cell surface glycoprotein Mac-1 (CD11b/CD18) mediates neutrophil adhesion and modulates degranulation independently of its quantitative cell surface expression. *J Immunol* 1989;142:3537–3545.

19. Barnett CC, Jr., Moore EE, Mierau GW, et al. ICAM-1-CD18 interaction mediates neutrophil cytotoxicity through protease release. *Am J Physiol* 1998;274:C1634–1644.

20. Kaneko M, Horie S, Kato M, et al. A crucial role for beta 2 integrin in the activation of eosinophils stimulated by IgG. *J Immunol* 1995;155:2631–2641.

21. Kato M, Abraham RT, Okada S, et al. Ligation of the beta 2 integrin triggers activation and degranulation of human eosinophils. *Am J Respir Cell Mol Biol* 1998;18:675–686.

22. Zimmerman GA, McIntyre TM, Prescott SM. Adhesion and signaling in vascular cell-cell interactions. *J Clin Invest* 1996;98:1699–1702.

23. Zimmerman G, McIntyre T, Prescott S. Cell-to-cell communication. In Crystal R, West J, eds: *The Lung: Scientific Foundations, 2nd ed.* Philadelphia: Lippincott-Raven; 1996:289–304.

24. McEver RP. Interactions of leukocytes with the vessel wall. In Loscalzo J, Schaffer AI, eds: *Thrombosis and Hemorrhage, 2nd ed.* Boston: Williams and Wilkins; 1998:321–336.

25. McEver R. Leukocyte adhesion through selectins under flow. *The Immunologist* 1998;6:61–67.

26. Crockett-Torabi E, Sulenbarger B, Smith CW, et al. Activation of human neutrophils through L-selectin and Mac-1 molecules. *J Immunol* 1995;154: 2291–2302.

27. Simon SI, Burns AR, Taylor AD, et al. L-selectin (CD62L) cross-linking signals neutrophil adhesive functions via the Mac-1 (CD11b/CD18) beta 2-integrin. *J Immunol* 1995;155:1502–1514.

28. Feldhaus MJ, Kessel JM, Zimmerman GA, et al. Engagement of ICAM-3 activates polymorphonuclear leukocytes: Aggregation without degranulation or beta 2 integrin recruitment. *J Immunol* 1998;161:6280–6287.

29. Oseas R, Yang HH, Baehner RL, et al. Lactoferrin: A promoter of polymorphonuclear leukocyte adhesiveness. *Blood* 1981;57:939–945.

30. Boxer LA, Haak RA, Yang HH, et al. Membrane-bound lactoferrin alters the surface properties of polymorphonuclear leukocytes. *J Clin Invest* 1982;70:1049–1057.

31. Plesner T, Ploug M, Ellis V, et al. The receptor for urokinase-type plasminogen activator and urokinase is translocated from two distinct intracellular compartments to the plasma membrane on stimulation of human neutrophils. *Blood* 1994;83:808–815.

32. Bianchi E, Bender JR, Blasi F, et al. Through and beyond the wall: Late steps in leukocyte transendothelial migration. *Immunol Today* 1997;18:586–591.

33. Chapman HA. Plasminogen activators, integrins, and the coordinated regulation of cell adhesion and migration. *Curr Opin Cell Biol* 1997;9:714–724.

34. Fehr J, Moser R, Leppert D, et al. Antiadhesive properties of biological surfaces are protective against stimulated granulocytes. *J Clin Invest* 1985; 76:535–542.

35. Granger DN, Kubes P. The microcirculation and inflammation: Modulation of leukocyte-endothelial cell adhesion. *J Leukoc Biol* 1994;55:662–675.

36. Zaoui P, Barro C, Morel F. Differential expression and secretion of gelatinases and tissue inhibitor of metalloproteinase-1 during neutrophil adhesion. *Biochim Biophys Acta* 1996;1290:101–112.

37. Lorant DE, Topham MK, Whatley RE, et al. Inflammatory roles of P-selectin. *J Clin Invest* 1993;92:559–570.

38. Zimmerman GA, McIntyre TM, Mehra M, et al. Endothelial cell-associated platelet-activating factor: A novel mechanism for signaling intercellular adhesion. *J Cell Biol* 1990;110:529–540.

39. Lorant DE, Patel KD, McIntyre TM, et al. Coexpression of GMP-140 and PAF by endothelium stimulated by histamine or thrombin: A juxtacrine system for adhesion and activation of neutrophils. *J Cell Biol* 1991;115:223–234.

40. Lorant D, McIntyre T, Prescott S, et al. Platelet-activating factor: A signaling molecule for leukocyte adhesion. In Pearson J, ed: *Vascular Adhesion Molecules and Inflammation.* Basel: Birkhauser; 1999:81–107.

41. Hidari KI, Weyrich AS, Zimmerman GA, et al. Engagement of P-selectin glycoprotein ligand-1 enhances tyrosine phosphorylation and activates mitogen-activated protein kinases in human neutrophils. *J Biol Chem* 1997;272:28750–28756.

42. Zimmerman G, Prescott S, McIntyre T. Platelet-activating factor: A fluid-phase and cell-associated mediator of inflammation. In Gallin J, Goldstein I, Snyderman R, eds: *Inflammation: Basic Principles and Clinical Correlates, 2nd ed.* New York: Raven Press; 1992:289–304.

43. Prescott S, McIntyre T, Zimmerman G. Platelet-activating factor: A phospholipid mediator of inflammation. In Gallin J, Snyderman R, eds: *Inflammation: Basic Principles and Clinical Correlates, 3rd ed.* Philadelphia: Lippincott Williams & Wilkins; 1999:387–396.

44. Vercellotti GM, Wickham NW, Gustafson KS, et al. Thrombin-treated endothelium primes neutrophil functions: Inhibition by platelet-activating factor receptor antagonists. *J Leukoc Biol* 1989;45:483–490.
45. Owen CA, Campbell MA, Boukedes SS, et al. Cytokines regulate membrane-bound leukocyte elastase on neutrophils: A novel mechanism for effector activity. *Am J Physiol* 1997;272:L385–393.
46. Dewald B, Baggiolini M. Platelet-activating factor as a stimulus of exocytosis in human neutrophils. *Biochim Biophys Acta* 1986;888:42–48.
47. Weber C, Springer TA. Neutrophil accumulation on activated, surface-adherent platelets in flow is mediated by interaction of Mac-1 with fibrinogen bound to alphaII beta3 and stimulated by platelet-activating factor. *J Clin Invest* 1997;100:2085–2093.
48. Ostrovsky L, King AJ, Bond S, et al. A juxtacrine mechanism for neutrophil adhesion on platelets involves platelet-activating factor and a selectin-dependent activation process. *Blood* 1998;91:3028–3036.
49. Imaizumi T, Albertine KH, Jicha DL, et al. Human endothelial cells synthesize ENA-78: Relationship to IL-8 and to signaling of PMN adhesion. *Am J Respir Cell Mol Biol* 1997;17:181–192.
50. Modur V, Feldhaus MJ, Wyerich AS, et al. Oncostatin M is a proinflammatory mediator: In vitro effects correlate with endothelial cell expression of inflammatory cytokines and adhesion molecules. *J Clin Invest* 1997;100: 158–168.
51. Green SP, Chuntharapai A, Curnutte JT. Interleukin-8 (IL-8), melanoma growth-stimulatory activity, and neutrophil-activating peptide selectively mediate priming of the neutrophil NADPH oxidase through the type A or type B IL-8 receptor. *J Biol Chem* 1996;271:25400–25405.
52. Harlan JM, Killen PD, Harker LA, et al. Neutrophil-mediated endothelial injury: In vitro mechanisms of cell detachment. *J Clin Invest* 1981;68:1394–1403.
53. Harlan JM, Schwartz BR, Reidy MA, et al. Activated neutrophils disrupt endothelial monolayer integrity by an oxygen radical-independent mechanism. *Lab Invest* 1985;52:141–150.
54. Varani J, Ginsburg I, Schuger L, et al. Endothelial cell killing by neutrophils: Synergistic interaction of oxygen products and proteases. *Am J Pathol* 1989;135:435–438.
55. Smedly LA, Tonnesen MG, Sandhaus RA, et al. Neutrophil-mediated injury to endothelial cells: Enhancement by endotoxin and essential role of neutrophil elastase. *J Clin Invest* 1986;77:1233–1243.
56. Zimmerman BJ, Granger DN. Reperfusion-induced leukocyte infiltration: Role of elastase. *Am J Physiol* 1990;259:H390–394.
57. Jochum M, Gippner-Steppert C, Machleidt W, et al. The role of phagocyte proteinases and proteinase inhibitors in multiple organ failure. *Am J Respir Crit Care Med* 1994;150:S123–130.
58. Pyo R, Lee JK, Shipley JM, et al. Targeted gene disruption of matrix metalloproteinase-9 (gelatinase B) suppresses development of experimental abdominal aortic aneurysms. *J Clin Invest* 2000;105:1641–1649.
59. Sundy J, Haynes B. Vasculitis: Pathogenic mechanisms of vessel damage. In Gallin J, Snyderman R, eds: *Inflammation: Basic Principles and Clinical Correlates, 3rd ed.* Philadelphia: Lippincott Williams & Wilkins; 1999:995–1016.
60. McColl S, Naccache P. Crystal-induced arthropathies. In Gallin J, Synderman R, eds: *Inflammation: Basic Principles and Clinical Correlates, 3rd ed.* Philadelphia: Lippincott Williams & Wilkins; 1999:1039–1046.

Chapter 16

Leukocyte Adhesion and Emigration in the Lung

S. Bradley Forlow, PhD, C. Edward Rose, MD, and Klaus Ley, MD

Introduction

Leukocyte recruitment to sites of infection or injury is essential for the immune response and healing, but is damaging when uncontrolled. Leukocyte adhesion is a hallmark of a number of inflammatory diseases including those of the vascular system and the pulmonary circulation. Ischemia-reperfusion injury, for example, after acute coronary occlusion followed by aggressive and successful recanalization therapy, is exacerbated by the influx of neutrophils into the myocardial tissue.[1] Acute lung injury (acute respiratory distress syndrome, ARDS) is largely mediated by neutrophils that migrate into the lung parenchyma and airspace in response to an inflammatory stimulus.[2-5] Asthma is characterized by the influx of lymphocytes and eosinophils into the airway wall and lumen.[6] During pneumonia, neutrophils accumulate in the alveolar spaces of the lungs.[7,8]

To design effective therapeutic interventions aimed at curbing leukocyte recruitment, a solid understanding of the molecular basis of leukocyte recruitment in vivo is necessary. Significant insight into the mediators and mechanisms of leukocyte recruitment has been gained through various in vitro and in vivo models. The use of specific monoclonal antibodies and the generation of leukocyte adhesion molecule-deficient mice have provided valuable information in elucidating the

Supported by NIH HL10447-01 to SBF and NIH HL54136 and HL64381 to KL.

From: Weir EK, Reeve HL, Reeves JT (eds). *Interactions of Blood and the Pulmonary Circulation*. Armonk, NY: Futura Publishing Company, Inc.; ©2002.

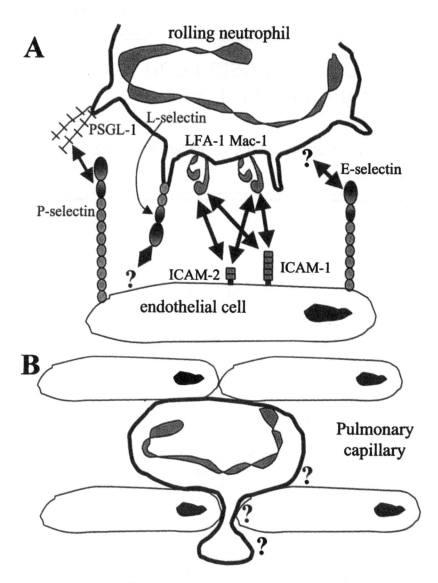

Figure 1. Recruitment of leukocytes in response to inflammatory mediators in the systemic microcirculation is mediated by specific leukocyte adhesion molecules, including P-, E-, and L-selectins, PSGL-1 and other selectin ligands, integrins like LFA-1 and Mac-1, and immunoglobulin-like molecules including ICAM-1 and ICAM-2 (A). Leukocyte sequestration in the pulmonary circulation may be independent of leukocyte adhesion molecules due to the biomechanical properties of leukocytes and the spatial constraints of pulmonary capillaries (B). It is unclear whether this sequestration is sufficient for transmigration (?).

mechanisms of leukocyte recruitment to sites of inflammation. As these insights are used to develop new therapeutics, it is important to consider the balance between anti-inflammatory effects with the requirements of effective host defense.

Leukocyte Recruitment in the Systemic Microcirculation

In the systemic microcirculation, leukocyte recruitment in response to an inflammatory mediator usually occurs in postcapillary venules.[9–11] Leukocyte recruitment to sites of inflammation requires leukocyte capture, rolling, and adhesion on activated endothelial cells. This cascade of events occurs through leukocyte/endothelial cell interactions mediated by several classes of adhesion molecules, including selectins, selectin ligands, integrins, and immunoglobulin-like molecules (Figure 1A).

Selectins

Selectin-Mediated Leukocyte Capture and Rolling

Recruitment of circulating leukocytes in postcapillary venules is initiated by specific adhesion molecule-dependent interactions. Leukocyte capture and rolling are largely mediated by selectins and their ligands.[12–14] The selectin family of adhesion molecules includes P-selectin, E-selectin, and L-selectin. P-selectin and E-selectin are expressed on activated endothelial cells (Figure 1A) in response to various thrombogenic and inflammatory mediators.[15–18] P-selectin is rapidly expressed (within minutes) on the endothelial cell surface following histamine or thrombin.[16,17] In mice, but not in humans, P-selectin is also upregulated by a transcriptional mechanism in response to cytokines. E-selectin expression requires de novo protein synthesis and is maximum between 2 and 6 hours in cultured endothelial cells.[15,19,20] L-selectin is constitutively expressed on most peripheral blood leukocytes, including neutrophils, eosinophils, monocytes, naïve lymphocytes, some natural killer cells, T cells, and B cells.[14]

Mice lacking one or more selectins have revealed unique and overlapping functions of P-, E-, and L-selectin. P-selectin-deficient mice show no leukocyte rolling after trauma-induced inflammation (times <1 hour) and a reduced rolling flux (number of rolling cells/min) after cytokine-stimulated inflammation.[21–26] However, neutrophil recruitment in models of peritonitis (thioglycollate- or *Streptococcus pneumoniae*-induced) is delayed only at 2, 4, and 8 hours and returns to wild-type levels at later times (24–48 hours).[21,26–29] Neutrophil recruitment to the skin is also delayed, not abolished, in the absence of P-selectin.[30,31] Mice lacking E-selectin show elevated leukocyte rolling velocities, increased leukocyte rolling flux, reduced leukocyte adhesion in response to chemoattractants, and impairment of inflammatory function in at least 3 different models.[24,32–34] L-selectin-deficient mice show significant reductions in neutrophil recruitment in several models of inflammation. Leukocyte rolling is impaired in trauma-induced inflammation[22] and cytokine-induced inflammation.[24,25,35] Neutrophil recruitment in thioglycollate-induced peritonitis at 4, 24, and 48 hours is reduced but not eliminated in L-selectin-deficient mice.[36–39] Blocking L-selectin function reduces neutrophil recruitment into sites of acute inflammation in the peritoneal cavity[40,41] and the skin.[42]

In cytokine-induced inflammation, leukocyte rolling is reduced by approximately 90% in E- and P-selectin-deficient mice compared to wild-type mice.[23,25,26,29,35] E- and P-selectin-deficient mice show significantly reduced neutrophil recruitment in *Streptococcus pneumoniae*- and thioglycollate-induced peritonitis models of inflammation at 4 and 8 hours,[23,26,29] but are not different from wild-type mice at 24 hours.[29] P- and L-selectin-deficient mice also show a severe reduction of leukocyte rolling[25,26] and neutrophil accumulation in a peritonitis model.[26] Mice lacking all 3 selectins have a 95% reduction in leukocyte rolling in a cytokine-induced model of inflammation.[25,26] The small population of rolling in E-, P-, and L-selectin triple knockout mice is α_4 integrin-dependent.[25] Mice deficient in all 3 selectins show the most pronounced reduction in neutrophil recruitment in a thioglycollate-induced model of inflammation,[26] indicating that there is a cumulative effect of selectins on efficient neutrophil recruitment.

Distinctive selectin functions are further revealed by the characteristic leukocyte rolling velocities of P-, E-, and L-selectin-mediated leukocyte rolling. Leukocyte rolling mediated by P-selectin occurs at much higher velocities (~20–50 μm/s) than rolling through E-selectin (<10 μm/s).[24,25] L-selectin-mediated leukocyte rolling is very fast, with velocities over 100 μm/s.[43] However, after long-term cytokine treatment, L-selectin can mediate leukocyte rolling at approximately 20 μm/s.[25,35] Rolling velocity is increased by continuous proteolytic shedding of L-selectin.[44,45]

Taken together, these data show that L-selectin and P-selectin largely mediate leukocyte capture in postcapillary venules of the systemic microcirculation. P-selectin is critical for efficient leukocyte rolling during early inflammation (<4 hours). L-selectin largely mediates leukocyte capture, but also has a rolling function after long-term cytokine treatment (>4 hours). E-selectin mediates slow leukocyte rolling, which appears necessary for efficient conversion to firm adhesion in response to chemokines. The selectin-mediated events of leukocyte recruitment are summarized in Table 1.

Table 1

Role of Leukocyte Adhesion Molecules in the Systemic Microcirculation

	Cytokine-Induced Inflammation
P-selectin	Leukocyte capture, stable leukocyte rolling
L-selectin	Leukocyte capture, leukocyte rolling after 4 hours
E-selectin	Slow leukocyte rolling, conversion to firm adhesion
CD18 integrins	Slow leukocyte rolling, conversion to adhesion, firm adhesion, transmigration (?)

Selectin Ligands

P-selectin glycoprotein ligand-1 (PSGL-1) is a well-characterized selectin ligand. PSGL-1 is a type I surface glycoprotein expressed on the tips of microvilli of most leukocytes.[46–49] PSGL-1 binds all 3 selectins in various in vitro assays[47,49–53]; however, it functions predominantly as a P-selectin ligand in vivo[54,55] (Figure 1A). PSGL-1-deficient mice show significant reductions in leukocyte rolling after trauma-induced inflammation, indicating that PSGL-1 is the dominant P-selectin ligand during early inflammation.[55] Leukocyte rolling in mice lacking PSGL-1 is only slightly reduced after cytokine stimulation, and this rolling is E-selectin-dependent.[55] These data show that under in vivo physiological conditions, PSGL-1 is the predominant P-selectin ligand and is not required for leukocyte rolling through E-selectin. The relevant physiological ligands for E-selectin and L-selectin have remained elusive.

Integrins

Integrin-Mediated Firm Adhesion and Transmigration

Firm adhesion and transmigration of leukocytes, following leukocyte activation by chemokines and other chemoattractants, require β_2 integrins (Table 1). The β_2 integrins are heterodimeric molecules composed of an α chain (CD11a, b, c, or d) and a common β chain. LFA-1 (CD11a/CD18) is expressed on all leukocytes.[56] Mac-1 (CD11b/CD18) is expressed exclusively on monocytes and granulocytes.[57] Both LFA-1 and Mac-1 bind to ICAM-1 and ICAM-2 on the endothelium[58,59] (Figure 1A). β_2 integrins change conformation upon cellular activation by a chemokine or chemoattractant. This conformation change is necessary for ligand binding.[60]

CD18 integrins play a vital role in leukocyte adhesion and transmigration in the systemic microcirculation. Leukocyte adhesion deficiency syndrome (LAD I) results from impaired leukocyte adhesion and transmigration due to a lack of CD18 expression.[61] Individuals with LAD I show severe neutrophilia, skin and mucosal lesions, impaired response to infections, and an absence of extravascular neutrophils in infected tissues.[61-63] In animal models, neutrophil emigration into the peritoneum or skin induced by *Streptococcus pneumoniae* or C5a complement fragments is CD18-dependent.[64,65] Neutrophil emigration from the systemic circulation is inhibited using CD18 integrin-blocking antibodies in various models of inflammation.[64-67]

CD18 null mice show severe defects in neutrophil recruitment to the skin, in neutrophil recruitment in thioglycollate-induced peritonitis, and in adhesion in response to chemoattractants.[68-70] LFA-1-deficient mice also show significant reductions in neutrophil accumulation in thioglycollate-induced peritonitis.[71] Neutrophil recruitment in thioglycollate-induced peritonitis in Mac-1-deficient mice is not reduced, indicating that LFA-1 can mediate efficient neutrophil emigration even in the absence of Mac-1.[72]

Immunoglobulin Adhesion Receptors

Intercellular adhesion molecule-1 (ICAM-1, CD54) is constitutively expressed on endothelial cells and is upregulated by cytokine stimulation[73] (Figure 1A). ICAM-1-deficient mice have impaired neutrophil accumulation in thioglycollate- or *Streptococcus pneumoniae*-induced peritonitis models of inflammation.[27,38,39,74] Leukocyte extravasation is attenuated in ICAM-1 mutant mice in the skin in response to an inflammatory challenge.[74] ICAM-2 (CD102) is expressed on resting endothelial cells and not upregulated by inflammatory cytokines. ICAM-2 also is a ligand for LFA-1 and Mac-1[75] (Figure 1A). ICAM-2-deficient mice have no obvious defect in neutrophil recruitment, suggesting that ICAM-2 is not strictly required for leukocyte recruitment in most models.[76]

Platelet-endothelial cell adhesion molecule-1 (PECAM-1, CD31), expressed on platelets, most leukocytes, and at intercellular junctions of endothelial cells,[77,78] is involved in leukocyte emigration through the endothelial cell layer and the perivascular basement membrane.[78,79] Leukocyte extravasation in IL-1β-treated mesenteric microcirculation is reduced by 67% with monoclonal antibody blockade of PECAM-1.[80] These data show that antibodies to PECAM-1 can inhibit the migration of neutrophils through the subendothelial basement membrane. PECAM-1-deficient mice show arrested leukocytes between the vascular endothelium and the basement membrane of mesenteric venules in response to

IL-1β but normal neutrophil recruitment into the peritoneal cavity in response to IL-1β or thioglycollate.[81]

Overlapping Functions of Adhesion Molecules

Recent evidence shows that the functions of selectins and integrins overlap to mediate efficient leukocyte recruitment. CD18-deficient mice have increased leukocyte rolling velocities, which shows that CD18 integrins also participate in leukocyte rolling[82] (Table 1). Leukocyte rolling velocities in these mice are further increased following the administration of an E-selectin antibody, indicating a cooperative function between E-selectin and CD18 integrins.[82] Leukocyte rolling velocities are drastically elevated and strongly influenced by increased wall shear rates in mice deficient in both E-selectin and CD18.[83] These mice show almost no neutrophil adhesion or emigration in the cremaster muscle after cytokine stimulation.[83]

Mice deficient in P-selectin and ICAM-1 show no leukocyte rolling in untreated cremaster venules,[84] have significantly reduced leukocyte rolling and increased rolling velocities after TNF-α treatment compared to mice lacking ICAM-1 and wild-type mice,[84] and lack neutrophil recruitment in a short-term peritonitis model (4 hours).[27] L-selectin/ICAM-1 double mutants also show increased rolling velocities and decreased neutrophil recruitment in various experimental models of inflammation.[38,39] These data suggest that ICAM-1 can be synergistic with the selectins in mediating efficient leukocyte recruitment.

Many models of inflammation have been used to elucidate the mediators and mechanisms of efficient leukocyte recruitment from the systemic microcirculation, including cytokine-induced inflammation of the mouse cremaster muscle and mesentery, bacterially and chemically induced peritonitis, and chemically induced inflammation of skin. It is evident that the mediators and mechanisms of leukocyte recruitment depend on the organ system and the inflammatory stimulus. However, the paradigm of leukocyte recruitment developed from data obtained in model organs such as the mesentery or cremaster muscle does not directly translate to leukocyte recruitment from the pulmonary circulation.

Leukocyte Recruitment in the Pulmonary Circulation

Like the systemic microcirculation, the pulmonary microvasculature is composed of arterioles, venules, and capillaries. Histological studies estimate that the human pulmonary vasculature contains 2.8 ×

10^{11} individual capillary segments.[85] This complex network of individual capillaries contains many interconnecting segments whose diameter is usually smaller than that of spherical neutrophils.[86]

The small diameter of pulmonary capillaries results in increased neutrophil transit times through the pulmonary capillary bed (~26 s) compared to plasma or red blood cells (1.4 s).[86–89] Neutrophils must deform, elongate, and at times stop in order to pass through capillary segments less than approximately 5.3 μm.[86–91] Therefore, even in normal lungs, neutrophil concentrations are 40–100 times higher within the pulmonary capillaries (marginated pool) compared to the systemic microcirculation.[88,92,93]

Despite the importance of selectins and integrins in leukocyte trafficking in the systemic microcirculation, margination of neutrophils in pulmonary capillaries appears to be largely independent of selectins and CD18 integrins, although P-selectin, but not E-selectin, is constitutively expressed on pulmonary arteries, arterioles, venules, and veins.[27,94] Neither P-selectin nor E-selectin are constitutively expressed in pulmonary capillaries or upregulated in response to *Streptococcus pneumoniae* or complement activation by cobra venom factor.[27,94] Levels of marginated neutrophils in the pulmonary circulation are unaffected in mice lacking E- and P-selectin or L-selectin.[95,96] Dogs show no difference in neutrophil margination in the absence of CD18 integrin function.[97]

Unlike the systemic microcirculation, the biomechanical characteristics of pulmonary capillaries and neutrophils allow intimate con-

Table 2

Leukocyte Recruitment in the Pulmonary Microcirculation

Recruitment Process	Mechanism
Margination	Independent of leukocyte adhesion molecules; occurs due to biomechanical properties of neutrophils and physical constraints of capillaries
Initial neutrophil sequestration in response to chemoattractant	Independent of leukocyte adhesion molecules; occurs due to biomechanical properties of neutrophils and physical constraints of capillaries
Continued neutrophil sequestration/ neutrophil adhesion	Partially dependent on L-selectin and CD18 integrins
Neutrophil emigration	Independent of L-selectin; CD18-independent or CD18-mediated, depending on inflammatory stimuli

tact between neutrophils and capillary endothelium via mechanisms other than leukocyte adhesion molecules (Figure 1B). Therefore, margination of neutrophils in the lungs most likely results from restricted neutrophil passage through the pulmonary circulation due to the physical characteristics of neutrophils and the space constraints of the capillaries (Table 2).

Leukocyte Adhesion Molecules in Lung Inflammation

After placement of a thoracic window, neutrophils can be seen to roll in pulmonary arterioles and venules.[90,98] Fucoidin, a carbohydrate inhibitor of P- and L-selectin, inhibits neutrophil rolling in arterioles and venules, indicating that selectins mediate rolling in pulmonary microvessels other than capillaries.[90] Despite leukocyte rolling in pulmonary venules and arterioles, no leukocyte rolling occurs within the pulmonary capillaries,[90,98] likely due to spatial constraints of the capillaries and the lack of E- and P-selectin expression.[86,99] However, in contrast to the systemic microcirculation, where leukocyte adhesion and emigration occur in postcapillary venules, neutrophil adhesion and emigration in the pulmonary microcirculation occur primarily within the capillaries.[8,9,100–102]

Adhesion Molecule-Independent Neutrophil Sequestration

In the pulmonary circulation, the first response to inflammatory mediators such as complement fragment C5a, IL-8, PAF, LTB4, fMLP, LPS, or TNF-α is the sequestration of neutrophils within pulmonary capillaries.[103–106] Neutrophil sequestration occurs very rapidly (within less than 1 minute) following the administration of an inflammatory mediator. This initial inflammatory event is independent of leukocyte adhesion molecules that mediate rolling, adhesion, and emigration in the systemic microcirculation.[107] Neutrophil sequestration in response to complement C5a is not altered by inhibition or absence of selectins (monoclonal antibodies, fucoidin, selectin-deficient mice) or CD18 integrins, but sequestration in response to fMLP requires L-selectin.[95,96,108,109,141]

Leukocyte adhesion molecule-independent neutrophil sequestration in pulmonary capillaries induced by inflammation is thought to be mediated by the biomechanical and physical properties that affect neutrophil trafficking in narrow capillaries. Neutrophils stimulated with inflammatory mediators transiently stiffen and lose their ability to deform.[93,110,111]

Neutrophil stiffening in response to inflammatory mediators results from increased polymerization of actin.[91,93,110] Ultrastructural immunohistochemical studies show a redistribution of actin from the central, perinuclear regions of intracapillary neutrophils to the peripheral regions under the cell membrane in response to complement C5a.[91] In vitro, the pressure required to pass neutrophils through 5-μm pores is increased following C5a stimulation.[110,112,113] Rabbit neutrophils show a lack of shape change (loss of deformability) in pulmonary capillaries immediately following C5a treatment.[91] The biomechanical changes that decrease neutrophil deformability do not allow neutrophil passage through pulmonary capillaries and appear to mediate the initial sequestration in response to inflammatory mediators (Figure 1B). Neutrophils regain increased deformability even in the continued presence of inflammatory stimuli after 15–20 minutes.[91,114] Although it is clear that these transient biomechanical changes contribute to immediate neutrophil sequestration, the process of subsequent emigration is not well understood (Table 2).

Neutrophil Adhesion and Emigration in the Pulmonary Microcirculation

Although in most cases leukocyte adhesion molecules do not play a role in the initial sequestration of neutrophils in the pulmonary capillaries, this may depend on the chemoattractant used. Recently, we have found that L-selectin is required for the sequestration of neutrophils in the lung in response to formyl peptide, but not C5a.[141] In addition, adhesion molecules partially mediate the continued sequestration. The initial neutrophil sequestration in response to complement fragments is not altered in mice treated with fucoidin or an anti-CD18 antibody; however, circulating neutrophil numbers recover more rapidly than in untreated mice.[108] L-selectin-deficient mice show decreased intracapillary neutrophil numbers after 5 minutes following complement fragment injection.[96] These data show that interactions of CD18 integrins and L-selectin with their endothelial ligands are necessary to maintain prolonged sequestration of neutrophils in the pulmonary capillaries.[96,97,108,115] Following neutrophil sequestration, neutrophil adhesion and emigration in the pulmonary circulation occur largely through the pulmonary capillaries.[8,9,100–102] L-selectin function is necessary for sustained intracapillary accumulation of neutrophils but is not required for emigration of neutrophils.[96]

In the pulmonary microcirculation, the role of CD18 integrins in neutrophil adhesion and emigration is strongly stimulus-dependent (Table 3). The complex role of CD18 integrins as mediators of neutrophil re-

Table 3

Role of CD18 Integrins in Leukocyte Recruitment to the Lung

CD18-Mediated Neutrophil Adhesion and Emigration	CD18-Independent Neutrophil Adhesion and Emigration
Escherichia coli	*Streptococcus pneumoniae*
Pseudomonas aeruginosa	group B *Streptococcus*
E. coli lipopolysaccharide (LPS)	*Staphylococcus aureus*
IgG immune complexes	hydrochloric acid
interleukin-1α	hyperoxia
phorbol myristate acetate	complement C5a

cruitment is shown by LAD I patients who show no neutrophil emigration into infected skin lesions, but some can recruit neutrophils to alveolar spaces.[64,116,117] CD18-mediated neutrophil adhesion and emigration occur in response to *Escherichia coli*, *Pseudomonas aeruginosa*, *E. coli* lipopolysaccharide (LPS), IgG immune complexes, interleukin-1α, and phorbol myristate acetate.[64,65,118–123] However, neutrophil adhesion and emigration initiated by *Streptococcus pneumoniae*, group B *Streptococcus*, *Staphylococcus aureus*, hydrochloric acid, hyperoxia, and C5a elicit CD18-independent adhesion and emigration mechanisms.[64,65,118–123] Recent in vitro assays show that neutrophil migration across human pulmonary artery endothelial cells is CD18-independent in response to IL-8 and leukotriene B$_4$, but CD18-dependent in response to formyl-methionyl-leucyl-phenylalanine (fMLP).[124] The induction of CD18-dependent or CD18-independent pathways of neutrophil adhesion and emigration may be linked to the differential effects of inflammatory stimuli on ICAM-1 expression. *E. coli*- or *Pseudomonas aeruginosa*-induced pneumonias increase ICAM-1 mRNA by 2 hours; however, no upregulation occurs when *S. pneumoniae* is administered.[125] Likewise, ICAM-1 expression is enhanced on pulmonary capillary endothelial cells in response to *E. coli* LPS but not *S. pneumoniae*.[125]

The molecular mechanisms mediating CD18-independent adhesion and emigration pathways remain unknown. Neutrophil adhesion and emigration independent of CD18 integrins do not depend on selectins. Neutrophil emigration is unchanged in response to *S. pneumoniae* in E- and P-selectin-deficient mice or following fucoidin administration to block L- and P-selectin function.[95] Upregulation of CD18-independent neutrophil adhesion and emigration possibly requires cytokines and/or chemokines produced by alveolar macrophages. A CD18-independent adhesion and recruitment mechanism is also observed in peritoneum primed 1–2 days previously by thioglycollate administration.[126] However, it is unclear whether this mechanism is similar to the CD18-independent recruitment mechanism in the lung.

Selectin-Mediated Leukocyte Recruitment in the Pulmonary Circulation

Unlike the systemic microcirculation, selectins are not required for the initiation of the inflammatory response in the pulmonary vasculature. However, selectins may play an important role in lung inflammation through mechanisms other than leukocyte capture and rolling. Antibody studies in rats show that CD18, ICAM-1, L-selectin, and P-selectin are required for full development of acute lung injury induced by complement activation in response to cobra venom factor.[94,127–130] Selectin inhibitors may diminish neutrophil emigration to the alveolar space in response to alveolar deposition of IgG immune complexes.[131,132]

The mechanisms of selectin-mediated leukocyte recruitment in the pulmonary circulation are not well defined, but might involve the small population of leukocytes recruited through pulmonary venules and/or arterioles. L-selectin is required for neutrophil accumulation within noncapillary microvessels after complement fragment injection.[96] The requirement of selectins in neutrophil accumulation depends on the inflammatory stimulus. Neutrophil accumulation within noncapillary microvessels is decreased in L-selectin-deficient mice in response to *E. coli* or *S. pneumoniae* and within pulmonary capillaries in response to *E. coli* but not *S. pneumoniae*.[96] In response to *S. pneumoniae*, mice deficient in E- and P-selectin show increased neutrophil tethering and spreading in noncapillary microvessels, suggesting that these events can be mediated independent of selectins.[95] Neutrophil emigration into the alveoli is unaffected in response to *S. pneumoniae* in mice lacking E-selectin and P-selectin with L-selectin function blocked.[95] However, selectins appear to be necessary for maximal pulmonary emigration of neutrophils in response to alveolar deposition of IgG immune complexes in rats,[132] bacterial LPS or IL-1 in rats,[133] and phorbol ester in rabbits.[134] Interestingly, these mediators elicit a CD18-independent pathway while *S. pneumoniae* elicits a CD18-dependent pathway. The extent of selectin involvement in lung inflammation processes might, therefore, also be dependent on the inflammatory stimuli.

Leukocyte adhesion molecules have been investigated largely in animal models of pneumonia induced by intratracheal administration of LPS or live bacteria.[27,95,96,118,135] Only a few studies have investigated leukocyte adhesion molecule function in animal models of systemic endotoxemia.[37,136,137] Kamochi et al. investigated the role of P-selectin and

ICAM-1 in a model of systemic endotoxemia resulting from intraperitoneal LPS.[137] In this model, lung injury is attenuated and mortality delayed in mice deficient in P-selectin and ICAM-1,[137] suggesting that P-selectin and ICAM-1 contribute significantly to lung injury after systemic endotoxemia. However, P-selectin/ICAM-1 double mutant mice are not protected from lung vascular albumin leak in response to intratracheal administration of *S. pneumoniae*[27] or intravenous administration of cobra venom factor.[94]

It appears that both the stimulus and the model of inflammation invoke recruitment mechanisms that are regulated by differential leukocyte adhesion molecule expression and/or function. Cytokine upregulation in the lung also varies depending on the mode of administration. *Salmonella typhosa* LPS administered intratracheally to rats induces a progressive increase in lung IL-1β mRNA 1, 2, and 4 hours after administration.[138] In contrast, IL-1β expression in the lung peaks at 1 hour after IV *S. typhosa* LPS.[138] Intratracheal injection of *S. typhosa* LPS results in significant accumulation of neutrophils 4 hours after administration and maximum neutrophil accumulation at 12 hours.[138] However, neutrophils do not appear in the bronchoalveolar lavage fluid until 24 hours after interperitoneal or intravenous injection of LPS.[139,140] These data show that the adhesion molecule-dependent leukocyte recruitment pathways used are dependent on the inflammatory stimulus and the mode of administration, both of which influence cytokine expression.

Conclusion

Despite the expression and involvement of identical leukocyte adhesion molecules, the mechanisms of leukocyte recruitment in the systemic microcirculation and pulmonary circulation differ greatly. Site- and stimulus-specific leukocyte adhesion molecule-mediated inflammatory pathways add complexity to inflammation in the pulmonary circulation. Although the existence of CD18-independent pathways of neutrophil recruitment have been known for more than 10 years,[64] and selectin-independent pathways were shown as early as 1996,[95] no significant progress has been made in defining the molecular mechanisms of neutrophil recruitment in the lung. It is possible that neutrophil recruitment in the lung to some stimuli may not require adhesion molecules at all, but it is equally likely that other adhesion pathways remain to be discovered. Interestingly, beneficial effects of selectin blockade, CD18 blockade, or ICAM-1 blockade have been observed in models of ARDS and pathological lung inflammation. These findings suggest that intervention with these adhesion molecules can curb lung damage although their mechanism of action remains unknown.

Acknowledgments: We thank Tim Olson for critically reviewing the manuscript. We would like to acknowledge funding provided by National Institutes of Health Grants HL10447–01 to SBF and HL54136 and HL64381 to KL.

References

1. Lefer AM. Role of the beta2-integrins and immunoglobulin superfamily members in myocardial ischemia-reperfusion. *Ann Thorac Surg* 1999;68: 1920–1923.

2. Downey GP, Granton JT. Mechanisms of acute lung injury. *Curr Opinion Pulmon Med* 1997;3:234–241.

3. Sachdeva RC, Guntupalli KK. Acute respiratory distress syndrome. *Crit Care Clin* 1997;13:503–521.

4. Weiland JE, Davis WB, Holter JF, et al. Lung neutrophils in the adult respiratory distress syndrome: Clinical and pathophysiologic significance. *Am Rev Respir Dis* 1986;133:218–225.

5. Brigham KL, Meyrick B. Interactions of granulocytes with the lungs. *Circ Res* 1984;54:623–635.

6. MacLean JA, Ownbey R, Luster AD. T cell-dependent regulation of eotaxin in antigen-induced pulmonary eosinophila. *J Exp Med* 1996;184:1461–1469.

7. Gunn FD, Nungester WJ. Pathogenesis and histopathology of experimental pneumonia in rats. *Arch Pathol* 1936;21:813–830.

8. Downey GP, Worthen GS, Henson PM, et al. Neutrophil sequestration and migration in localized pulmonary inflammation: Capillary localization and migration across the interalveolar septum. *Am Rev Respir Dis* 1993;147:168–176.

9. Marchesi VT. The site of leucocyte emigration during inflammation. *Q J Exp Physiol* 1961;46:115–118.

10. Atherton A, Born GV. Quantitative investigations of the adhesiveness of circulating polymorphonuclear leucocytes to blood vessel walls. *J Physiol* 1972;222:447–474.

11. Ley K, Gaehtgens P. Endothelial, not hemodynamic, differences are responsible for preferential leukocyte rolling in rat mesenteric venules. *Circ Res* 1991;69:1034–1041.

12. Butcher EC. Leukocyte-endothelial cell recognition: Three (or more) steps to specificity and diversity. *Cell* 1991;67:1033–1036.

13. Ley K, Tedder TF. Leukocyte interactions with vascular endothelium: New insights into selectin-mediated attachment and rolling. *J Immunol* 1995;155:525–528.

14. Kansas GS. Selectins and their ligands: Current concepts and controversies. *Blood* 1996;88:3259–3287.

15. Bevilacqua MP, Stengelin S, Gimbrone MAJ, et al. Endothelial leukocyte adhesion molecule 1: An inducible receptor for neutrophils related to complement regulatory proteins and lectins. *Science* 1989;243:1160–1165.

16. Hattori R, Hamilton KK, Fugate RD, et al. Stimulated secretion of endothelial von Willebrand factor is accompanied by rapid redistribution to the cell surface of the intracellular granule membrane protein GMP-140. *J Biol Chem* 1989;264:7768–7771.

17. Lorant DE, Patel KD, McIntyre TM, et al. Coexpression of GMP-140 and PAF by endothelium stimulated by histamine or thrombin: A juxtacrine system for adhesion and activation of neutrophils. *J Cell Biol* 1991;115:223–234.

18. Patel KD, Zimmerman GA, Prescott SM, et al. Oxygen radicals induce human endothelial cells to express GMP-140 and bind neutrophils. *J Cell Biol* 1991;112:749–759.

19. Subramaniam M, Koedam JA, Wagner DD. Divergent fates of P- and E-selectins after their expression on the plasma membrane. *Molec Biol Cell* 1993;4:791–801.

20. Henseleit U, Steinbrink K, Goebeler M, et al. E-selectin expression in experimental models of inflammation in mice. *J Pathol* 1996;180:317–325.

21. Mayadas TN, Johnson RC, Rayburn H, et al. Leukocyte rolling and extravasation are severely compromised in P-selectin-deficient mice. *Cell* 1993;74:541–554.

22. Ley K, Bullard DC, Arbones ML, et al. Sequential contribution of L- and P-selectin to leukocyte rolling in vivo. *J Exp Med* 1995;181:669–675.

23. Frenette PS, Mayadas TN, Rayburn H, et al. Susceptibility to infection and altered hematopoiesis in mice deficient in both P- and E-selectins. *Cell* 1996;84:563–574.

24. Kunkel EJ, Ley K. Distinct phenotype of E-selectin-deficient mice: E-selectin is required for slow leukocyte rolling in vivo. *Circ Res* 1996;79:1196–1204.

25. Jung U, Ley K. Mice lacking two or all three selectins demonstrate overlapping and distinct functions for each selectin. *J Immunol* 1999;162:6755–6762.

26. Robinson SD, Frenette PS, Rayburn H, et al. Multiple, targeted deficiencies in selectins reveal a predominant role for P-selectin in leukocyte recruitment. *Proc Natl Acad Sci USA* 1999;96:11452–11457.

27. Bullard DC, Qin L, Lorenzo I, et al. P-selectin/ICAM-1 double mutant mice: Acute emigration of neutrophils into the peritoneum is completely absent but is normal into pulmonary alveoli. *J Clin Invest* 1995;95:1782–1788.

28. Johnson RC, Mayadas TN, Frenette PS, et al. Blood cell dynamics in P-selectin-deficient mice. *Blood* 1995;86:1106–1114.

29. Bullard DC, Kunkel EJ, Kubo H, et al. Infectious susceptibility and severe deficiency of leukocyte rolling and recruitment in E-selectin and P-selectin double mutant mice. *J Exp Med* 1996;183:2329–2336.

30. Subramaniam M, Saffaripour S, Watson SR, et al. Reduced recruitment of inflammatory cells in a contact hypersensitivity response in P-selectin-deficient mice. *J Exp Med* 1995;181:2277–2282.

31. Staite ND, Justen JM, Sly LM, et al. Inhibition of delayed-type contact hypersensitivity in mice deficient in both E-selectin and P-selectin. *Blood* 1996;88:2973–2979.

32. Munoz FM, Hawkins EP, Bullard DC, et al. Host defense against systemic infection with *Streptococcus pneumoniae* is impaired in E-, P-, and E-/P-selectin-deficient mice. *J Clin Invest* 1997;100:2099–2106.

33. Ley K, Allietta M, Bullard DC, et al. Importance of E-selectin for firm leukocyte adhesion in vivo. *Circ Res* 1998;83:287–294.

34. Milstone DS, Fukumura D, Padgett RC, et al. Mice lacking E-selectin show normal numbers of rolling leukocytes but reduced leukocyte stable arrest on cytokine-activated microvascular endothelium. *Microcirculation* 1998; 5:153–171.

35. Jung U, Ramos CL, Bullard DC, et al. Gene-targeted mice reveal importance of L-selectin-dependent rolling for neutrophil adhesion. *Am J Physiol* 1998;274:H1785–H1791.

36. Arbones ML, Ord DC, Ley K, et al. Lymphocyte homing and leukocyte rolling and migration are impaired in L-selectin-deficient mice. *Immunity* 1994;1:247–260.

37. Tedder TF, Steeber DA, Pizcueta P. L-selectin-deficient mice have impaired leukocyte recruitment into inflammatory sites. *J Exp Med* 1995;181: 2259–2264.

38. Steeber DA, Tang ML, Green NE, et al. Leukocyte entry into sites of inflammation requires overlapping interactions between the L-selectin and ICAM-1 pathways. *J Immunol* 1999;163:2176–2186.

39. Steeber DA, Campbell MA, Basit A, et al. Optimal selectin-mediated rolling of leukocytes during inflammation in vivo requires intercellular adhesion molecule-1 expression. *Proc Natl Acad Sci USA* 1998;95:7562–7567.

40. Jutila MA, Berg EL, Kishimoto TK, et al. Inflammation-induced endothelial cell adhesion to lymphocytes, neutrophils, and monocytes: Role of homing receptors and other adhesion molecules. *Transplantation* 1989;48:727–731.

41. Watson SR, Fennie C, Lasky LA. Neutrophil influx into an inflammatory site inhibited by a soluble homing receptor-IgG chimaera. *Nature* 1991; 349:164–167.

42. Lewinsohn DM, Bargatze RF, Butcher EC. Leukocyte-endothelial cell recognition: Evidence of a common molecular mechanism shared by neutrophils, lymphocytes, and other leukocytes. *J Immunol* 1987;138:4313–4321.

43. Jung U, Bullard DC, Tedder TF, et al. Velocity differences between L- and P-selectin-dependent neutrophil rolling in venules of mouse cremaster muscle in vivo. *Am J Physiol* 1996;271:H2740–H2747.

44. Walcheck B, Kahn J, Fisher JM, et al. Neutrophil rolling altered by inhibition of L-selectin shedding in vitro. *Nature* 1996;380:720–723.

45. Hafezi-Moghadam A, Ley K. Relevance of L-selectin shedding for leukocyte rolling in vivo. *J Exp Med* 1999;189:939–948.

46. Moore KL, Stults NL, Diaz S, et al. Identification of a specific glycoprotein ligand for P-selectin (CD62) on myeloid cells. *J Cell Biol* 1992;118:445–456.

47. Sako D, Chang XJ, Barone KM, et al. Expression cloning of a functional glycoprotein ligand for P-selectin. *Cell* 1993;75:1179–1186.

48. Laszik Z, Jansen PJ, Cummings RD, et al. P-selectin glycoprotein ligand-1 is broadly expressed in cells of myeloid, lymphoid, and dendritic lineage and in some nonhematopoietic cells. *Blood* 1996;88:3010–3021.

49. Moore KL, Patel KD, Bruehl RE, et al. P-selectin glycoprotein ligand-1 mediates rolling of human neutrophils on P-selectin. *J Cell Biol* 1995;128: 661–671.

50. Guyer DA, Moore KL, Lynam EB, et al. P-selectin glycoprotein ligand-1 (PSGL-1) is a ligand for L-selectin in neutrophil aggregation. *Blood* 1996; 88:2415–2421.

51. Alon R, Fuhlbrigge RC, Finger EB, et al. Interactions through L-selectin between leukocytes and adherent leukocytes nucleate rolling adhesions on selectins and VCAM-1 in shear flow. *J Cell Biol* 1996;135:849–865.

52. Walcheck B, Moore KL, McEver RP, et al. Neutrophil-neutrophil interactions under hydrodynamic shear stress involve L-selectin and PSGL-1: A mechanism that amplifies initial leukocyte accumulation of P-selectin in vitro. *J Clin Invest* 1996;98:1081–1087.

53. Goetz DJ, Greif DM, Ding H, et al. Isolated P-selectin glycoprotein ligand-1 dynamic adhesion to P- and E-selectin. *J Cell Biol* 1997;137:509–519.

54. Borges E, Eytner R, Moll T, et al. The P-selectin glycoprotein ligand-1 is important for recruitment of neutrophils into inflamed mouse peritoneum. *Blood* 1997;90:1934–1942.

55. Yang J, Hirata T, Croce K, et al. Targeted gene disruption demonstrates that P-selectin glycoprotein ligand-1 (PSGL-1) is required for P-selectin-

mediated but not E-selectin-mediated neutrophil rolling and migration. *J Exp Med* 1999;190:1769–1782.

56. Krensky AM, Sanchez-Madrid F, Robbins E, et al. The functional significance, distribution, and structure of LFA-1, LFA-2, and LFA-3: Cell surface antigens associated with CTL-target interactions. *J Immunol* 1983;131: 611–616.

57. Springer T, Galfre G, Secher DS, et al. Mac-1: A macrophage differentiation antigen identified by monoclonal antibody. *Eur J Immunol* 1979;9:301–306.

58. Marlin SD, Springer TA. Purified intercellular adhesion molecule-1 (ICAM-1) is a ligand for lymphocyte function-associated antigen 1 (LFA-1). *Cell* 1987;51:813–819.

59. Staunton DE, Dustin ML, Springer TA. Functional cloning of ICAM-2, a cell adhesion ligand for LFA-1 homologous to ICAM-1. *Nature* 1989;339:61–64.

60. Hughes PE, Pfaff M. Integrin affinity modulation. *Trends Cell Biol* 1998;8: 359–364.

61. Anderson DC, Springer TA. Leukocyte adhesion deficiency: An inherited defect in the Mac-1, LFA-1, and p150,95 glycoproteins. *Annu Rev Med* 1987;38:175–194.

62. Anderson DC, Schmalsteig FC, Finegold MJ, et al. The severe and moderate phenotypes of heritable Mac-1, LFA-1 deficiency: Their quantitative definition and relation to leukocyte dysfunction and clinical features. *J Infectious Dis* 1985;152:668–689.

63. Harlan JM. Leukocyte adhesion deficiency syndrome: Insights into the molecular basis of leukocyte emigration. *Clin Immunol Immunopathol* 1993; 67:S16–S24.

64. Doerschuk CM, Winn RK, Coxson HO, et al. CD18-dependent and -independent mechanisms of neutrophil emigration in the pulmonary and systemic microcirculation of rabbits. *J Immunol* 1990;144:2327–2333.

65. Hellewell PG, Young SK, Henson PM, et al. Disparate role of the beta 2-integrin CD18 in the local accumulation of neutrophils in pulmonary and cutaneous inflammation in the rabbit. *Am J Respir Cell Mol Biol* 1994;10:391–398.

66. Arfors KE, Lundberg C, Lindbom L, et al. A monoclonal antibody to the membrane glycoprotein complex CD18 inhibits polymorphonuclear leukocyte accumulation and plasma leakage in vivo. *Blood* 1987;69:338–340.

67. Price TH, Beatty PG, Corpuz SR. In vivo inhibition of neutrophil function in the rabbit using monoclonal antibody to CD18. *J Immunol* 1987;139: 4174–4177.

68. Scharffetter-Kochanek K, Lu H, Norman K, et al. Spontaneous skin ulceration and defective T cell function in CD18 null mice. *J Exp Med* 1998;188: 119–131.

69. Walzog B, Scharffetter-Kochanek K, Gaehtgens P. Impairment of neutrophil emigration in CD18-null mice. *Am J Physiol* 1999;276:G1125–G1130.

70. Mizgerd JP, Kubo H, Kutkoski GJ, et al. Neutrophil emigration in the skin, lungs, and peritoneum: Different requirements for CD11/CD18 revealed by CD18-deficient mice. *J Exp Med* 1997;186:1357–1364.

71. Schmits R, Kundig TM, Baker DM, et al. LFA-1-deficient mice show normal CTL responses to virus but fail to reject immunogenic tumor. *J Exp Med* 1996;183:1415–1426.

72. Lu H, Smith CW, Perrard J, et al. LFA-1 is sufficient in mediating neutrophil emigration in Mac-1-deficient mice. *J Clin Invest* 1997;99:1340–1350.

73. Dustin ML, Rothlein R, Bhan AK, et al. Induction by IL-1 and interferon-

gamma: Tissue distribution, biochemistry, and function of a natural adherence molecule (ICAM-1). *J Immunol* 1986;137:245–254.

74. Sligh JE, Ballantyne CM, Rich SS, et al. Inflammatory and immune responses are impaired in mice deficient in intercellular adhesion molecule 1. *Proc Natl Acad Sci USA* 1993;90:8529–8533.

75. Issekutz AC, Rowter D, Springer TA. Role of ICAM-1 and ICAM-2 and alternate CD11/CD18 ligands in neutrophil transendothelial migration. *J Leuk Biol* 1999;65:117–126.

76. Gerwin N, Gonzalo JA, Lloyd C, et al. Prolonged eosinophil accumulation in allergic lung interstitium of ICAM-2-deficient mice results in extended hyperresponsiveness. *Immunity* 1999;10:9–19.

77. Newman PJ, Berndt MC, Gorski J, et al. PECAM-1 (CD31) cloning and relation to adhesion molecules of the immunoglobulin gene superfamily. *Science* 1990;247:1219–1222.

78. Simmons DL, Walker C, Power C, et al. Molecular cloning of CD31, a putative intercellular adhesion molecule closely related to carcinoembryonic antigen. *J Exp Med* 1990;171:2147–2152.

79. Vaporciyan AA, DeLisser HM, Yan HC, et al. Involvement of platelet-endothelial cell adhesion molecule-1 in neutrophil recruitment in vivo. *Science* 1993;262:1580–1582.

80. Thompson RD, Wakelin MW, Larbi KY, et al. Divergent effects of platelet-endothelial cell adhesion molecule-1 and beta 3 integrin blockade on leukocyte transmigration in vivo. *J Immunol* 2000;165:426–434.

81. Duncan GS, Andrew DP, Takimoto H, et al. Genetic evidence for functional redundancy of platelet/endothelial cell adhesion molecule-1 (PECAM-1): CD31-deficient mice reveal PECAM-1-dependent and PECAM-1-independent functions. *J Immunol* 1999;162:3022–3030.

82. Jung U, Norman KE, Scharffetter-Kochanek K, et al. Transit time of leukocytes rolling through venules controls cytokine-induced inflammatory cell recruitment in vivo. *J Clin Invest* 1998;102:1526–1533.

83. Forlow SB, White EJ, Lu H, et al. Severe inflammatory defect and reduced viability in CD18 and E-selectin double mutant mice. 2000;106:1457–1466.

84. Kunkel EJ, Jung U, Bullard DC, et al. Absence of trauma-induced leukocyte rolling in mice deficient in both P-selectin and intercellular adhesion molecule 1. *J Exp Med* 1996;183:57–65.

85. Weibel ER. *Morphometry of the Human Lung.* New York: Academic; 1963: 73–89.

86. Doerschuk CM, Beyers N, Coxson HO, et al. Comparison of neutrophil and capillary diameters and their relation to neutrophil sequestration in the lung. *J Appl Physiol* 1993;74:3040–3045.

87. Martin BA, Wright JL, Thommasen H, et al. Effect of pulmonary blood flow on the exchange between the circulating and marginating pool of polymorphonuclear leukocytes in dog lungs. *J Clin Invest* 1982;69:1277–1285.

88. Lien DC, Wagner WWJ, Capen RL, et al. Physiological neutrophil sequestration in the lung: Visual evidence for localization in capillaries. *J Appl Physiol* 1987;62:1236–1243.

89. Hogg JC, McLean T, Martin BA, et al. Erythrocyte transit and neutrophil concentration in the dog lung. *J Appl Physiol* 1988;65:1217–1225.

90. Gebb SA, Graham JA, Hanger CC, et al. Sites of leukocyte sequestration in the pulmonary microcirculation. *J Appl Physiol* 1995;79:493–497.

91. Motosugi H, Graham L, Noblitt TW, et al. Changes in neutrophil actin and shape during sequestration induced by complement fragments in rabbits. *Am J Pathol* 1996;149:963–973.

92. Hogg JC. Neutrophil kinetics and lung injury. *Physiol Rev* 1987;67:1249–1295.
93. Hogg JC, Doerschuk CM. Leukocyte traffic in the lung. *Annu Rev Physiol* 1995;57:97–114.
94. Doerschuk CM, Quinlan WM, Doyle NA, et al. The role of P-selectin and ICAM-1 in acute lung injury as determined using blocking antibodies and mutant mice. *J Immunol* 1996;157:4609–4614.
95. Mizgerd JP, Meek BB, Kutkoski GJ, et al. Selectins and neutrophil traffic: Margination and *Streptococcus pneumoniae*-induced emigration in murine lungs. *J Exp Med* 1996;184:639–645.
96. Doyle NA, Bhagwan SD, Meek BB, et al. Neutrophil margination, sequestration, and emigration in the lungs of L-selectin-deficient mice. *J Clin Invest* 1997;99:526–533.
97. Yoder MC, Checkley LL, Giger U, et al. Pulmonary microcirculatory kinetics of neutrophils deficient in leukocyte adhesion-promoting glycoproteins. *J Appl Physiol* 1990;69:207–213.
98. Kuebler WM, Kuhnle GE, Groh J, et al. Leukocyte kinetics in pulmonary microcirculation: Intravital fluorescence microscopic study. *J Appl Physiol* 1994;76:65–71.
99. Wiggs BR, English D, Quinlan WM, et al. Contributions of capillary pathway size and neutrophil deformability to neutrophil transit through rabbit lungs. *J Appl Physiol* 1994;77:463–470.
100. Loosli CG, Baker RF. Acute experimental pneumococcal (type I) pneumonia in the mouse: The migration of leucocytes from the pulmonary capillaries into the alveolar spaces as revealed by the electron microscope. *Trans Am Clin Climatol Assoc* 1962;74:15–28.
101. Shaw JO. Leukocytes in chemotactic-fragment-induced lung inflammation: Vascular emigration and alveolar surface migration. *Am J Pathol* 1980;101:283–302.
102. Doerschuk CM, Markos J, Coxson HO, et al. Quantitation of neutrophil migration in acute bacterial pneumonia in rabbits. *J Appl Physiol* 1994;77: 2593–2599.
103. Doerschuk CM. Neutrophil rheology and transit through capillaries and sinusoids. *Am J Respir Crit Care Med* 1999;159:1693–1695.
104. Kubo H, Graham L, Doyle NA, et al. Complement fragment-induced release of neutrophils from bone marrow and sequestration within pulmonary capillaries in rabbits. *Blood* 1998;92:283–290.
105. Doerschuk CM, Allard MF, Hogg JC. Neutrophil kinetics in rabbits during infusion of zymosan-activated plasma. *J App Physiol* 1989;67:88–95.
106. Gupta S, Feng L, Yoshimura T, et al. Intra-alveolar macrophage-inflammatory peptide 2 induces rapid neutrophil localization in the lung. *Am J Respir Cell Mol Biol* 1996;15:656–663.
107. Gebb SA, Graham JA, Hanger CC, et al. Sites of leukocyte sequestration in the pulmonary microcirculation. *J Appl Physiol* 1995;79:493–497.
108. Kubo H, Doyle NA, Graham L, et al. L- and P-selectin and CD11/CD18 in intracapillary neutrophil sequestration in rabbit lungs. *Am J Respir Crit Care Med* 1999;159:267–274.
109. Lundberg C, Wright SD. Relation of the CD11/CD18 family of leukocyte antigens to the transient neutropenia caused by chemoattractants. *Blood* 1990;76:1240–1245.
110. Worthen GS, Schwab B, Elson EL, et al. Mechanics of stimulated neutrophils: Cell stiffening induces retention in capillaries. *Science* 1989;245:183–186.
111. Westlin WF, Kiely JM, Gimbrone MA, Jr. Interleukin-8 induces changes in human neutrophil actin conformation and distribution: Relationship to

inhibition of adhesion to cytokine-activated endothelium. *J Leuk Biol* 1992; 52:43–51.

112. Downey GP, Worthen GS. Neutrophil retention in model capillaries: Deformability, geometry, and hydrodynamic forces. *J Appl Physiol* 1988;65: 1861–1871.

113. Selby C, Drost E, Wraith PK, et al. In vivo neutrophil sequestration within lungs of humans is determined by in vitro "filterability." *J Appl Physiol* 1991;71:1996–2003.

114. Pecsvarady Z, Fisher TC, Fabok A, et al. Kinetics of granulocyte deformability following exposure to chemotactic stimuli. *Blood Cells* 1992;18:333–352.

115. Doerschuk CM. The role of CD18-mediated adhesion in neutrophil sequestration induced by infusion of activated plasma in rabbits. *Am J Respir Cell Mol Biol* 1992;7:140–148.

116. Hawkins HK, Heffelfinger SC, Anderson DC. Leukocyte adhesion deficiency: Clinical and postmortem observations. *Pediatr Pathol* 1992;12:119–130.

117. van Garderen E, Muller KE, Wentink GH, et al. Post-mortem findings in calves suffering from bovine leukocyte adhesion deficiency (BLAD). *Veterinary Quarterly* 1994;16:24–26.

118. Qin L, Quinlan WM, Doyle NA, et al. The roles of CD11/CD18 and ICAM-1 in acute *Pseudomonas aeruginosa*-induced pneumonia in mice. *J Immunol* 1996;157:5016–5021.

119. Ramamoorthy C, Sasaki SS, Su DL, et al. CD18 adhesion blockade decreases bacterial clearance and neutrophil recruitment after intrapulmonary *E. coli*, but not after *S. aureus*. *J Leuk Biol* 1997;61:167–172.

120. Motosugi H, Quinlan WM, Bree M, et al. Role of CD11b in focal acid-induced pneumonia and contralateral lung injury in rats. *Am J Respir Crit Care Med* 1998;157:192–198.

121. Sherman MP, Johnson JT, Rothlein R, et al. Role of pulmonary phagocytes in host defense against group B streptococci in preterm versus term rabbit lung. *J Infect Dis* 1992;166:818–826.

122. Keeney SE, Mathews MJ, Haque AK, et al. Oxygen-induced lung injury in the guinea pig proceeds through CD18-independent mechanisms. *Am J Respir Crit Care Med* 1994;149:311–319.

123. Mulligan MS, Wilson GP, Todd RF, et al. Role of beta 1, beta 2 integrins and ICAM-1 in lung injury after deposition of IgG and IgA immune complexes. *J Immunol* 1993;150:2407–2417.

124. Mackarel AJ, Russell KJ, Brady CS, et al. Interleukin-8 and leukotriene-B4, but not formylmethionyl leucyphenylalanine, stimulate CD18-independent migration of neutrophils across human pulmonary endothelial cells in vitro. *Am J Respir Cell Mol Biol* 2000;23:154–161.

125. Burns AR, Takei F, Doerschuk CM. Quantitation of ICAM-1 expression in mouse lung during pneumonia. *J Immunol* 1994;153:3189–3198.

126. Mileski W, Harlan J, Rice C, et al. *Streptococcus pneumoniae*-stimulated macrophages induce neutrophils to emigrate by a CD18-independent mechanism of adherence. *Circ Shock* 1990;31:259–267.

127. Mulligan MS, Varani J, Warren JS, et al. Roles of beta 2 integrins of rat neutrophils in complement- and oxygen radical-mediated acute inflammatory injury. *J Immunol* 1992;148:1847–1857.

128. Mulligan MS, Smith CW, Anderson DC, et al. Role of leukocyte adhesion molecules in complement-induced lung injury. *J Immunol* 1993;150:2401–2406.

129. Mulligan MS, Polley MJ, Bayer RJ, et al. Neutrophil-dependent acute lung injury: Requirement for P-selectin (GMP-140). *J Clin Invest* 1992;90:1600–1607.
130. Albelda SM, Smith CW, Ward PA. Adhesion molecules and inflammatory injury. *FASEB J* 1994;8:504–512.
131. Mulligan MS, Miyasaka M, Tamatani T, et al. Requirements for L-selectin in neutrophil-mediated lung injury in rats. *J Immunol* 1994;152:832–840.
132. Mulligan MS, Varani J, Dame MK, et al. Role of endothelial-leukocyte adhesion molecule 1 (ELAM-1) in neutrophil-mediated lung injury in rats. *J Clin Invest* 1991;88:1396–1406.
133. Ulich TR, Howard SC, Remick DG, et al. Intratracheal administration of endotoxin and cytokines: VIII. LPS induces E-selectin expression; Anti-E-selectin and soluble E-selectin inhibit acute inflammation. *Inflammation* 1994;18:389–398.
134. Shimaoka M, Ikeda M, Iida T, et al. Fucoidin, a potent inhibitor of leukocyte rolling, prevents neutrophil influx into phorbol-ester-induced inflammatory sites in rabbit lungs. *Am J Respir Crit Care Med* 1996;153:307–311.
135. Kumasaka T, Quinlan WM, Doyle NA, et al. Role of the intercellular adhesion molecule-1 (ICAM-1) in endotoxin-induced pneumonia evaluated using ICAM-1 antisense oligonucleotides, anti-ICAM-1 monoclonal antibodies, and ICAM-1 mutant mice. *J Clin Invest* 1996;97:2362–2369.
136. Xu H, Gonzalo JA, St. Pierre Y, et al. Leukocytosis and resistance to septic shock in intercellular adhesion molecule 1-deficient mice. *J Exp Med* 1994; 180:95–109.
137. Kamochi M, Kamochi F, Kim YB, et al. P-selectin and ICAM-1 mediate endotoxin-induced neutrophil recruitment and injury to the lung and liver. *Am J Physiol* 1999;277:L310–L319.
138. Ulich TR, Watson LR, Yin SM, et al. The intratracheal administration of endotoxin and cytokines: I. Characterization of LPS-induced IL-1 and TNF mRNA expression and the LPS-, IL-1-, and TNF-induced inflammatory infiltrate. *Am J Pathol* 1991;138:1485–1496.
139. Chang JC, Lesser M. Quantitation of leukocytes in bronchoalveolar lavage samples from rats after intravascular injection of endotoxin. *Am Rev Respir Dis* 1984;129:72–75.
140. Rinaldo JE, Dauber JH, Christman J, et al. Neutrophil alveolitis following endotoxemia: Enhancement by previous exposure to hyperoxia. *Am Rev Respir Dis* 1984;130:1065–1071.
141. Olson TS, Singbartl K, Ley K. L-selectin is required for fMLP but not C5a-induced sequestration of neutrophils in the pulmonary circulation. *Am J Physiol: Regulatory, Integrative and Comparative Physiology.* In press.

Chapter 17

In Vitro Regulation of Leukocyte Diapedesis by the Endothelial Cell Contractile Apparatus

Keri N. Jacobs, BS, Irina Petrache, MD, Joe G.N. Garcia, MD

Introduction

The vascular endothelium has historically been viewed as a passive, inert barrier to circulating macromolecules and leukocytes. However, over the past 2 decades, the characterization of the remarkable role of the endothelium in cytokine release, barrier regulation, and the elaboration of key components involved in both coagulation and fibrinolytic cascades has been recognized. In this regard, a key feature of both acute and chronic inflammatory processes is the coordinated migration of leukocytes across the vascular endothelium into inflamed or infected tissues. This neutrophil diapedesis occurs in response to the spatially defined elaboration of a wide array of chemotactic factors including leukotriene B_4 (LTB$_4$), C5A, interleukin-8 (IL-8), etc., within interstitial areas that attract leukocytes to specific sites within the affected organ. The interaction of circulating leukocytes with the vascular endothelium under dynamic conditions of flow within vessels of varying size is a highly complex process and has proven exceptionally difficult to precisely model. However, the development of intravital microscopy allowing in situ visualization of leukocyte-endothelial cell interaction, the ready availability of cultured endothelial cells, and the easy isolation of blood-derived human polymorphonuclear leukocytes has greatly facilitated our understanding of these important events.

From: Weir EK, Reeve HL, Reeves JT (eds). *Interactions of Blood and the Pulmonary Circulation*. Armonk, NY: Futura Publishing Company, Inc.; ©2002.

Circulating neutrophils adhere to the endothelium, which allows them to be activated, flatten, and emigrate across the vascular endothelium. Most aspects of leukocyte-endothelial cell interaction with attendant rolling, adhesion, and transendothelial migration have been characterized in the systemic vasculature, but are also referable to the unique pulmonary circulation. However, work by Hogg and Doerschuk[9,26] has clearly demonstrated that unlike the systemic circulation, where neutrophil extravasation occurs in the postcapillary venules, leukocyte diapedesis in the pulmonary circulation occurs predominantly through the capillary walls where the average diameter is ~ 10 μM, suggesting an additional physical barrier to neutrophil rolling and adhesion with a significant emphasis on the stiffness of the circulating polymorphonuclear leukocytes (PMNs) as well as the recipient endothelial cells. Indeed, neutrophil trafficking in the pulmonary circulation appears to involve both adhesion molecule-dependent and -independent pathways.[4] The latter pathway, coupled to the intimate cell-cell interaction between leukocyte and endothelial cell, clearly suggested to a number of investigators that the endothelial cell might actively participate in this essential feature of inflammation. Indeed, within the past decade, both eosinophil and lymphocyte diapedesis have likewise been appreciated to be highly dependent on endothelial cell responsiveness and activation.

While the molecular determinants that regulate neutrophil-endothelial cell adhesion interaction have been extensively evaluated, there is actually very little information on the mechanisms by which neutrophils actually traverse the endothelial cell barrier. While it would appear that neutrophils are capable of initiating this process by the insertion of filopodia-like processes into forming endothelial cell caveolae or vesiculo-vacuolar organelles,[12,33] a paracellular route for diapedesis is the predominant opinion at this time with migration through endothelial cell-cell junctions. Regardless of whether this occurs via paracellular or transcellular mechanisms, the regulation of endothelial-specific paracellular gap regulation and barrier responses is now recognized as dependent on the signal transduction pathways that modulate the activity of the endothelial cell cytoskeleton (Figure 1), a complex array of structural filaments. The key components include (1) actin/myosin-containing microfilaments, (2) the hollow, rigid microtubule structures that are dependent on tubulin assembly/disassembly, and (3) desmin- and vimentin-enriched intermediate filaments. Although recent studies also implicate microtubule dynamic rearrangement in regulation of leukocyte trafficking,[7] in this brief review, we will focus on the role of the endothelial cell microfilamentous cytoskeleton (for which the greatest information is known) in the regulation of leukocyte diapedesis.

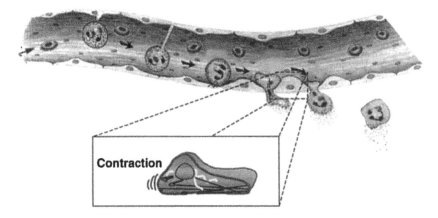

Figure 1. Mechanisms of PMN-induced endothelial cell contraction. After the initial phases of neutrophil rolling and adhesion, the PMNs cause activation of the endothelial cell cytoskeleton, resulting in an increase in actin stress fibers (black), rearrangement of the microtubules (white), and activation of the actin-myosin contractile apparatus with subsequent endothelial cell contraction and rounding.

Role of Neutrophil-Evoked Endothelial Ca^{2+} Transients in Leukocyte Migration

That endothelium can be an active participant in leukocyte trafficking was not always a widely held view and, in our opinion, Vercellotti et al. advanced the initial observation that suggested an active role for the vascular endothelium in leukocyte migration into tissues.[47,48] This was significantly extended subsequently by the Silverstein laboratory, where a rise in endothelial cell cytosolic Ca^{2+} in response to fMLP-mediated PMN migration was first described.[27] In this latter study, this Ca^{2+} transient was demonstrated to be a critical signaling event to subsequent PMN migration, as Ca^{2+} chelation of the PMN-induced endothelial cell Ca^{2+} response abolished the subsequent endothelium chemoattractant-induced neutrophil migration.[27] The mechanism by which PMN interaction with the surface of the endothelium elicits this increase in endothelial cell cytosolic Ca^{2+} was unclear, and the exact endothelial signaling pathways evoked in response to PMN-mediated increases in endothelial cell Ca^{++}, which would facilitate PMN diapedesis, were not defined. However, this group[13] and others[43] reasoned that PMN-endothelial cell interaction in the presence of a chemotactic gradient could produce a Ca^{2+}-dependent opening of the intercellular junction, a phenomenon first reported by Majno[6,31] and later Simionescu,[40] in response to bioactive agents. In situ light microscopy studies subsequently clearly confirmed paracellular functional endothelial permeability in response to substance

P.[24,32] Using primarily in vitro techniques, we had initially demonstrated similar paracellular gap formation in response to thrombin,[14,18] reactive oxygen species,[23] phorbol esters,[41] and pertussis toxin,[34,35] and had implicated actomyosin contractile properties in paracellular gap formation and subsequent enhanced vascular permeability.[17,42] Furthermore, since we demonstrated that the level of myosin light chain phosphorylation in endothelial cells was a key determinant of centripetal tension development and cell contraction/retraction,[14] we and others speculated that in PMN-stimulated endothelium, the activation of the endothelial cell contractile apparatus by Ca^{2+}-dependent pathways would be a primary determinant of paracellular gap formation and hence leukocyte diapedesis.

Role of Endothelial Contractile Elements in Leukocyte Diapedesis

A key bioregulatory molecule of smooth muscle and nonmuscle contraction is the Ca^{2+}/calmodulin-dependent Ser/Thr kinase known as myosin light chain kinase (MLCK). We previously cloned the 214 kD myosin light chain kinase from human endothelium EC MLCK,[15] subsequently identifying several EC MLCK splice variants in human tissues, which we have extensively characterized biochemically.[3,21,30,39,49] To assess the role of endothelial cell myosin light chain (MLC) phosphorylation in PMN diapedesis, we first enhanced the level of EC MLCK phosphorylation using thrombin, a potent activator of EC MLCK,[14,39] and calyculin, a Ser/Thr phosphatase inhibitor that produces marked increases in phosphorylated MLC[50] (Figure 2). Both strategies resulted in marked paracellular gap formation and significantly enhanced transendothelial cell PMN migration in response to the abluminally placed neutrophil chemoattractant LTB_4.[19] Alternatively, strategies to reduce MLC phosphorylation, either by direct EC MLCK inhibition or indirectly by elevation in intracellular cAMP concentrations, produced marked attenuation of the PMN chemotactic response (Figure 2). These results were highly consistent with the notion that the level of MLC phosphorylation as determined by PMN-mediated EC MLCK activation served as a key determinant of junctional integrity and hence PMN migration.[38] We next determined that the actual physical PMN-endothelial cell interaction, in the presence of LTB_4, substantially increased MLC phosphorylation in endothelium from a basal stoichiometry of 0.4 mol PO_4/mol MLC to ~1.1 mol/mol in the presence of LTB_4-stimulated transendothelial neutrophil migration, whereas LTB_4 alone did not alter basal levels of MLC phosphorylation in endothelium.[19] These results were subsequently confirmed by Saito et al. (Figure 3), using immunofluorescent microscopy, which demonstrated a marked increase in PMN-mediated

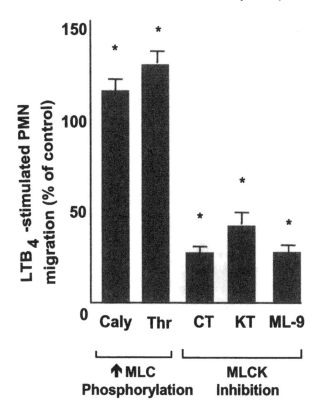

Figure 2. Role of MLC phosphorylation in PMN migration. Calyculin (10 nM) and thrombin (100 ng/mL) significantly increase PMN migration in response to chemotactic stimuli, both of which increase MLC phosphorylation by inhibiting Ser/Thr phosphatases and by activating MLCK, respectively. Cholera toxin (1 μg/mL), KT-5926 (4 μM), and ML-9 (10 μM) attenuate the increase in PMN migration through inactivation of MLCK.

endothelial cell actin and myosin rearrangement in conjunction with prominent stress fiber formation (in the presence of LTB$_4$),[38] which is very consistent with the increase in MLC phosphorylation we noted. Furthermore, the role of EC MLCK activation was substantiated by pharmacological studies utilizing MLCK inhibitors, Ca^{2+} chelation, and calmodulin antagonists.[19,38] The Silverstein laboratory provided highly convincing biophysical confirmation of the hypothesis that the endothelial cell contractile apparatus is activated by PMN-endothelial cell interaction. Specifically, they demonstrated that endothelial cell contraction occurs as a consequence of fMLP-stimulated PMN interaction by actual measurements of endothelial cell tension development as well as increased MLC phosphorylation.[25] Interestingly, the biochemical and biophysical events present in fMLP-stimulated PMN-endothelial cell inter-

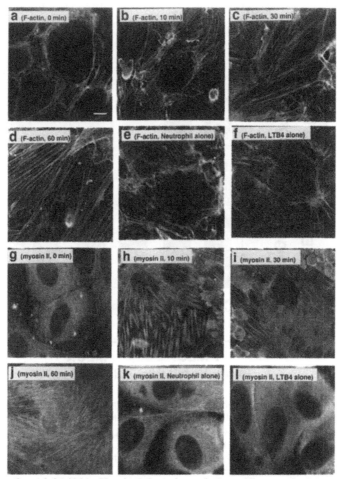

Copyright 1998. The American Association of Immunologists.

Figure 3. Immunofluorescence labeling of endothelial F-actin and myosin II during neutrophil transendothelial migration. Time course of redistribution of F-actin (a-f) and myosin (g-l) is shown. F-actin was visualized by rhodamine-phalloidin staining. Myosin II was visualized by indirect immunostaining with anti-M II pAb followed by rhodamine-labeled anti-rabbit IgG pAb. Panels a and g were images obtained in the absence of neutrophils and LTB_4 (controls). Panels e and k show effects of neutrophils alone; f and l show effects of LTB_4 alone. Panels b and h, c and i, d and j depict the image at 10, 30, and 60 minutes, respectively. A rim of F-actin staining was present at the margins of control cells with a few randomly disoriented stress fibers within the cytoplasm (a). Myosin II was diffusely localized within the cytoplasm and exhibited no organized pattern in control cells (g). Neutrophils alone and LTB_4 alone caused a slight increase in actin filaments (e and f), but did not cause any change in the distribution of myosin II (k and l). During neutrophil transendothelial migration, both F-actin (b-d) and myosin II (h-j) underwent progressive redistribution forming organized filamentous networks. Bar, 10 μm. Reprinted with permission of *The Journal of Immunology,* 1998;161:1533–1540.

actions occurred with a nearly identical time course to the increases in endothelial cell MLC phosphorylation that we observed in the course of LTB$_4$-mediated PMN-transendothelial migration.

Adherent Neutrophils Induce Endothelial Cell Stiffness After Tumor Necrosis Factor Pretreatment

Additional studies have confirmed a vital role for the endothelial cell contractile apparatus in regulating PMN diapedesis. For example, Wang et al., in the Doerschuk laboratory, measured endothelial cell stiffness as reflected by twisting magnetic cytometry and found that PMN interaction with tumor necrosis factor (TNF)-stimulated endothelial cells produces prompt increases in endothelial cell stiffness,[51,52] a putative reflection of cytoskeletal reorganization. In this biophysical model, a significant role for ICAM ligation was determined,[52] findings that are similar to studies of transendothelial lymphocyte diapedesis.[45] Furthermore, the PMN-induced endothelial cell stiffness was dependent on reactive oxygen species (ROS) generation and required an intact endothelial cell cytoskeleton.[52] Comparisons between the TNF-treated endothelial cell stiffened model were made to the LTB$_4$- or fMLP-stimulated PMN model of transendothelial migration described above, where endothelial cell MLC phosphorylation and MLCK activity were increased and critically involved in transendothelial PMN migration. Unlike the LTB$_4$ or fMLP diapedesis models, PMN interactions with TNF-treated endothelium failed to elicit an increase in endothelial cell MLC phosphorylation, and endothelial cell MLCK inhibition did not alter PMN-mediated endothelial cell stiffness[51] although they unequivocally confirm the requirement of an intact cytoskeleton for the cell-cell contractile response.

These intriguing data appear to conflict with the role of MLC phosphorylation in leukocyte diapedesis in the LTB$_4$ and fMLP models. We have considered this conflict and have identified obvious important differences in these models of leukocyte-endothelial cell interaction and chemotaxis, which may explain the discrepant results. One difference is that, in general, in both the LTB$_4$ and fMLP chemoattractant models, PMNs are migrating in response to a specified chemoattractant gradient. In contrast, the biophysical-defined cell stiffness that occurs in the TNF-pretreated endothelial cell model, after PMN exposure, does not utilize a chemoattractant gradient but rather measures the direct effects of PMN-endothelial cell interaction by use of integrin-coated magnetic beads. A second important and relevant confounder in the TNF-pretreated biophysical model is the direct effect of TNF on the endothelium. In addition to its induction of ICAM expression, we recently determined that TNF directly stimulates significant

EC MLCK activity beginning at 1 hour and persisting for up to 5 hours,[36] subsequently declining to basal levels. The rise in MLC phosphorylation elicited by TNF was abolished by either MLCK or Rho kinase inhibition. The role of Rho GTPases in endothelial cell MLC phosphorylation and cytoskeletal rearrangement is well recognized.[11,20,46] Rho kinase, an effector for Rho GTPase, phosphorylates the regulatory subunit of myosin phosphatase, thereby enhancing the level of MLC phosphorylation.[28,29] Rho kinase can also directly phosphorylate MLC at Ser-19.[1,28] The role of Rho GTPases in cytoskeletal rearrangement was confirmed by studies using toxin B, a cell-permeable agent that inhibits Rho family GTPases (Rho, Rac, and CDC42) by glycosylation of the enzyme. Thus, the likelihood exists that PMN-endothelial cell interaction in endothelium treated with TNF for 20 hours differs considerably from the acute response of untreated endothelium to LTB_4- or fMLP-mediated PMN migration. What is clear is that both models provide relevant information on contractile/cytoskeletal involvement in leukocyte diapedesis. Further studies examining the regulation of the PMN-stimulated endothelial cell contractile apparatus will undoubtedly lead to better understanding of the role of the endothelial cell cytoskeleton as gatekeeper of inflammation.

Potential Cytoskeletal Targets for Paracellular Gap Formation After PMN-Mediated Endothelial Cell Activation

While the Ca^{2+}-dependent activation of the contractile apparatus is crucial for PMN-induced EC paracellular gap formation, another key feature of this phenomenon is the loss of adherens junction stability (Figure 4). Endothelial cell barrier integrity is mediated primarily by the homotypic binding of VE-cadherin between adjacent endothelial cells, which is associated with a complex of actin binding proteins including β-catenin, α-catenin, and γ-catenin (plakoglobin). This complex binds to and anchors the actin network, allowing the cells to maintain shape and barrier function under normal conditions. Modulation of the phosphorylation status of these proteins alters barrier function and consequently the cadherins and catenins serve as key targets for numerous signaling pathways. Several known barrier disrupting agents, such as thrombin and histamine, have been shown to increase β-catenin or VE-cadherin phosphorylation,[2,37] as well as producing cell contraction through activation of the actomyosin contractile apparatus.[16,17,22] However, the increased permeability that occurs after vascular endothelial growth factor stimulation, through MLC-independent pathways, also produces an increase in adherens junction protein phosphorylation, suggesting the im-

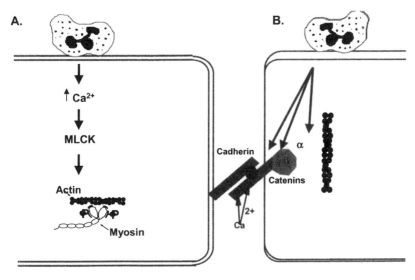

Figure 4. Hypothetical pathways of leukocyte-dependent endothelial cell activation and paracellular gap formation. Panel A demonstrates the PMN-induced Ca^{2+}-dependent signaling cascade involving the rapid increase in cyotsolic calcium, activation of MLCK, followed by MLC phosphorylation and EC contraction. Panel B demonstrates the processes involved in dissociation of adherens junctions and subsequent loss of barrier function after stimulation with chemotractant-stimulated PMNs.

portance of this pathway in EC barrier dysfunction.[5,10] Interestingly, activated PMNs cause a profound increase in β-catenin and VE-cadherin tyrosine phosphorylation[44] and a loss of adherens junction complexes as determined by immunofluorescence and immunoprecipitation studies,[8] occurring in a time frame consistent with increased albumin flux and activation of the contractile apparatus previously discussed. These data suggest that the endothelial cell cytoskeleton and associated proteins play an even more prominent role in PMN diapedesis and inflammation than initially hypothesized. The ability of neutrophils to induce multiple pathways leading to EC gap formation supports the paracellular versus transcellular pathway of PMN migration through the endothelium.

Summary

Vascular leak and tissue edema have been implicated in numerous disease states and have been the focus of a significant amount of scientific research; however, the mechanism by which the endothelial barrier becomes dysfunctional has yet to be completely elucidated. We have discussed here the essential role of the endothelium itself in the initiation and propagation of PMN diapedesis into underlying tissues as well as the fundamental role of the endothelial cell-neutrophil inter-action. These processes are critically dependent on the activity of the cytoskeleton and the activation of the actomyosin contractile appara-tus. It has been clearly demonstrated that attachment of chemotactic-stimulated PMNs to endothelial cell monolayers causes a rapid pro-gression of signaling cascades involving an increase in cytosolic Ca^{2+}, prompt activation of MLCK with subsequent MLC phosphorylation, and increased tension development. In addition, stress fiber formation and dissolution of the filamentous cortical actin ring accompany these events. Inhibitor studies utilizing Ca^{2+} chelators, direct and indirect mechanisms to block MLCK activation, and stabilization of the actin cy-toskeleton by phallocidin demonstrate a marked decline in PMN dia-pedesis, data that emphasize the importance of the cytoskeleton in the processes leading to inflammation.

It is now obvious that the coordinated events leading to PMN re-cruitment, attachment, activation, and extravasation rely heavily on the signaling pathways of the endothelium. Actomyosin-contractile appara-tus activation is an essential mechanism by which neutrophils cause paracellular gap formation; however, PMNs also exert their effects on cy-toskeletal adherens junction proteins, resulting in increased EC perme-ability. It is through these processes that leukocytes are able to transverse the endothelium and enter sites of infection or injury that may eventu-ally lead to edema or life-threatening organ damage if left uncontrolled. With a better understanding of the molecular in vitro mechanisms of PMN diapedesis, therapies and preventive measures to control the ad-verse effects of the inflammatory process may be forthcoming.

Acknowledgments: The authors gratefully acknowledge the contributions of Drs. Qin Wang and Claire M. Doerschuk.

References

1. Amano M, Ito M, Kimura K, et al. Phosphorylation and activation of myosin by Rho-associated kinase (Rho-kinase). *J Biol Chem* 1996;271:20246-20249.
2. Andriopoulou P, Navarro P, Zanetti A, et al. Histamine induces tyrosine phosphorylation of endothelial cell-to-cell adherens junctions. *Arterioscler Thromb Vasc Biol* 1999;19:2286-2297.
3. Birukov KG, Csortos C, Marzilli L, et al. Differential regulation of alter-natively spliced endothelial cell myosin light chain kinase isoforms by p60Src. *J Biol Chem* 2000;11:11.
4. Burns AR, Doerschuk CM. Quantitation of L-selectin and CD18 expression on rabbit neutrophils during CD18-independent and CD18-dependent emigration in the lung. *J Immunol* 1994;153:3177-3188.
5. Cohen AW, Carbajal JM, Schaeffer RC. VEGF stimulates tyrosine phos-phorylation of beta-catenin and small-pore endothelial barrier dysfunc-tion. *Am J Physiol* 1999;277:H2038-2049.

6. Cotran RS, Majno G. Studies on the intercellular junctions of mesothelium and endothelium. *Protoplasma* 1967;63:45–51.

7. Cronstein BN, Molad Y, Reibman J, et al. Colchicine alters the quantitative and qualitative display of selectins on endothelial cells and neutrophils. *J Clin Invest* 1995;96:994–1002.

8. Del Maschio A, Zanetti A, Corada M, et al. Polymorphonuclear leukocyte adhesion triggers the disorganization of endothelial cell-to-cell adherens junctions. *J Cell Biol* 1996;135:497–510.

9. Doerschuk CM, Beyers N, Coxson HO, et al. Comparison of neutrophil and capillary diameters and their relation to neutrophil sequestration in the lung. *J Appl Physiol* 1993;74:3040–3045.

10. Esser S, Lampugnani MG, Corada M, et al. Vascular endothelial growth factor induces VE-cadherin tyrosine phosphorylation in endothelial cells. *J Cell Sci* 1998;111:1853–1865.

11. Essler M, Hermann K, Amano M, et al. Pasteurella multocida toxin increases endothelial permeability via Rho kinase and myosin light chain phosphatase. *J Immunol* 1998;161:5640–5646.

12. Feng D, Flaumenhaft R, Bandeira-Melo C, et al. Ultrastructural localization of vesicle-associated membrane protein(s) to specialized membrane structures in human pericytes, vascular smooth muscle cells, endothelial cells, neutrophils, and eosinophils. *J Histochem Cytochem* 2001;49: 293–304.

13. Furie MB, Naprstek BL, Silverstein SC. Migration of neutrophils across monolayers of cultured microvascular endothelial cells: An in vitro model of leucocyte extravasation. *J Cell Sci* 1987;88:161–175.

14. Garcia JG, Davis HW, Patterson CE. Regulation of endothelial cell gap formation and barrier dysfunction: Role of myosin light chain phosphorylation. *J Cell Physiol* 1995;163:510–522.

15. Garcia JG, Lazar V, Gilbert-McClain LI, et al. Myosin light chain kinase in endothelium: Molecular cloning and regulation. *Am J Respir Cell Mol Biol* 1997;16:489–494.

16. Garcia JG, Pavalko FM, Patterson CE. Vascular endothelial cell activation and permeability responses to thrombin. *Blood Coagul Fibrinolysis* 1995;6: 609–626.

17. Garcia JG, Schaphorst KL. Regulation of endothelial cell gap formation and paracellular permeability. *J Investig Med* 1995;43:117–126.

18. Garcia JG, Siflinger-Birnboim A, Bizios R, et al. Thrombin-induced increase in albumin permeability across the endothelium. *J Cell Physiol* 1986;96:104.

19. Garcia JG, Verin AD, Herenyiova M, English D. Adherent neutrophils activate endothelial myosin light chain kinase: Role in transendothelial migration. *J Appl Physiol* 1998;84:1817–1821.

20. Garcia JG, Verin AD, Schaphorst K, et al. Regulation of endothelial cell myosin light chain kinase by Rho, cortactin, and p60(src). *Am J Physiol* 1999;276:L989–998.

21. Gilbert-McClain LI, Verin AD, Shi S, et al. Regulation of endothelial cell myosin light chain phosphorylation and permeability by vanadate. *J Cell Biochem* 1998;70:141–155.

22. Goeckeler ZM, Wysolmerski RB. Myosin light chain kinase-regulated endothelial cell contraction: The relationship between isometric tension, actin polymerization, and myosin phosphorylation. *J Cell Biol* 1995;130:613–627.

23. Hart CM, Andreoli SP, Patterson CE, Garcia JG. Oleic acid supplementation

reduces oxidant-mediated dysfunction of cultured porcine pulmonary artery endothelial cells. *J Cell Physiol* 1993;156:24–34.

24. Hirata A, Baluk P, Fujiwara T, McDonald DM. Location of focal silver staining at endothelial gaps in inflamed venules examined by scanning electron microscopy. *Am J Physiol* 1995;269:L403–418.

25. Hixenbaugh EA, Goeckeler ZM, Papaiya NN, et al. Stimulated neutrophils induce myosin light chain phosphorylation and isometric tension in endothelial cells. *Am J Physiol* 1997;273:H981–988.

26. Hogg JC, Doerschuk CM. Leukocyte traffic in the lung. *Annu Rev Physiol* 1995;57:97–114.

27. Huang AJ, Manning JE, Bandak TM, et al. Endothelial cell cytosolic free calcium regulates neutrophil migration across monolayers of endothelial cells. *J Cell Biol* 1993;120:1371–1380.

28. Kawano Y, Fukata Y, Oshiro N, et al. Phosphorylation of myosin-binding subunit (MBS) of myosin phosphatase by Rho-kinase in vivo. *J Cell Biol* 1999;147:1023–1038.

29. Kimura K, Ito M, Amano M, et al. Regulation of myosin phosphatase by Rho and Rho-associated kinase (Rho-kinase). *Science* 1996;273:245–248.

30. Lazar V, Garcia JG. A single human myosin light chain kinase gene (MLCK; MYLK). *Genomics* 1999;57:256–267.

31. Majno G, Joris I. Endothelium 1977: A review. *Adv Exp Med Biol* 1978;104: 169–225.

32. McDonald DM. Endothelial gaps and permeability of venules in rat tracheas exposed to inflammatory stimuli. *Am J Physiol* 1994;266:L61–83.

33. Minshall RD, Tiruppathi C, Vogel SM, et al. Endothelial cell-surface gp60 activates vesicle formation and trafficking via G(i)-coupled Src kinase signaling pathway. *J Cell Biol* 2000;150:1057–1070.

34. Patterson CE, Garcia JG. Regulation of thrombin-induced endothelial cell activation by bacterial toxins. *Blood Coagul Fibrinolysis* 1994;5:63–72.

35. Patterson CE, Stasek JE, Schaphorst KL, et al. Mechanisms of pertussis toxin-induced barrier dysfunction in bovine pulmonary artery endothelial cell monolayers. *Am J Physiol* 1995;268:L926–934.

36. Petrache I, Verin AD, Crow MT, et al. Differential effect of MLC kinase in TNF-α-induced endothelial cell apoptosis and barrier dysfunction. *Am J Physiol Lung Cell Mol Physiol* 2001;280:L1168–1178.

37. Rabiet MJ, Plantier JL, Rival Y, et al. Thrombin-induced increase in endothelial permeability is associated with changes in cell-to-cell junction organization. *Arterioscler Thromb Vasc Biol* 1996;16:488–496.

38. Saito H, Minamiya Y, Kitamura M, et al. Endothelial myosin light chain kinase regulates neutrophil migration across human umbilical vein endothelial cell monolayer. *J Immunol* 1998;161:1533–1540.

39. Shi S, Verin AD, Schaphorst KL, et al. Role of tyrosine phosphorylation in thrombin-induced endothelial cell contraction and barrier function. *Endothelium* 1998;6:153–171.

40. Simionescu M, Simionescu N. Proatherosclerotic events: Pathobiochemical changes occurring in the arterial wall before monocyte migration. *Faseb J* 1993;7:1359–1366.

41. Stasek JE, Garcia JG. The role of protein kinase C in alpha-thrombin-mediated endothelial cell activation. *Semin Thromb Hemost* 1992;18:117–125.

42. Stasek JE, Patterson CE, Garcia JG. Protein kinase C phosphorylates caldesmon77 and vimentin and enhances albumin permeability across cultured bovine pulmonary artery endothelial cell monolayers. *J Cell Physiol* 1992;153:62–75.

43. Su WH, Chen HI, Huang JP, Jen CJ. Endothelial [Ca(2+)](i) signaling during transmigration of polymorphonuclear leukocytes. *Blood* 2000;96:3816–3822.
44. Tinsley JH, Wu MH, Ma W, et al. Activated neutrophils induce hyperpermeability and phosphorylation of adherens junction proteins in coronary venular endothelial cells. *J Biol Chem* 1999;274:24930-24934.
45. Vachula M, Van Epps DE. In vitro models of lymphocyte transendothelial migration. *Invasion Metastasis* 1992;12:66–81.
46. van Nieuw Amerongen GP, Vermeer MA, van Hinsbergh VW. Role of RhoA and Rho kinase in lysophosphatidic acid-induced endothelial barrier dysfunction. *Arterioscler Thromb Vasc Biol* 2000;20:E127–133.
47. Vercellotti GM, McCarthy J, Furcht LT, et al. Inflamed fibronectin: An altered fibronectin enhances neutrophil adhesion. *Blood* 1983;62:1063–1069.
48. Vercellotti GM, Wickham NW, Gustafson KS, et al. Thrombin-treated endothelium primes neutrophil functions: Inhibition by platelet-activating factor receptor antagonists. *J Leukoc Biol* 1989;45:483–490.
49. Verin AD, Lazar V, Torry RJ, et al. Expression of a novel high molecular weight myosin light chain kinase in endothelium. *Am J Respir Cell Mol Biol* 1998;19:758–766.
50. Verin AD, Patterson CE, Day MA, Garcia JG. Regulation of endothelial cell gap formation and barrier function by myosin-associated phosphatase activities. *Am J Physiol* 1995;269:L99–108.
51. Wang Q, Chiang ET, Lim M, et al. Changes in the biomechanical properties of neutrophils and endothelial cells during adhesion. *Blood* 2001;97:660–668.
52. Wang Q, Doerschuk CM. Neutrophil-induced changes in the biomechanical properties of endothelial cells: Roles of ICAM-1 and reactive oxygen species. *J Immunol* 2000;164:6487–6494.

Chapter 18

Neutrophil Sequestration and Migration in Lung Microvessels:
Influence of Neutrophil Heterogeneity

Stephan F. van Eeden MD, PhD

Introduction

Neutrophils are essential for host defense, but they also mediate tissue injury and have been implicated in the pathogenesis of several important diseases, including those that may trigger acute lung injury and the acute respiratory distress syndrome.[1,2] In these conditions, activated neutrophils accumulate in lung microvessels and cause endothelial damage, increased vascular permeability, and produce tissue injury.[3] The neutrophils that mediate these changes come either from those already in the vascular space where they circulate or marginate along vessel walls, or from those released from the bone marrow into the vascular space.[4]

The factors controlling the number of circulating neutrophils, their sequestration in different vascular beds, and their migration into the tissues have been a topic of interest and also controversy for nearly a century. The number of circulating neutrophils is influenced by their rate of production in the bone marrow, the release from the bone marrow into the circulation, the exchange between the circulating and the marginated pool of intravascular neutrophils, and their permanent removal from the circulation (Figure 1). The neutrophil levels change rapidly during stress, with moderate stimuli such as exercise, causing cells marginated along vessel walls to enter the circulation, but such stimuli do not increase the

This work was supported by the Medical Research Council of Canada (grant #4219) and the B.C. Lung Association. Stephan F. van Eeden is the recipient of a Career Investigators Award of the American Lung Association.

From: Weir EK, Reeve HL, Reeves JT (eds). *Interactions of Blood and the Pulmonary Circulation*. Armonk, NY: Futura Publishing Company, Inc.; ©2002.

291

Granulocyte Pools and Kinetics

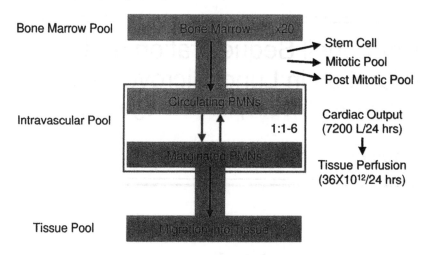

Figure 1. The different pools that granulocytes reside in during their lifespan. The bone marrow pool consists of a stem cell pool, a mitotic pool committed to granulopoiesis, and a postmitotic or maturation pool. The maturation pool is ~×20 larger than the circulating pool of granulocytes. The intravascular neutrophil pool consists of a circulating and a marginated pool. The marginated pool is between 1 and 6 times the size of the circulating pool. The size of the tissue pool of neutrophils is unknown. The delivery of neutrophils to the lung is $36 \times 10^{12}/24$ hours in a subject with a cardiac output of 5 L/min.

total number of cells in the vascular pool. Stronger stimuli cause a release of neutrophils from the bone marrow,[4] which increases the total number of cells that are circulating as well as the size of the pool marginated along vessel walls. The importance of the lung as a site where neutrophils leave the circulating pool but remain in the vascular space has been well established.[5] This sequestration of neutrophils in the lung microvessels provides a pool of cells that can be mobilized into the circulation in times of stress. This pool has been calculated to be between 1 and 6 times the size of the circulating pool of neutrophils. Activation of neutrophils sequestered in the pulmonary microvessels may damage the endothelium by releasing enzymes and oxygen-free radicals[6,7] and is crucially important in the pathogenesis of neutrophil-induced tissue damage in conditions such as acute respiratory distress syndrome and emphysema. Factors that control the sequestration of neutrophils in the lung and their subsequent migration into the tissues have been shown to be critically important in determining this neutrophil-induced tissue injury. This chapter focuses on the phenotypic and functional characteristics of neutrophils that determine their sequestration and migration in lung microvessels with an emphasis on the bone marrow response as an important determinant of neutrophil behavior in the lung.

Neutrophil Traffic Through the Pulmonary Capillaries

The average adult human with a cardiac output of 5 L/min delivers ~7200 L of blood to the pulmonary circulation in 24 hours. Each liter of blood contains ~5×10^9 leukocytes or ~2.5×10^9 neutrophils with a calculated 18×10^{12} neutrophils delivered to the lung microvessels in 24 hours, emphasizing the extent of the neutrophil traffic through the lung (Figure 1). The alveolar capillaries consist of a network of interconnecting segments (Figure 2) and quantitative histological studies have shown that the pulmonary vascular bed contains 2.8×10^{11} individual capillary segments or an estimated 1000 capillary segments/alveolus.[8] The interconnecting network of capillary segments provides a large number of parallel routes for cell traffic (Figure 2). Red blood cells (RBCs) have a discoid shape and an average diameter similar to spherical neutrophils[5] but can rapidly reduce their maximum diameter by folding when they en-

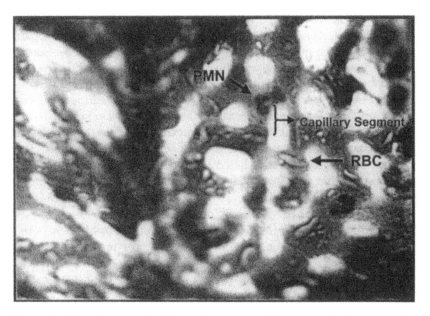

Figure 2. Microphotograph of the pulmonary capillary network demonstrating the multiple short capillary segments. Neutrophils (PMN) trapped in a capillary segment allow red blood cells (RBC) to stream around them. The micrograph is of a 10-μm thick section of normal rabbit lung.

counter a narrow capillary segment. Several studies have shown that RBC transit time through the pulmonary vascular bed is about 1 second,[9-11] whereas neutrophils take between 60 and 100 times longer to make the same journey.[9,11] The interconnecting nature of the pulmonary capillary bed allows the faster moving RBCs to flow around slower moving neutrophils. This discrepancy between the transit time of RBCs and neutrophils results in a concentration of neutrophils in pulmonary capillary blood up to 60–65 times that in circulating blood[5,10,12] and accounts for the majority of the so-called marginated pool of neutrophils in the lung.[5] Important phenotypic characteristics of neutrophils that determine their concentration in the pulmonary capillaries are their size, their ability to deform, and their adhesiveness to endothelium.

Neutrophil Size and Traffic Through the Lung

The discrepancy between the diameter of the circulating neutrophil (range 5–8 :m, mean 7.03 :m) and the capillary segments (range 1–16 :m, mean 5 :m) mandates that a large number of neutrophils must deform to negotiate the pulmonary vascular bed.[13,14] Hogg has calculated that the average pathway for a neutrophil from the arterial to the venous site of the pulmonary bed consists of ~60 capillary segments[5] with a high likelihood that it will encounter a capillary segment smaller than itself. Therefore, the majority of neutrophils must deform to pass through the pulmonary capillary bed just because of the size discrepancy between themselves and the capillary segments. The effect of gravity on capillary segment size accounts for the difference in retention of neutrophils in the upper and lower regions of the lung.[5,15,16] The mean capillary diameter has been calculated to be ~2 μm in zone II and 5.78 μm in zone III in rat lung,[17] and any reduction in this capillary size will enhance the neutrophil retention in the lung microvessels. The change in capillary size associated with gravitational forces changes vascular transmural pressures and predicts a shorter transit time and a lower neutrophil retention in dependent lung regions.[5,13,14,17] Markos and colleagues have shown that an increase in alveolar pressure causes an immediate arteriovenous (AV) difference in neutrophils across the lung that rapidly reverses when the capillary pressure is removed.[18] Subsequent studies show that with prolonged elevations of alveolar pressure this AV difference disappears, suggesting a new steady state is eventually achieved in a chronically compressed capillary bed.[19] The size of the marginated pool of neutrophils is also sensitive to the level of pulmonary blood flow, with mobilization of neutrophils[12,20] from the marginated pool in the lung during high flow states such as exercise.[21-23] The preferential location of the marginated pool of neutrophils in the lung, as opposed to the systemic microvasculature, may be due to the relatively low flow found within in the pulmonary system and the slightly smaller size of pulmonary capillaries compared with the systemic capillaries.

Neutrophil Deformability and Traffic Through the Lung

The importance of neutrophil deformability in passage through the lung microcirculation has been explored by several workers.[24–27] Direct measurements of pulmonary capillary segments and neutrophil diameters showed that ~60% of capillary segments are narrower than the spherical neutrophils and that neutrophils deform from a spherical to an elliptic shape to negotiate the capillary bed under normal physiological conditions.[27] Doerschuk and colleagues showed that glutaraldehyde-stiffened neutrophils are nearly all (1% circulate after 1 minute) trapped in the lung during their first pass through the pulmonary capillary bed[12] compared to native neutrophils (43% ± 5% circulate after 1 minute), demonstrating that neutrophil transit through the lung is inversely related to cell stiffness. Neutrophil stiffness has also been determined by measuring the pressure needed to insert micropipettes with different diameters[28] or by using a cell poker where the measurement is independent of cell adhesion.[24] All of these studies have clearly shown that, in addition to size, cell viscoelastic properties or deformability determine in part their ability to transit the pulmonary capillaries and influence the magnitude of the marginated pool of neutrophils in the lung.

An important variable in these elegant studies of neutrophil deformability is the need to purify the neutrophils, which has been shown to mildly activate neutrophils using sensitive parameters of cell activation such as F-actin assembly and calcium signaling.[29,30] Our laboratory has recently developed a method to label neutrophils in whole blood using a fluorescent labeling technique. Using these labeled cells in whole blood, we could show that just ~30% of neutrophils are retained during their first pass through the lung in contrast to ~60% using purified neutrophils labeled with radioisotopes (Figure 3).

Mechanical deformation of PMNs has been observed in pulmonary microvessels,[31] but whether this deformation is an active or passive process remains to be determined. Using an in vitro system of passing PMNs through 5- and 3-μm pore size polycarbonate filters and flow rates simulating pulmonary capillary flow, Kitagawa and colleagues showed that the magnitude of deformation and the length of time cells remain deformed were dependent on the pore size of the filter used.[32] The delayed recovery of neutrophils to a rounded shape is also consistent with recent studies from our laboratory using isolated perfused rabbit lungs where

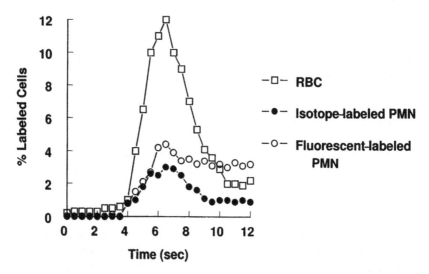

Figure 3. The first pass of red blood cells (RBC) and neutrophils (PMN) labeled either with indium[111] or by a fluorescent label (DiL, Molecular Probes) through the lung. Recirculation occurs at about 12 seconds following intravenous injection of the labeled cells, and ~60% of indium[111] cells are retained in contrast to ~30% of cells labeled with the fluorescent label.

neutrophils deformed in the capillaries maintained this elongated shape as they exited the pulmonary capillary bed.[31] Varying the flow rates produced different driving pressures and shear stress on the neutrophils, but did not affect the degree to which the cells deform or their recovery time to a spherical shape. Therefore, we conclude that the degree of deformation is determined mainly by pore size. These studies also established that mechanical deformation of neutrophils causes functional changes in the neutrophils that include reorganization and stabilization of the cytoskeleton that could contribute to their passage through small restrictions in the pulmonary capillary bed. An increase in intracellular free calcium and upregulation of the surface expression of CD18/CD11b were also observed following cell deformation. Subsequent studies showed that these deformation-induced changes in CD18/CD11b result in an increased adhesion of neutrophils to a surface coated with the endothelial adhesion molecule, intercellular adhesion molecule 1 (ICAM-1) (Figure 4). This increased adhesiveness of deformed cells suggests that deformation of neutrophils in the pulmonary capillary bed has downstream functional consequences. Passage of neutrophils through smaller capillary segments will trap neutrophils longer in these capillaries and induce enhanced neutrophil adhesiveness, therefore increasing the likelihood for migration into lung tissues. These studies also show that priming neutrophils can enhance this increase in CD18/CD11b induced by cell deformation.[32]

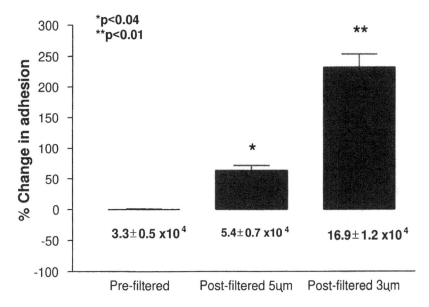

Figure 4. The adhesion of neutrophils deformed by filtration through 5- and 3-μm pore size polycarbonate filters at a constant flow rate (1 mL/min) to ICAM-1-coated wells. Significantly more deformed neutrophils adhere to the ICAM-1-coated wells than prefiltered neutrophils (*$P<0.05$). More neutrophils deformed through 3-μm filters than 5-μm filters adhere to the ICAM-1-coated wells. The numbers represent the absolute number of adherent neutrophils.

This observation suggests that primed neutrophils are more likely to be activated during mechanical stress and we speculate that mechanically stressed cells could enhance the inflammatory response by potentiating their function at the inflammatory sites. These functional changes in PMNs induced by deformation may be of relatively little importance under normal physiological conditions but could enhance neutrophil sequestration in the pulmonary capillary beds compressed by positive end expiratory pressure induced by either external sources in mechanically ventilated patients or internal sources in patients with chronic airway obstruction. Similarly, priming of circulating neutrophils by inflammatory mediators during sepsis could enhance their sequestration, adhesiveness, and recruitment, contributing to neutrophil-mediated lung injury.

Neutrophil Adhesiveness and Traffic Through the Lung

The cell adhesion molecules, which are expressed on the surface of leukocytes and endothelial cells, play a pivotal role in leukocyte-endothelial interaction.[33–35] This interaction is an early and requisite event in inflammation, contributing to the margination of neutrophils and their activation and recruitment into the tissues. Both L-selectin (CD62L) and the β_2-integrins on the surface of leukocytes play an important role in this leukocyte-endothelial interaction.[35] The concepts of neutrophil-endothelial interaction have been dominated by studies in systemic microvessels. These studies show that the first step in neutrophil recruitment is rolling or tethering of neutrophils to the endothelial surface induced by members of the selectin group of adhesion molecules (L-selectin on neutrophils with E- and P-selectin on the endothelial surface).[34,36] This allows close contact between neutrophils and chemokines on the surface of endothelium that activates the neutrophil, initiating subsequent firm adhesion mediated via the integrin group of molecules (mainly CD18/CD11b in neutrophils). The integrins interact with adhesion molecules of the immunoglobulin superfamily (ICAM-1 and ICAM-2) expressed on the endothelial surface, and this interaction is essential for migration of neutrophils into the tissues. Another member of the immunoglobulin superfamily, PECAM-1, is preferentially expressed at endothelial cell corners and, via homotypic binding with PECAM-1 on neutrophils, assists migration into the tissues. These adhesion molecules undergo quantitative and qualitative changes in response to various inflammatory stimuli that are a prerequisite for neutrophil-endothelial interactions that contribute to margination and recruitment of cells. This proadhesive condition that initiates adhesion and promotes migration is regulated by a network of inflammatory mediators. Tumor necrosis factor-α (TNF-α), interferon-γ, and IL-1 activate endothelium and also stimulate the production of chemotactic cytokines such as IL-8 and GM-CSF.[37-39] A major function of the α chemokine, IL-8, is as a chemoattractant for neutrophils but it is also an important stimulus that results in shedding of L-selectin, translocation of CD18/CD11b (Mac-1) from intracellular storage pools to the cell surface, and activation of the integrins to firmly adhere to the endothelium. The fact that neutrophils are in prolonged contact with the capillary endothelium in the lung[9-11] suggests that the sequential cascade of events proposed for the systemic capillaries may not be similar in pulmonary capillaries. The tight contact of neutrophils with the endothelium of the pulmonary capillaries makes rolling of cells to slow them down redundant. Although this phenomenon occurs in pulmonary postcapillary venules, most sequestration and migration of neutrophils in the lung occurs in pulmonary capillaries.[40,41] Blocking of either L-selectin or CD18 on neutrophils does not reduce the rapid sequestration of neutrophils in pulmonary capillaries induced by complement fragments.[42,43] However, prolonged sequestration of neutrophils in capillaries is partially dependent on both L-selectin and CD18.[42,44,45] Evidence that endothelial-associated adhesion molecules such as E-selectin, P-selectin, and ICAM-1 enhance neutrophil sequestration in the lung is lacking. In a model of focal pneumococcal pneumonia, ICAM-1 expression increased on endothelium in the pneumonic region but not in the adjacent normal lung,[46] making it unlikely that ICAM-1 is responsible for the sequestration of neutrophils in normal lung tissue.

The influence of cell adhesion molecules on either neutrophils or the endothelium on sequestration and migration of neutrophils in lung capillaries is still unclear. The migration of neutrophils also appears to be distinctly different between the systemic and the pulmonary capillaries. Two pathways mediate neutrophil migration in pulmonary capillaries, one that requires CD11/CD18 and one that does not, whereas all neutrophil migration from systemic capillaries appears to require CD11/CD18.[47,48] Stimuli such as *Streptococcus pneumoniae*, hydrochloric acid, and complement fragments in the alveolar space are associated with CD18-independent migration of neutrophils, in contrast to *E. coli* endotoxin, live *E. coli*, or phorbol ester-induced neutrophil migration that is largely CD18-dependent. The mechanisms for the CD18-independent migration of neutrophils are still elusive. Most recognized adhesion molecules such as E-, P-, and L-selectin or ICAM-1 have been excluded in mediating the CD18-independent migration of neutrophils. Recent studies suggest that this migration is dependent on the chemoattractant present, with IL-8 and LTB_4 involved in CD18-independent migration and fMLP-mediated migration requiring CD18.[49] These studies were conducted in an in vitro model and still need to be confirmed in vivo.

The concept of neutrophil margination based on cells leaving the circulating pool of leukocytes by rolling on endothelium of postcapillary venules is not applicable to the pulmonary circulation because neutrophils normally are in close contact with endothelium in the pulmonary capillaries. Therefore, adhesion interaction between neutrophils and endothelium normally plays a small role in margination of neutrophils in the lung. In conditions leading to neutrophil or endothelial cell activation, it may be responsible for prolonged retention of neutrophils in the lung. Furthermore, the emigration of neutrophils into the alveolar space in many inflammatory and infectious lung conditions is independent of CD18/CD11, in contrast to emigration into the systemic vascular bed.

Neutrophil Heterogeneity

Circulating neutrophils are heterogeneous in nature. They may differ in their size, their deformability, expression of surface receptors, granular content, and response toward stimulation with an agonist.

Differences in cell age and their activation state are responsible for the majority of these differences in phenotypic and functional characteristics of circulating neutrophils.

Neutrophil Activation and Traffic Through the Lung

Activation of neutrophils causes an increase in cell stiffness characterized by conversion of G-actin to F-actin,[50,51] an increase in expression of CD18/CD11 and a shedding of L-selectin.[34,52] These changes will cause cell sequestration in microvessels and promote cell adhesion to endothelium, preparing the cell for migration into the tissues. The sequestration of activated neutrophils in microvessels removes them from the circulating pool. Using complement fragments to activate circulating neutrophils, Doerschuk and colleagues have shown that the majority of these neutrophils sequester in the lung microvessels and return to the circulating pool with removal of the inciting activation stimulus.[12] They also showed that the immediate sequestration of neutrophils in the lung is largely dependent on changes in cell deformability but that prolonged sequestration is dependent on neutrophil surface adhesion molecules such as L-selectin and CD18.[46] Recent studies from our laboratory have shown that neutrophils that demarginate from the lung express high levels of CD18/CD11b,[23] suggesting that cells with high surface expression of CD11b preferentially sequester in lung microvessels. We tested the hypothesis that neutrophils in the circulation that express high levels of CD11b are less deformable than those that express low levels of CD11b in subjects during heart catheterization performing a Valsalva maneuver. The increase in transmural pressure across the alveolar wall causes an immediate drop in the neutrophil counts across the lung that is accompanied by a removal of neutrophils from the circulating pool that express high levels of CD11b. Both the neutrophil count and the CD11b expression return to baseline with termination of the forced expiratory maneuver. This immediate retention and release of these circulating neutrophils expressing high levels of CD18/CD11b suggest that neutrophils in the circulation that express high levels of CD18/ CD11b are stiffer than their counterparts expressing lower levels of CD18/CD11b.

Activation-induced changes in the deformability of neutrophils have been shown to result in sequestration of neutrophils in pulmonary capillaries.[12,24–26] This activation may occur during prolonged cell transit through the pulmonary capillary bed primed by a focal inflammatory lung condition, such as pneumonia, or by an intravascular stimulus such as bacteremia or endotoxemia. Interestingly, bacteremia following a focal subcutaneous or lung infection caused more sequestration than bacteremia alone, suggesting that the focal infection primed the circulating neutrophils or the vascular endothelium of the lung to enhance neutrophil sequestration.[53,54]

Neutrophil Age and Traffic Through the Lung

One of the well-established systemic responses to a localized inflammatory reaction is the change in the age distribution of neutrophils in peripheral blood with a shift toward younger, more immature cells. These younger immature neutrophils are released from the bone marrow.

Neutrophil Traffic Through the Bone Marrow

The bone marrow is a hematopoietic factory weighing approximately 2600 g, or 4.5% of the body weight of a normal adult. The bone marrow as a single organ is larger than the liver, and about 55–60% of the bone marrow is dedicated to the production of a single cell type, the neutrophil. In normal adults, the life of neutrophils is spent in 3 environments: the bone marrow, blood, and tissue (Figure 1). Bone marrow is the site of proliferation, terminal differentiation, and maturation of neutrophilic granulocytes. Proliferation consists of approximately 5 divisions and takes place only during the first 3 stages of neutrophil development (myeloblast, promyelocyte, and myelocyte stages). After the myelocyte stage, the cells become "end cells" that are no longer capable of dividing.[55] They then enter a large storage pool where they mature to segmented neutrophils for ~5 days before being released into the blood.[55-57] Figure 5 illustrates the neutrophils' lifespan and stages of maturation in the marrow.[56-58] Neutrophils spend only a small proportion of their lifespan in the vascular space, and circulating cells turn over ~2.5 times per day to replace the circulating pool. To accomplish this, the bone marrow produces $\pm850 \times 10^6$ cells/kg/day in humans. These cells come from the postmitotic granulocyte pool in the bone marrow (5.6×10^9 cells/kg), which is the largest storage pool of neutrophils and is ~10 times the size of the intravascular pool.[59] Inflammation and stress increase the rate of neutrophil production from the precursors, shorten the maturation time, decrease the time mature neutrophils reside in the marrow, and stimulate mature and immature neutrophils to enter the circulation.[60] The turnover of neutrophils may increase from 100 billion per day at baseline to over a trillion per day during a serious infection.[61] Faster transit times of neutrophils through the marrow with infections suggests that segmented neutrophils in these conditions are younger or more immature, compatible with the "shift to the left" or cytoplasmic "toxic granulation" seen on differen-

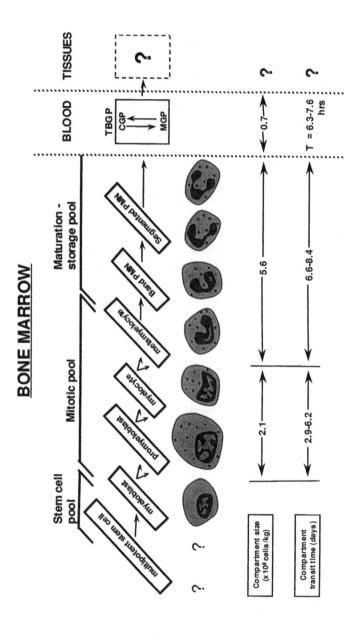

Figure 5. Compartment size and transit time of neutrophils in the bone marrow, blood, and tissue of humans. Cells in the mitotic pool in the marrow divide an average of 5 times before entering the postmitotic pool, where they reside to mature before their release into the circulation. Note the maturation pool size is nearly 3 times the mitotic pool and ~20 times the circulating pool. The transit time of neutrophils is between 3 and 6 days in the mitotic pool, between 6 and 8 days in the maturation pool, and just 6–8 hours in the blood. The size and transit time of neutrophils in tissues are not known but it has been suggested that they live for days at an inflammatory site. For more details, see references 55–63.

tial counts.[62] Whether these younger cells released into the circulation have different kinetic and functional properties is currently a topic of active investigation.

Earlier studies have utilized tritiated thymidine (H^3TDR) to determine the myelocyte-to-blood transit times,[62,63] which are shorter in patients with infections, suggesting that mature segmented neutrophils are either released earlier than usual or that more immature cells are released from the bone marrow.[64] We have recently developed a method to label neutrophils in the bone marrow and follow them during their lifespan in the circulation by using the thymidine analog, 5'-bromo-2'-deoxyuridine (BrdU).[65] The method used is similar to that of Maloney and Pratt, who used tritiated thymidine to label dividing neutrophils in dogs.[63] This method allows us to measure the transit time of neutrophils through the mitotic and the postmitotic pools in the bone marrow and also study the behavior of these newly released neutrophils in the circulation.

Release of Immature Neutrophil from the Marrow

Inflammatory stimuli increase the rate of neutrophil production from the precursors, shorten their maturation time, decrease the time they reside in the marrow, and cause both mature and immature neutrophils to enter the circulation. Using BrdU to label dividing cells in the marrow, we could demonstrate that the stimulation of the marrow produced by pneumococcal pneumonia shortens the transit time of PMNs through both the mitotic and the postmitotic or maturation pool in the bone marrow.[65] The release of these neutrophils from the marrow was also dependent on the nature of the stimulus, with more intense or systemic stimuli causing a more rapid release of neutrophils into the circulation pool (Figure 6). These neutrophils also have a shortened transit time through the bone marrow that is probably mediated by soluble factors released from the inflammatory site in the lung. The alveolar macrophages are an important source of these mediators,[66] and we suspect that they may play an important part in regulating the transit time of neutrophils through the bone marrow during lung inflammation. Mediators capable of stimulating the marrow to release neutrophils are hematopoietic growth factors such as G-CSF and GM-CSF, as well as cytokines such as IL-1, IL-3, IL-6, and IL-8, complement fragments, and leukotrines.[67,68] Release of these mediators from the lung into the circulation may be responsible for the bone marrow response associated with lung inflammation. Using BrdU to label dividing cells in the marrow, we could show that the individual inflammatory mediators each have a distinct pattern of release of neutrophils

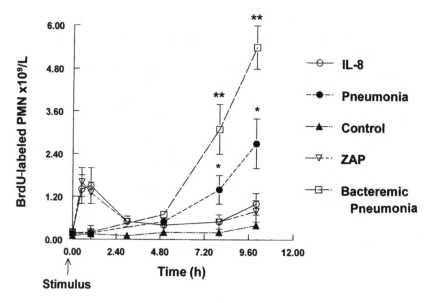

Figure 6. The release of neutrophils from the bone marrow with different stimuli. 5'-Bromo-2'-deoxyuridine (BrdU) was used to pulse label all dividing myeloid cells in the bone marrow of rabbits and their release was measured in the circulation using immunocytochemistry.[64,65] Interleukin-8 and complement fragments (ZAP) caused a rapid (minutes) release of cells from the marrow in contrast with pneumococcal pneumonia or pneumonia complicated by bacteremia that caused a more gradual release of neutrophils. At 8 and 10 hours following the stimulus, significantly more labeled neutrophils were in the circulation in the pneumonia groups than in controls or the IL-8 and ZAP groups (*P<0.01). At 8 and 10 hours, more labeled neutrophils were in the circulation in the bacteremic group compared to the pneumonia group (**P<0.05).

from the marrow (Figure 7). IL-8 causes a rapid release of neutrophils from the bone marrow sinusoidal pool of cells but does not change the overall transit time of neutrophils through either the mitotic or the post-mitotic pool and it also fails to increase the immature (band cells) in the circulation.[69] In contrast, IL-6 causes a slower but a more prolonged release of neutrophils from the bone marrow and significantly shortens the transit time of neutrophils through both the mitotic and postmitotic pools in the marrow.[70] This rapid bone marrow transit time was also associated with an increase in circulating band cells. G-CSF has an effect similar to IL-6[71] and an inflammatory stimulus in the lung such as pneumococcal pneumonia. Interestingly, chronic stimulation of the bone marrow, with cigarette smoke or particulate matter air pollutants, has a very small effect on the bone marrow transit times but a large effect on increasing the size of the bone marrow pool of neutrophils.[72] These chronic stimuli also release immature cells into the circulation

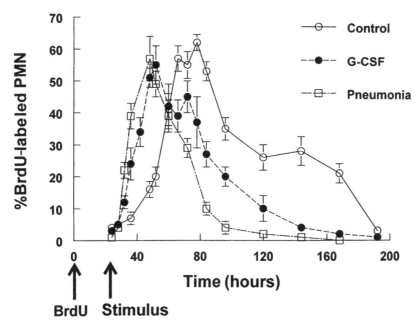

Figure 7. The transit of 5'-bromo-2'-deoxyuridine (BrdU)-labeled neutrophils through the bone marrow. BrdU was used to pulse label all dividing myeloid cells in the bone marrow of rabbits and their release was measured in the circulation over time using immunocytochemistry.[64,65] Using these curves, the transit time of neutrophils through the different pools in the marrow can be calculated by grading the intensity of staining for BrdU.[65] G-CSF and pneumonia caused a rapid release of BrdU-labeled neutrophils from the marrow and significantly shortened their transit time, through both the mitotic and the postmitotic pools in the bone marrow.[65,71]

and support the results of human studies in smokers, showing a leukocytosis with a bandemia in chronic smokers.[73]

Phenotypic and Functional Characteristics of Immature Neutrophils

Normally only fully differentiated neutrophils enter the circulation, but stimulation of the bone marrow during an inflammatory reaction results in the release of more immature neutrophils such as band cells into the circulation.[59–62] Immature neutrophils harvested from the bone marrow have been shown to be less deformable, have reduced motility, and are less phagocytic if compared to mature cells in peripheral blood[74] (Figure 8). These immature neutrophils are also larger than their mature counterparts,[74,75] which may promote their sequestration in lung microvessels. With the advent of flow cytometric analysis of cell surface re-

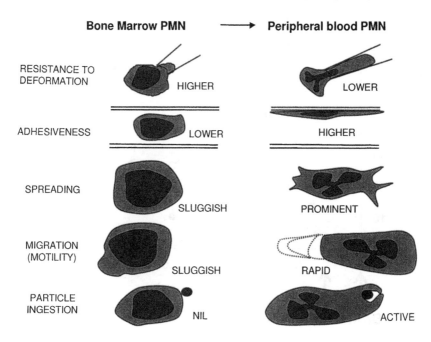

Figure 8. Differences in neutrophil functions between neutrophils harvested from the bone marrow and peripheral blood. Bone marrow neutrophils are less deformable, are slow to spread, are less adhesive to plastic, are slow to migrate, and reluctant to ingest particles in vitro.[74] Studies on neutrophils newly released from the bone marrow show that they are more likely to sequester in lung microvessels,[78,82] suggesting that they are less deformable, slow to migrate[78,82,85] into lung tissues, and are less chemotactic.[88]

ceptors, heterogeneity in the expression of several surface receptors such as the LPS receptor CD14, CD16, and CD18 on circulating neutrophils has been described.[76] Studies from our laboratory have shown that neutrophils newly released from the bone marrow express higher levels of L-selectin than their counterparts in the circulation, a molecule that contributes to the recruitment of neutrophils to a site of inflammation.[77,78] L-selectin is a neutrophil maturation receptor and neutrophils increase their levels in the bone marrow as they mature in the bone marrow postmitotic pool.[79,80] With bone marrow stimulation, neutrophils expressing high levels of L-selectin are rapidly released into the circulation.[77] We have also shown that the L-selectin on neutrophils decreases as they age in the circulation, with neutrophils in the circulation for more than 24 hours lacking L-selectin on their surface.[81] These unique L-selectin kinetics during the lifespan of the neutrophil are responsible for the heterogeneity of L-selectin expression on circulating neutrophils and we suspect they are critically important in determining which neutrophils participate in the inflammatory response and which are destined to be removed from the circulating pool for processing.

The primary granules in neutrophils are formed at a early stage (promyelocytic) in the mitotic pool in the marrow and the number of granules are reduced by mitosis as the cells pass through the mitotic stage.[56,57] Because these granules contain myeloperoxidase (MPO), which is critical for neutrophil reactive oxygen radical production as well as proteolytic enzymes, skipping divisions during the mitotic stage results in the production of neutrophils with a higher granule number and greater destructive capabilities.[64] This concept was supported by studies from our laboratory showing an increase in the MPO content of circulating neutrophils in chronic smokers with high levels of circulating immature neutrophils.[73] The neutrophil MPO correlated with the neutrophilia and bandemia in these smokers, suggesting that immature neutrophils released from stimulated bone marrow contain high levels of MPO. Several neutrophil granule proteolytic enzymes are formed early during the mitotic phase of development in the bone marrow and we suspect that bone marrow stimulation could release neutrophils into the circulation that are high in enzymes such as elastase, proteinase 3, cathepsin G, and metaloproteinases. We have shown that neutrophils released from stimulated bone marrow preferentially sequester in lung microvessels,[78,82–84] and if these neutrophils contain large amounts of these potentially destructive proteolytic enzymes, they could play a pivotal role in inappropriate neutrophil-mediated lung injury associated with infection and sepsis.

Sequestration of Neutrophils Released from the Bone Marrow

The molecular mechanisms responsible for sequestration and migration of neutrophils in the pulmonary vascular bed are different from those in the systemic vascular bed. First, the longer transit time of neutrophils through the lung capillaries than through systemic capillaries[9,10] increases their exposure to inflammatory mediators on activated capillary endothelium in infected lung tissue. Second, mechanical deformation of neutrophils in pulmonary capillaries causes F-actin assembly and upregulation of CD11b, both events involved in their sequestration and recruitment. Third, the many alveolar macrophages in the lungs are capable of releasing cytokines that stimulate the bone marrow and activate both circulating neutrophils and capillary endothelium. These factors may contribute to more sequestration of neutrophils in lung capillaries and enhanced migration into lung tissue.[54,85] Doerschuk and colleagues showed that a focal pneumococcal pneumonia causes sequestration of neutrophils in the infectious site but also causes sequestration of neutrophils in the contralateral noninfected lung, compared to control noninfected animals.[86] Studies from our laboratory have shown that neutrophils released from the bone marrow during a focal pneumococcal pneumonia preferentially sequester in both infected and noninfected lung tissue.[82] This observation was supported by similar findings in models of bacteremic pneumococcal pneumonia,[85] endotoxemia,[78] and when the bone marrow was stimulated with G-CSF[84] and IL-6.[87] All of these stimuli cause an accelerated release of neutrophils from the bone marrow and preferential sequestration of these newly released cells in the lung microvessels. The similar findings with different stimuli suggest that the sequestration is due to age-related phenotypic characteristics of these younger neutrophils. Filtration of these newly released neutrophils through polycarbonate filters with different pore sizes showed preferential retention of these cells in the filter,[88] suggesting that newly released neutrophils are less deformable than their counterparts already in the circulation. Studies from our laboratory have also shown that PMNs newly released from the bone marrow express higher levels of L-selectin than their counterparts in the circulation,[77,78] a molecule that contributes to prolonged sequestration of PMNs in lung microvessels.[45]

Taken together, these results suggest that younger PMNs released from the bone marrow stimulated by an inflammatory condition in the lung or by a systemic stimulus preferentially sequester in lung capillaries, indicating that these cells have unique characteristics that result in a long transit time through pulmonary capillaries. This longer transit time of younger neutrophils through the lung will expose them longer to activating inflammatory mediators, such as IL-8, on the endothelium. We suspect that activation and degranulation of these sequestered neutrophils are 2 of the key steps in the pathogenesis of acute and chronic alveolar wall damage in adult respiratory disease syndrome and emphysema.

Migration of Neutrophils Released from the Bone Marrow

Several studies from our laboratory as well as others have demonstrated that neutrophils sequester in the lung during a focal inflammatory condition such as pneumococcal pneumonia.[12,42,45,82–86] Neutrophils released from the bone marrow contribute significantly to this sequestration. That raises the question of whether these newly released neutrophils also preferentially migrate into the tissues to assist with clearing of offending micro-organisms. However, studies in animals show that these younger neutrophils are slow to migrate into the alveoli during focal pneumococcal pneumonia.[82,84] Similar results were obtained in a model of bacteremic pneumococcal pneumonia or focal pneumococcal pneumonia treated with G-CSF.[85] To test whether this is unique to the pulmonary vascular bed, we infected subcutaneous tissue with pneumococci and demonstrated that newly released neutrophils are also slow to emigrate out of systemic microvessels.[54] The reason for this slow migration of neutrophils newly released from the bone marrow is still not clear. In vitro studies comparing neutrophils in the bone marrow with neutrophils in peripheral blood showed that bone marrow neutrophils are less motile and do not migrate and phagocytose as well as neutrophils obtained from the circulation.[74,75,89,90] We tested chemotaxis in neutrophils newly released from the bone marrow and showed that their chemotactic ability is reduced compared to their older counterparts in the circulation (Figure 9). Recent studies from our laboratory showed lower baseline levels of CD18 expression on bone marrow neutrophils than that of neutrophils in the peripheral blood.[91] Stimulation of these younger neutrophils from the bone marrow also cause less upregulation of CD18. Neutrophils use the CD18 receptor to firmly adhere and crawl on the endothelium toward cell corners where they emigrate into the tissues. An attenuated CD18 response and reduced chemotactic ability could both contribute to the slow migration of newly released neutrophils. Neutrophil migration into lung tissue is CD18-independent in several inflammatory lung conditions and we suspect the reduced CD18 response of younger neutrophils is not the only reason for their slow migration into lung tissue. We speculate that the preferential

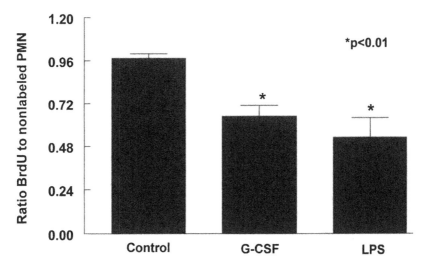

Figure 9. Chemotaxis of BrdU-labeled neutrophils released from the bone marrow by intravenous G-CSF (12.5 µg/kg) and LPS (5 µg/kg) toward IL-8. Cells were harvested 8 hours following stimulation and placed in a Boyden chamber on 5-µm pore size polycarbonate filters. The results are expressed as the ratio of BrdU-labeled to nonlabeled cells that have migrated. Significantly fewer BrdU-labeled neutrophils have migrated toward the chemotactic stimulus.

sequestration and slow migration of the newly released neutrophils provide these cells with a greater opportunity to injure the capillary endothelium. Younger neutrophils released from stimulated bone marrow contain higher levels of granules enzymes, such as MPO, and could play a major role in injuring the capillary endothelium if they were activated during their prolonged transit through the lung capillaries.

Summary

The data presented here show that circulating neutrophils are a heterogeneous population of cells with different phenotypic and functional characteristics. Activation and age-related characteristics are the main reasons for this heterogeneity. Stimulation of the bone marrow induced by lung inflammation stimulates the release of younger and more immature neutrophils into the circulation. These younger PMNs preferentially sequester in the lung and are slow to migrate into the site of inflammation. These observations suggest that they still possess immature functional characteristics. It also suggests that younger PMNs newly released from the bone marrow could play an important role in the pathogenesis of widespread lung injury.

Acknowledgments: The scientific contributions and support of many technicians, students, postdoctoral fellows, colleagues, and mentors were invaluable in generating these data, especially my longtime mentors and friends Jim Hogg and Claire Doerschuk for inspiration, advice, and ideas. I also want to thank the B.C. Lung Association and Canadian Institute for Health Research for financial support.

References

1. Sibille Y, Reynolds HY. Macrophages and polymorphonuclear neutrophils in lung defense and injury. *Am Rev Respir Dis* 1990;141(2):471–501.
2. Tate RM, Repine JE. Neutrophils and the adult respiratory distress syndrome. *Am Rev Respir Dis* 1983;128(3):552–559.
3. Weiss SJ. Tissue destruction by neutrophils. *N Engl J Med* 1989;320 (6):365–376.
4. Boggs DR. The kinetics of neutrophilic leukocytes in health and in disease. *Sem Hematol* 1967;4(4):359–386.
5. Hogg JC. Neutrophil kinetics and lung injury. *Physiol Rev* 1987;67(4): 1249–1295.
6. Cochrane CG. Cellular injury by oxidants. *Am J Med* 1991;91(3C):23S–30S.
7. Janoff A. Elastases and emphysema. Current assessment of the protease-antiprotease hypothesis. *Am Rev Respir Dis* 1985;132(2):417–433.
8. Weibel ER. *Morphometry of the Human Lung.* New York: Academic; 73–89.
9. Hogg JC, McLean T, Martin BA, Wiggs B. Erythrocyte transit and neutrophil concentration in the dog lung. *J Appl Physiol* 1988;65(3):1217–1225.
10. Hogg JC, Coxson HO, Brumwell ML, et al. Erythrocyte and polymor-

phonuclear cell transit time and concentration in human pulmonary capillaries. *J Appl Physiol* 1994;77(4):1795–1800.

11. Lien DC, Wagner WW Jr, Capen RL, et al. Physiological neutrophil sequestration in the lung: Visual evidence for localization in capillaries. *J Appl Physiol* 1987;62(3):1236–1243.

12. Doerschuk CM, Allard MF, Martin BA, et al. Marginated pool of neutrophils in rabbit lungs. *J Appl Physiol* 1987;63(5):1806–1815.

13. Schmid-Schonbein GW, Shih YY, Chien S. Morphometry of human leukocytes. *Blood* 1980;56(5):866–875.

14. Weibel ER. Lung cell biology. Handbook of Physiology: The Respiratory System. Bethesda, MD: American Physiology Society; 47–91.

15. MacNee W, Wiggs B, Belzberg AS, Hogg JC. The effect of cigarette smoking on neutrophil kinetics in human lungs. *N Engl J Med* 1989;321 (14):924–928.

16. Martin BA, Wiggs BR, Lee S, Hogg JC. Regional differences in neutrophil margination in dog lungs. *J Appl Physiol* 1987;63(3):1253–1261.

17. Glazier JB, Hughes JM, Maloney JE, West JB. Measurements of capillary dimensions and blood volume in rapidly frozen lungs. *J Appl Physiol* 1969;26(1):65–76.

18. Markos J, Hooper RO, Kavanagh-Gray D, et al. Effect of raised alveolar pressure on leukocyte retention in the human lung. *J Appl Physiol* 1990;69 (1):214–221.

19. Markos J, Doerschuk CM, English D, et al. Effect of positive end-expiratory pressure on leukocyte transit in rabbit lungs. *J Appl Physiol* 1993;74(6): 2627–2633.

20. Martin BA, Wright JL, Thommasen H, Hogg JC. Effect of pulmonary blood flow on the exchange between the circulating and marginating pool of polymorphonuclear leukocytes in dog lungs. *J Clin Invest* 1982;69 (6):1277–1285.

21. Larrabee RC. Leukocytosis after violent exercise. *J Med Res* 1992;7:76–82.

22. Foster NK, Martyn JB, Rangno RE, et al. Leukocytosis of exercise: Role of cardiac output and catecholamines. *J Appl Physiol* 1986;61:2218–2223.

23. van Eeden SF, Granton J, Hards JM, et al. Expression of the cell adhesion molecules on leukocytes that demarginate during acute maximal exercise. *J Appl Physiol* 1999;86(3):970–976.

24. Downey GP, Doherty DE, Schwab B 3d, et al. Retention of leukocytes in capillaries: Role of cell size and deformability. *J Appl Physiol* 1990;69(5): 1767–1778.

25. Downey GP, Worthen GS. Neutrophil retention in model capillaries: Deformability, geometry, and hydrodynamic forces. *J Appl Physiol* 1988;65 (4):1861–1871.

26. MacNee W, Selby C. New perspectives on basic mechanisms in lung disease. Neutrophil traffic in the lungs: Role of haemodynamics, cell adhesion, and deformability. *Thorax* 1993;48(1):79–88.

27. Wiggs BR, English D, Quinlan WM, et al. Contributions of capillary pathway size and neutrophil deformability to neutrophil transit through rabbit lungs. *J Appl Physiol* 1994;77(1):463–470.

28. Meiselman HJ, Bauersachs RM, Hein HJ, et al. Rheological behavior of human PMN studied by micropipette aspiration and by micropore filtration. *Monographs on Atherosclerosis* 1990;15:181–185.

29. McAfee JG, Subramanian G, Gagne G. Technique of leukocyte harvesting and labeling: Problems and perspectives. *Semin Nucl Med* 1984;14(2):83–106.

30. Haslett C, Guthrie LA, Kopaniak MM, et al. Modulation of multiple neu-

trophil functions by preparative methods or trace concentrations of bacterial lipopolysaccharide. *Am J Pathol* 1985;119(1):101–110.

31. Redenbach DM, English D, Hogg JC. The nature of leukocyte shape changes in the pulmonary capillaries. *Am J Physiol* 1997;273(4 Pt 1):L733–740.

32. Kitagawa Y, van Eeden SF, Redenbach D, et al. The effect of mechanical deformation on the structure and function of polymorphonuclear leukocytes. *J Appl Physiol* 1997;82(5);1397–1405.

33. Springer TA. Adhesion receptors of the immune system. *Nature* 1990; 346(6283):425–434.

34. Carlos TM, Harlan JM. Leukocyte-endothelial adhesion molecules. *Blood* 1994;84(7):2068–2101.

35. Adams DH, Shaw S. Leucocyte-endothelial interactions and regulation of leucocyte migration. *Lancet* 1994;343(8901):831–836.

36. Bevilacqua MP, Nelson RM. Selectins. *J Clin Invest* 1993;91(2):379–387.

37. Pober JS. Cytokine-mediated activation of vascular endothelium: Physiology and pathology. *Am J Pathol* 1988;133(3):426–433.

38. Mulligan MS, Vaporciyan A, Miyasaka M, et al. Tumor necrosis factor alpha regulates in vivo intrapulmonary expression of ICAM-1. *Am J Pathol* 1993;142(6):1739–1749.

39. Ward PA, Mulligan MS. Molecular mechanisms in acute lung injury. *Adv Pharmacol (New York)* 1993;24:275–292.

40. Downey GP, Worthen GS, Henson PM, Hyde DM. Neutrophil sequestration and migration in localized pulmonary inflammation: Capillary localization and migration across the interalveolar septum. *Am Rev Respir Dis* 1993;147(1):168–176.

41. Marchesi VT. The site leukocyte migration during inflammation. *Q J Exp Physiol* 1961;46;115–118.

42. Doerschuk CM. The role of CD18-mediated adhesion in neutrophil sequestration induced by infusion of activated plasma in rabbits. *Am J Respir Cell Mol Biol* 1992;7(2):140–148.

43. Lundberg C, Wright SD. Relation of the CD11/CD18 family of leukocyte antigens to the transient neutropenia caused by chemoattractants. *Blood* 1990;76(6):1240–1245.

44. Yoder MC, Checkley LL, Giger U, et al. Pulmonary microcirculatory kinetics of neutrophils deficient in leukocyte adhesion-promoting glycoproteins. *J Appl Physiol* 1990;69(1):207–213.

45. Doyle NA, Bhagwan SD, Meek B, et al. Neutrophil margination, sequestration, and emigration in the lungs of L-selectin-deficient mice. *J Clin Invest* 1997;99(3):526–533.

46. Burns AR, Takei F, Doerschuk CM. Quantitation of ICAM-1 expression in mouse lung during pneumonia. *J Immunol* 1994;153(7):3189–3198.

47. Doerschuk CM, Winn RK, Coxson HO, Harlan JM. CD18-dependent and -independent mechanisms of neutrophil emigration in the pulmonary and systemic microcirculation of rabbits. *J Immunol* 1990;144(6):2327–2333.

48. Doerschuk CM, Tasaka S, Wang Q. CD11/CD18-dependent and -independent emigration in the lung: How do neutrophils know which route to take. *Am J Respir Cell Mol Biol* 2000;23:133–136.

49. Mackarel AJ, Russel KJ, Brady CS, et al. IL-8 and LTB$_4$ but not fMLP stimulate CD18-independent migration of neutrophils across pulmonary endothelium in vitro. *Am J Respir Cell Mol Biol* 2000;23;154–161.

50. Klut ME, Whalen BA, Hogg JC. Activation-associated changes in blood and bone marrow neutrophils. *J Leukoc Biol* 1997;62:187.

51. Packman CH, Lichtman MA. Activation of neutrophils, measurement of actin conformational changes by flow cytometry. *Blood Cells* 1990;16:193.
52. Kishimoto TK, Jutila MA, Berg EL, Butcher EC. Neutrophil Mac-1 and MEL-14 adhesion proteins inversely regulated by chemotactic factors. *Science* 1989;245:1238.
53. Hallett MB, Lloyds D. Neutrophil priming: The cellular signals that say amber but not green. *Immunol Today* 1995;16(6):264–268.
54. Sato Y, Van Eeden SF, English D, Hogg JC. Pulmonary sequestration of polymorphonuclear leukocytes released from bone marrow in bacteremic infection. *Am J Physiol* 1998;275(Pt 1):L255–261.
55. Bainton DF, Ullyot JL, Farquhar MG. The development of neutrophilic polymorphonuclear leukocytes in human bone marrow. *J Exp Med* 1971;134(4):907–934.
56. Bainton DF, Friedlander LM, Shohet SB. Abnormalities in granule formation in acute myelogenous leukemia. *Blood* 1977;49(5):693–704.
57. Bainton DF. Neutrophil granules. *Br J Haematol* 1975;29(1):17–22.
58. Beckstead JH, Halverson PS, Ries CA, Bainton DF. Enzyme histochemistry and immunohistochemistry on biopsy specimens of pathologic human bone marrow. *Blood* 1981;57(6):1088–1098.
59. Finch CA, Harker LA, Cook JD. Kinetics of the formed elements of human blood. *Blood* 1977;50:699–707.
60. Cronkite EP. Analytic review of the structure and regulation of hematopoiesis. *Blood Cells* 1988;14:313–328.
61. Walker RI, Willemze R. Neutrophil kinetics and the regulation of granulopoiesis. *Rev Infect Dis* 1980;2:282–292.
62. Fliender TM, Cronkite EP, Killman SA, Bond VP. Granulopoiesis II: Emergence and patterns of labeling neutrophilic granulocytes in humans. *Blood* 1964;24:683–700.
63. Maloney MA, Pratt HM. Granulocyte transit from bone marrow to blood. Blood 1968;31:195–201.
64. Terashima T, Wiggs B, English D, et al. Polymorphonuclear leukocyte transit times in bone marrow during Streptococcal pneumonia. *Am J Physiol* 1996;271:L587-L592.
65. Bicknell S, van Eeden SF, English D, et al. A non-isotopic method to trace leukocytes with 5′-bromo-2′-deoxyuridine in vivo. *Am J Respir Cell Mol Biol* 1994;8:16–23.
66. Lohmann-Matthes ML, Steinmuller C, Franke-Ullmann G. Pulmonary macrophages. *Europ Respir J* 1994;7:1678- 1689.
67. Rennick D, Yang G, Gemmell L, Lee F. Control of hematopoiesis by a bone marrow stromal cell clone: Lipopolysaccharides and interleukin-1 inducible production of colony stimulating factors G-CSF and GM-CSF. *Blood* 1987;69:682–691.
68. Lord BI, Bronchud MH, Owens S, et al. The kinetics of human granulopoiesis following granulocyte colony stimulating factor in vivo. *Proc Natl Acad Sci USA* 1989;86:9499–9503.
69. Terashima T, English D, Hogg JC, van Eeden SF. The release of polymorphonuclear leukocytes from the bone marrow by interleukin-8. *Blood* 1998;92:1062–1069.
70. Suwa T, Hogg JC, Englis D, van Eeden SF. Interleukin-6-induced neutrophilia: Contribution of bone marrow release and demargination of intravascular neutrophils. *Am J Physiol (Lung Mol Biol)*. In press.
71. Mukae H, Zamfir D, English D, et al. Polymorphonuclear leukocytes re-

leased from the bone marrow by granulocyte colony-stimulating factor: Intravascular behavior. *Hematol J* 2000;1(3):159–171.

72. Terashima T, Wiggs B, Hogg JC, van Eeden SF. The effect of cigarette smoking on the bone marrow. *Am J Respir Crit Care Med* 1997;155:1021–1026.

73. van Eeden SF, Hogg JC. Changes in peripheral blood polymorphonuclear leukocytes indicative of bone marrow stimulation in chronic smokers. *Eur J Respir* 2000;15;915–921.

74. Lichtman MA, Weed RI. Alterations of cell periphery during granulocyte maturation: Relationship to cell function. *Blood* 1972;39:301–316.

75. Lichtman MA, Kearney EA. The filterability of normal and leukemic human leukocytes. *Blood Cells* 1976;2:491.

76. van Eeden SF, Klut ME, Walker BAM, JC Hogg. The role of flow cytometry to measure neutrophil function. *J Immunol Methods* 1999;232:23–43.

77. van Eeden SF, Miyagashima R, Haley L, Hogg JC. L-selectin expression on peripheral blood polymorphonuclear leukocytes during active bone marrow release in humans. *Am J Respir Crit Care Med* 1995;151:500–507.

78. van Eeden SF, Klut EM, Lawrence E, Hogg JC. Bone marrow release is associated with sequestration of newly released PMNs in the lung microvessels. *Microcirculation* 1997;4:369–380.

79. Lund-Johansen F, Terstappen LW. Differential surface expression of cell adhesion molecules during granulocyte maturation. *J Leuk Biol* 1993;54:47.

80. van Eeden SF, Miyagashima R, Haley L, Hogg JC. A possible role for L-selectin in the release of polymorphonuclear leukocytes from the bone marrow. *Am J Physiol* 1997;272:H1717–1724.

81. van Eeden SF, Bicknell S, Walker BAM, Hogg JC. Polymorphonuclear leukocytes L-selectin expression decreases as they age in the circulation. *Am J Physiol* 1997;272:H401–408.

82. Lawrence E, van Eeden SF, English D, Hogg JC. Polymorphonuclear leukocyte migration of Streptococcal pneumonia: Evidence for slow migration of cells recently released from the bone marrow. *Am J Respir Cell Mol Biol* 1996;16:217–224.

83. Terashima T, Klut ME, English D, et al. Chronic cigarette smoking causes sequestration of polymorphonuclear leukocytes released from the bone marrow in pulmonary capillaries. *Am J Resp Cell Mol Biol* 1998;20; 171–177.

84. Van Eeden SF, Lawrence L, Sato Y, Hogg JC. The effect of granulocyte colony stimulating factor (G-CSF) on the sequestration and migration of neutrophils during pneumococcal pneumonia. *Eur Respir J* 2000;15;1079–1086.

85. Sato Y, van Eeden SF, English D, Hogg JC. Bacteremic pneumonia: Bone marrow release and pulmonary sequestration of polymorphonuclear leukocytes. *Crit Care Med* 1998;26:501–509.

86. Doerschuk CM, Markos J, Coxson HO, et al. Quantitation of neutrophil migration in acute bacterial pneumonia in rabbits. *J Appl Physiol* 1994;77 (6):2593–2599.

87. Suwa T, English D, Hogg JC, van Eeden SF. The effect of interleukin-6 on PMN in the circulation and bone marrow. *Am J Respr Crit Care Med* 2000;161;A684.

88. Van Eeden SF, Kitagawa Y, Sat Y, Hogg JC. Polymorphonuclear leukocytes released from the bone marrow and acute lung injury. *Chest* 1999 ;116;(S)43–46.

89. Berkow RL, Dodson RW. Purification and functional evaluation of mature neutrophils from human bone marrow. *Blood* 1986;68(4):853–860.

90. Glasser L, Fiederlein RL. Functional differentiation of normal human neutrophils. *Blood* 1987;69(3):937–944.
91. Klut ME, Whalen BA, Hogg JC. Activation-associated changes in blood and bone marrow neutrophils. *J Leuk Biol* 1997;62(2):186–194.

Chapter 19

Leukocyte and Erythrocyte Kinetics in the Pulmonary Microcirculation

Wiltz W. Wagner, Jr, PhD

Introduction

This focus of this chapter is on the technique of in vivo microscopy, a method developed by myself and many valuable colleagues in Denver while we were being trained by Bob Grover in the Cardiovascular Pulmonary Laboratory. This close relationship with Bob also led to many pleasant social occasions spent with Estelle Grover. At the conclusion of the chapter, I will have some comments to make on this very kind and scientifically influential couple.

With this focus, all of the data presented comes from our in vivo microscopy technique. During the same time period, very important observations were being made in other laboratories using different techniques. This was especially important during our work on leukocyte kinetics. Due to space limitations, the work of others will not be presented. But I certainly want to acknowledge the work of Claire Doerschuk and Jim Hogg and their colleagues in Vancouver.[1-7] Their investigations moved along fruitful and parallel tracks and had a continuous and important influence on what we did and how we thought about our results.

Supported by National Heart, Lung, and Blood Institute Grant HL-36033.

From: Weir EK, Reeve HL, Reeves JT (eds). *Interactions of Blood and the Pulmonary Circulation*. Armonk, NY: Futura Publishing Company, Inc.; ©2002.

Leukocyte Kinetics in the
Pulmonary Microcirculation

In 1935, Clark and Clark[8] used in vivo microscopy to show that white blood cells rolled along the margins of postcapillary venules in the systemic circulation, hence the term "marginated" pool. It was assumed that white blood cells behaved similarly in the pulmonary microcirculation. However, in vivo microscopic observations made in my laboratory showed that neutrophils sequestered in the pulmonary capillaries[9] (Table 1).

By videorecording the passage of fluorescently labeled neutrophils, the transit time through the capillary could be measured.[10] Almost half of the labeled cells traversed the capillaries rapidly without stopping. This population is shown by the group having a transit time of <10 s in Figure 1. Another group had longer transit times of 10–300 s, and a third group stopped in the capillaries for >300 s. Our observation period was limited to 1200 s, but it was clear that some of the cells sequestered in the capillaries for much longer periods than 20 minutes.

The long-transit-time neutrophils did not progress by a slow steady passage, but rather by rapid movements interrupted by sudden, long stops. The number of stops varied. The right panel of Figure 1 shows that about 20% stopped once, 30% stopped 2 or more times, while the remaining half of the cells moved through the capillaries without any stops. This stop-start characteristic gave many of the cells the appearance of jumping from one stopping point to another and suggested that the cells were being trapped by discrete obstructions in the capillary network.

If the cells were being trapped at specific locations, we were curious to learn how many obstructions would be necessary to trap half of the neutrophils as they crossed the capillary bed. A computer model was developed in which the number of obstructions could be varied between 0% and 100%.[11] The "neutrophils" in the model moved through a 28 × 28 hexagonal grid. We selected this size because it caused the

---

Table 1

Neutrophils in the Pulmonary Microcirculation

Observation Site	Arterioles	Capillaries	Venules
Lower lung	0	2997	0
Upper lung	0	1958	0

All fluorescently labeled neutrophils that stopped in the pulmonary microcirculation were exclusively in the pulmonary capillaries. In vivo microscopy was used to study the canine lung both in the upper (Zone 2) and lower (Zone 3) lung.

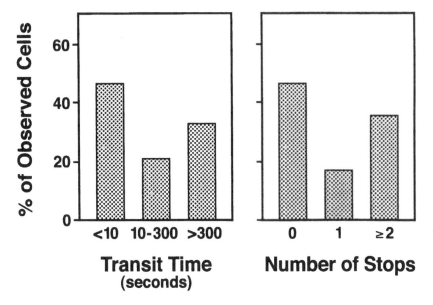

Figure 1. Direct measurements made of neutrophil kinetics in the pulmonary capillaries. Neutrophils with transit times <10 seconds do not stop in the capillaries. Longer transits can involve one or more stops at discrete sites. Used with permission.[10]

neutrophil to cross an average of 60 segments, a figure that Hogg[3] had calculated to be the average number of capillaries a blood cell would cross from arteriole to venule in the human lung. An example of the grid is shown in Figure 2. The heavy line shows the pathway of a neutrophil as it moves down the grid. The dots are obstructions. All observers who ran the computer model recognized that all of the cells would pass through the grid with 0% obstructions and none would pass through with 100% obstructions. The observer's job was to guess how many obstructions were needed to trap half of the cells as they passed through the grid. All observers started with a relatively large number of obstructions. If the initial guess was the typical 50%, all of the cells were trapped many times. Even if the number of obstructions was reduced to 10%, all of the cells were still trapped. To the surprise of all observers, whether they were scientists or lay persons, only between 1% and 2% obstructions, as shown in Figure 2, were needed to trap half of the cells and let the other half pass through unimpeded.

Of course, a hexagonal grid is not a true representation of the capillary bed. The computer, however, permitted the use of a wide range of grid designs. By changing to 4 segments per junction, a square model was generated. Again, 1–2% obstructions trapped half of the cells. Unrealistically exaggerated models of 8 and even 16 segments per junction

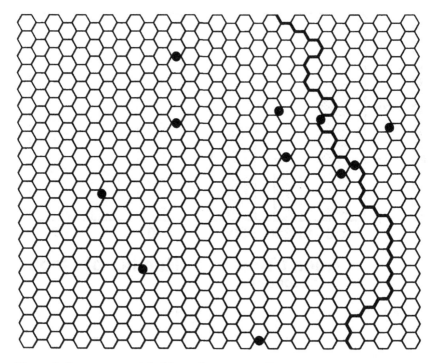

Figure 2. Computer model of the pulmonary capillary bed. In this case, 3 segments meet at each juncture forming a hexagonal grid. The heavy line shows typical pathway. The dots represent obstructions. Surprisingly, only 1–2% obstructions are required to trap half of the neutrophils. Used with permission.[11]

were tried with the same result, regardless of whether the obstructions were placed in the segments or in the junctions between segments. This consistency of results, shown in Figure 3, demonstrated that the model was robust. Even though we do not know how to model the pulmonary capillary network exactly, it does not matter because all of the geometric models produced identical results.

As a side note, the layout of the grid was based on the mathematical problem known as tiling the plane, i.e., how does one lay regularly shaped tiles on a plane without leaving spaces in between. That problem was solved and published by Leonhard Euler (1707–1783), an ancestor of U.S. von Euler of fame in the pulmonary circulation field for demonstrating that airway hypoxia caused a rise in pulmonary arterial pressure.[12]

The obstructions in these computer models were of an unspecified nature and simply trapped or passed the neutrophils in a binary way. To simulate anatomy more realistically, a hexagonal network was generated and neutrophils, chosen randomly from a published distribution

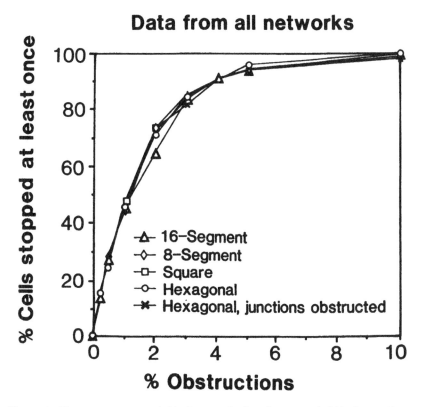

Figure 3. The computer model is impressively robust, as 1–2% obstructions trap half of the passing neutrophils whether the obstructions are placed in the segments or junctions or whether there are 3, 4, 8, or 16 segments meeting at each junction. Used with permission.[11]

of neutrophil diameters,[13] were passed through the network. The diameter of each capillary was picked randomly by the computer from published distributions of capillary diameters.[14] If a neutrophil became trapped in a segment because its diameter was larger than the segmental diameter, it was permitted to continue its transit across the network, but the computer counted how many times each neutrophil became trapped. After passing through an obstruction, the neutrophil resumed its original diameter. Runs with this model were made with 10,000 randomly selected neutrophils. From the published distributions of neutrophil and pulmonary capillary diameters, there were many combinations of small capillaries and large neutrophils that would result in trapping. The effects of these combinations were impressive: of the 10,000 neutrophils passed into the network, none made it across without being trapped. The run with the least number of stops was 12 times. The average was 36 stops. Even though the mean diameter of the selected neutrophils was less than that of the capillaries, 7.1 versus 7.5 μm, the standard deviations for the capillary diameters of 3.1 μm show that many small capillary segments would be in the 60-segment-long pathway that the neutrophil would cross.

For the half of the neutrophils to cross the network without stopping and a further quarter to stop only once, it appeared that the neutrophils had to elongate into sausage shapes. The program was altered so that a neutrophil could deform instantly up to 45% of its original diameter without being stopped when it reached a small capillary segment. Then it continued with its new diameter. If it entered a capillary that required >55% reduction of its original diameter, it would stop and be counted as a stop. After deforming sufficiently to pass through the small capillary, it would continue its journey while maintaining its newest diameter. The results reasonably approximated the direct in vivo observations.

Using in vivo microscopy, we were able to observe sausage-shaped leukocytes in the pulmonary capillaries. Although we could not quantify the shape changes in the capillaries, for the cells moved too rapidly, the shapes could be measured in the arterioles and venules that fed and drained the capillary bed. In that study,[15] the aspect ratio (major axis ÷ minor axis) was computed. Of the sample of leukocytes in arterioles (n = 1000), 94% had aspect ratios ≤1.25 and none was >1.53 (Figure 4). This narrow range demonstrated that the leukocytes were nearly circular (the aspect ratio of a circle is 1.0) as they reached the pulmonary capillaries from the feeding pulmonary arterioles. In contrast, 47% of the leukocytes in the venules (n = 1000) had aspect ratios ≤1.25, 37% were slightly elongated with aspect ratios of 1.5–2.0, and 16% were considerably elongated with aspect ratios of 2.0–4.0, showing that more than half of the cells were still altered in shape when they passed through the venules (Figure 4).

In summary, we think these data support the following model of leukocyte kinetics in the pulmonary microcirculation:

1. The capillaries are the site of sequestration for neutrophils in the pulmonary circulation.
2. Based on direct observations and on our computer modeling, we conclude that all white blood cells must deform to pass through the pulmonary capillaries.
3. Half of incoming neutrophils pass through the network without stopping.
4. The remainder stop 1 or more times at discrete locations in the capillaries.
5. Only 1% or 2% of the segments in a network can effectively trap half of the white cells. Because activated leukocytes become rigid, we conclude that activated cells would be

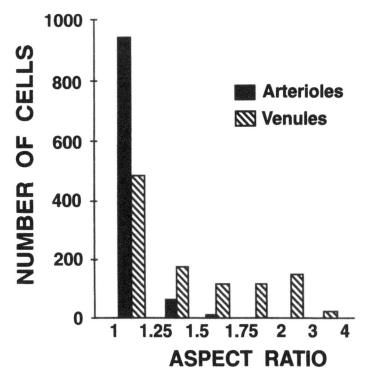

Figure 4. Direct measurement of leukocyte shapes coming into the capillaries (arterioles) or leaving the capillaries (venules). The incoming leukocytes are nearly round, because the aspect ratio (major axis ÷ the minor axis) of a circle is 1.0. Many leukocytes retain an elongated shape as they leave the capillaries, evidence that these cells must distort to pass through the capillaries. Used with permission.[15]

stopped by mechanical means in the pulmonary capillary bed. Following that trapping, there would be adequate time for the cell to upregulate its adhesion molecules and be held in place by those molecules.

Erythrocyte Kinetics in the Pulmonary Microcirculation

The first 15 years of work with my colleagues were devoted to the 2 problems that all in vivo microcirculationists must solve. First, the tissue must be held still so that the same vessels can be studied over time and thereby act as their own controls. Second, the local microphysiology as well as the physiology of the whole animal must be maintained in a normal condition. Throughout the history of microcirculatory studies, immobilizing the tissue was and still is being done at the expense of the micro- and macrophysiology. This is especially true of the pulmonary microcirculation. Investigators have resorted to breath-holds of absurd lengths of time or to tactics such as diffusion respiration during which the blood gas and hemodynamic values can deteriorate to morbid levels. Some give up on holding the vessels still and do not use vessels as their own controls, but compare measurements from whatever vessels come into view. It is often difficult to discern the true state of the micro- and macrophysiological in their manuscripts, or the validity of their control groups. Through the investment of considerable time and effort, we were able to devise methods that maintain reasonably normal physiology on both scales, as well as holding the surface of the lung still for many hours.[16,17]

Our first studies were designed to quantify how red blood cells moved through the capillaries. Although increases in cardiac output and elevation of pulmonary arterial or venous pressures caused obvious changes in capillary hemodynamics in the form of capillary recruitment and altered capillary transit times, the changes were difficult to quantitate. Initially we used high-speed photo- and cinemicrography, utilizing cameras and lighting systems developed for the space program.[18] Despite years of very interesting technical work, these approaches bore little biological fruit. With the advent of the Vietnam War, extremely sensitive solid-state and reasonably inexpensive television cameras became available. With these devices, we were able to measure the capillary transit time of fluorescent dye boluses. To our surprise, the transit times in the upper lung were much longer than expected.[19,20] This finding caused a controversy that was finally resolved when Hogg et al.[7] also found long transit times in the upper lung using independent techniques.

Later work by our group showed that several interesting changes occurred in capillary transit time as cardiac output was increased.[21] Because we were measuring the transit of dye boluses, we could compute the entire distribution of capillary transit times, and not just the mean. Of course the mean transit time became more rapid as pulmonary blood flow rose. There was, however, a much greater shift toward more rapid transits by the tail end of the distribution curves (Figure 5). This showed that there was a significant effect on the longest transit times, making for a more efficient passage. Although the head end of the curves also shifted to the left, even the most rapidly moving blood did not cross the capillaries in <0.25 seconds, the minimum time for complete saturation of the red cells.[22] Thus, with rising blood flow, the distribution of transit times became narrower, thereby approaching the ideal, which would be a spike at 0.25 seconds. That distribution would mean that all red cells became fully saturated exactly at the down-

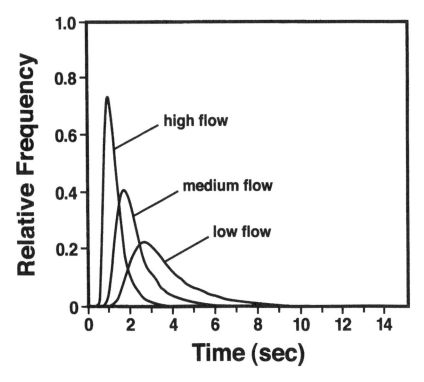

Figure 5. Mean capillary transit times shorten as pulmonary blood flow increases. The largest change is among the red cells with the longest transit times. The most rapid transit times become more rapid, but do not transit faster than 0.25 seconds and therefore still become fully saturated with oxygen. Used with permission.[21]

stream end of the capillary. Such a distribution is virtually an impossibility in a network with pathways of varying lengths and resistances, but the change in the shape of the curve is clearly heading in that more efficient direction.

These data were obtained for plasma transits. Later, when fluorescent dyes became available for labeling red cells, we were able to track their passage.[23] The fluorescent videomicrographs were intriguing to watch. Against a dark background, the bolus of brightly labeled red cells would suddenly appear in an arteriole (Figure 6, top) and then disperse rapidly into the capillary bed. The videos give the impression of fireworks exploding in the night sky. Following the capillary transit, the cellular stream would coalesce into venular pathways (Figure 6, bottom) and abruptly disappear from the field.

Red cell transits were more rapid than the plasma transits, measured across the same capillary bed under the same conditions (Fig-

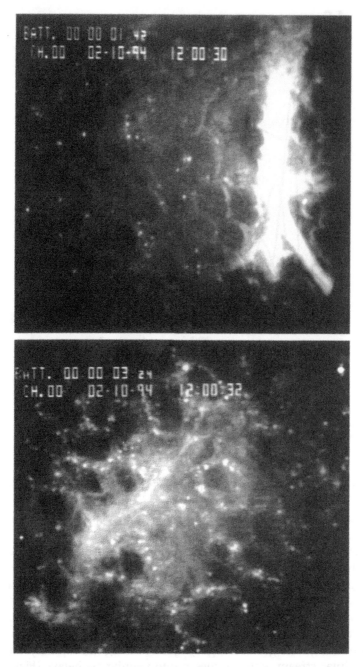

Figure 6. Red cells labeled with fluorescent dye make a dramatic appearance in an arteriole (upper panel). In the lower panel, 1.82 seconds later, the arteriole is empty of labeled cells, and many are in the venule having completed their capillary transit. Used with permission.[23]

ure 7). That observation, plus the fact that our maximum cardiac outputs in the experimental animals were less than the outputs during maximal exercise in the intact animal, suggests that the fastest moving red cells might become too rapid for complete saturation when maximal exercise was reached. The system is so well designed, however, that desaturation does not occur in the dog, our experimental animal in these studies, even during the heaviest exercise.[23]

The other obvious change that occurs in the pulmonary microcirculation during increased hemodynamics is the perfusion of previously unperfused capillaries. In fact, it was this capillary recruitment that was the first change we could quantitate.[24-26] One obvious question about recruitment was how rapidly it could occur. At first thought, it was not difficult to imagine that it would require many seconds for a new steady state to occur in capillary perfusion after a change in pulmonary blood flow. Consider what must happen when blood flow suddenly increases: the arterial vascular tree must distend and the many interconnected reserve capillaries must open and pressures throughout must equilibrate.

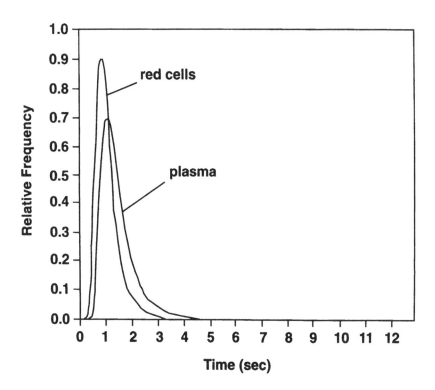

Figure 7. Red blood cells cross the capillaries more rapidly than plasma. These curves were obtained from the same capillary bed under identical hemodynamic conditions. Used with permission.[23]

To investigate how rapidly capillaries recruit, we used an isolated lung lobe perfused by 2 pumps running in parallel.[27] When one pump was turned off, flow rapidly halved; when it was turned on again, flow immediately (<0.3 seconds) doubled. Our observations of the capillary recruitment response were made on the surface of the lung, representing the most distant capillaries from the hilum and thus providing a longest-case response time. When flow was doubled in this experiment, capillary flow reached steady state in <4 seconds. When flow was halved, steady state was reached in ~8 seconds. These changes are shown in a series of computer-enhanced images in Figure 8 with an ensemble average of all data shown in Figure 9; a video clip of the videomicroscopic changes has been posted by the *Journal of Applied Physiology* on the internet.[28] These changes were surprisingly rapid, which again suggested the impressive design of the pulmonary circulation.

As red blood cells move from pulmonary arterioles to venules, they cross several alveolar walls, each of which contains an intricate network of capillaries. The total number of capillary segments crossed from arteriole to venule varies among species but generally ranges between 50 and 100 segments. Blood perfuses the capillaries in a complex manner; some segments are nearly always perfused and form interconnecting pathways across the alveolar wall,[29,30] while in other regions of the same alveolar wall, the blood frequently switches among segments, turning them on and off.[29,31] For decades, we considered the noisy-looking pattern of pulmonary capillary perfusion to be random, the result of highly flexible red blood cells coursing through complex capillary networks. Another possible cause of blood flow switching between segments could have been subtle alterations in pressure and flow into the capillary network. To test these ideas, we made a considerable effort in recent experiments to maintain stable conditions. Flows were held steady by a pump-perfusion system. The leukocyte counts fell as those cells adhered to the plastic tubing and were removed from the circulating blood. Pulmonary arterial and venous pressures were constant, indicating that pulmonary vascular resistance was stable. Blood gas values, blood temperatures, and airway pressures were stable as well. We expected that by achieving this level of stationarity, capillary perfusion would at last become stable.[32] As usual, we were wrong. In a typical example, shown in Figure 10, 3 adjacent alveoli, labeled A, B, and C, are shown along with their capillary segments, each of which is numbered. Despite our efforts to control hemodynamic variables, the path of the flowing blood switched frequently among capillary segments, causing the number of perfused segments to vary remarkably over time (Figure 11).

These findings came when a new analytic technique called fractal analysis had fortuitously been developed. This method permitted us to

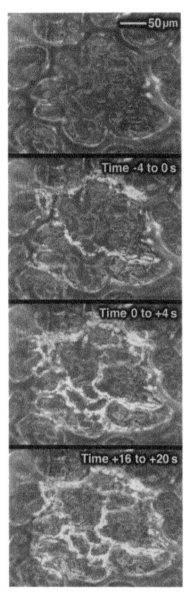

Figure 8. A large, subpleural alveolus is shown in the uppermost panel in an isolated, pump-perfused lung lobe preparation. The computer-enhanced image of the perfused capillaries in that alveolus is shown in the next panel over a 4-second-long period. At time zero, a second pump running in parallel with the first pump is suddenly turned on. In <4 seconds, many new capillaries have been recruited. In the lowest panel, the capillaries that are perfused 16–20 seconds later are shown and lead to the conclusion that capillary recruitment is remarkably rapid, reaching steady state in <4 seconds after a doubling of flow. Used with permission.[27]

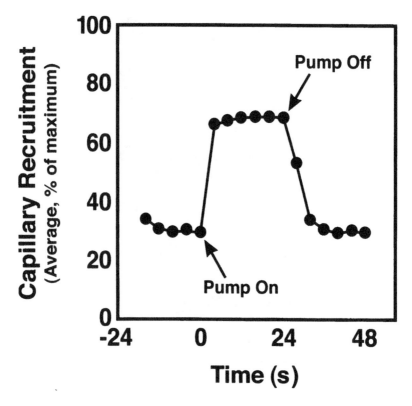

Figure 9. By ensemble averaging all data, the rapidity of the recruitment response is shown. The "derecruitment" is somewhat slower when the second pump is turned off and pulmonary blood flow halves. Used with permission.[27]

determine whether the fluctuations of flow within the capillary network were random or whether there was a pattern to the switching.[32] The analysis showed that the fluctuations were nonrandom and that the patterns were self-similar and repeated over time. The power of this kind of analysis is important for it demonstrates that there are strong repeating patterns in the datastreams shown in Figure 12 even though the data do not visually appear to be orderly.

Because the observed capillary networks lay in between a single feeding arteriole and a single draining venule and had perfusion patterns that repeated over time, it seemed reasonable to expect that the perfusion of neighboring alveoli would be correlated. One likely possibility was that perfusion of neighboring alveoli would be positively correlated. Even though overall pulmonary hemodynamics were stable, small regional alterations in the incoming arteriolar flow might cause the 3 neighbors to increase or decrease their level of perfusion in concert, thereby correlating positively with each other. Another possi-

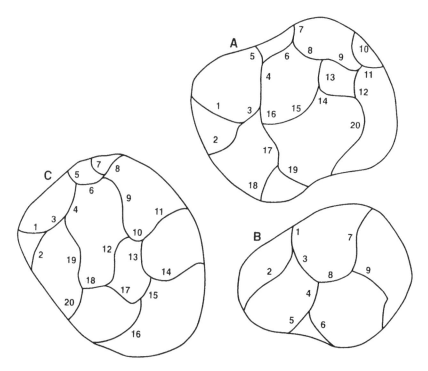

Figure 10. The capillary segments are numbered in 3 adjacent alveoli that are fed by a single arteriole and drained by a single venule. Used with permission.[32]

bility was a negative correlation; e.g., if flow increased in alveolus A, it might do so at the expense of alveolus B or C. Stealing of this kind would lead to a negative correlation. The possibility no one anticipated was that there would be virtually no correlation of the number of perfused segments in adjoining alveolar walls. That surprising and counterintuitive result, however, is what we found (Figure 13).

These data support the idea that the perfusion pattern within each alveolar wall is autonomous and independent; therein, we think, lie two important design features of the lung that provide robustness. First, fractal patterns are themselves robust, i.e., fractal patterns that repeat over time will, if perturbed, return to their original repeating pattern on their own. Thus, the fractal character of perfusion of an individual alveolar-capillary network is inherently robust. The second characteristic that is robust is the independence of neighbors. If there were dependence of neighboring alveolar perfusion patterns, especially if they were tightly correlated, then if the perfusion pattern of one alveolar wall were disrupted, the neighbors would likely be affected in a potentially disruptive way. The independent perfusion

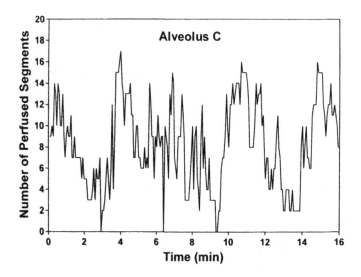

Figure 11. Even though the capillaries in the wall of alveolus C shown in Figure 10 are being perfused by a pump producing very steady pressure and flow, there is a very large variation in capillary perfusion in that alveolar wall over time. The number of perfused segments were counted every 4 seconds over a 16-minute-long interval. Used with permission.[32]

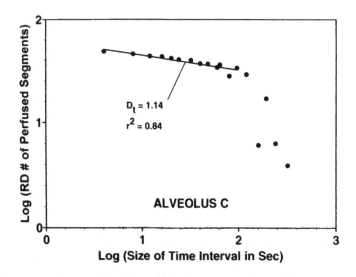

Figure 12. The fractal dimension (D_t) of the datastream in Figure 11 is 1.14 and lies reasonably close to a fractal dimension of 1.0. A value of 1.0 shows that a system has the characteristic of repeating in a self-similar manner, whereas a fractal dimension of 1.5 means that the system fluctuates in a random way. Used with permission.[32]

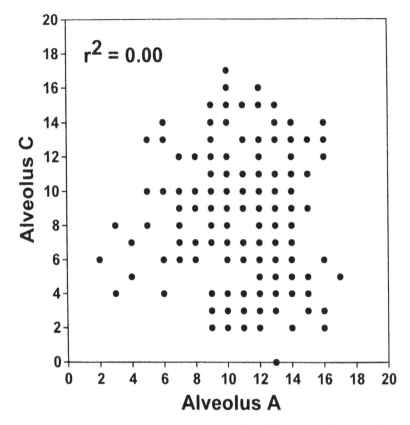

Figure 13. When the number of segments perfused in a given 4-second increment from one alveolus was plotted against the perfusion state of its adjacent neighbor, we were surprised to learn that the alveolar perfusion patterns were independent of each other with an average r^2 value of 0.06. These data show that the perfusion pattern of each alveolar-capillary network is independent of its neighbors. Used with permission.[32]

pattern displayed by alveolar capillaries makes them appear to be impervious to the behavior of their neighbors.

Ideally, a robust design must contain both a flexible component to adapt to new conditions and a more rigid component to provide long-term continuity. The functional independence of individual alveolar capillary networks, shown by the very low r^2 values, is the flexible component that can adapt to new conditions and is undisturbed by the perfusion state of its immediate neighbors. The fractal nature of perfusion, the automatically repeating component of perfusion within an individual capillary network, may serve as the more rigid component.

In both cases, the perfusion pattern of each alveolar wall is created by the unique characteristics of its own network. These patterns result in function that is independent of neighboring walls. If this reasoning is correct, then the capillary bed has, in addition to its delicate yet remarkably strong walls, an unsuspected elegance of design that imparts a robust character to the perfusion of pulmonary gas exchange vessels.

The Grovers

I was extremely fortunate to be hired by Bob Grover in October 1960 to work in his laboratory. My first job was the postmortem injec-

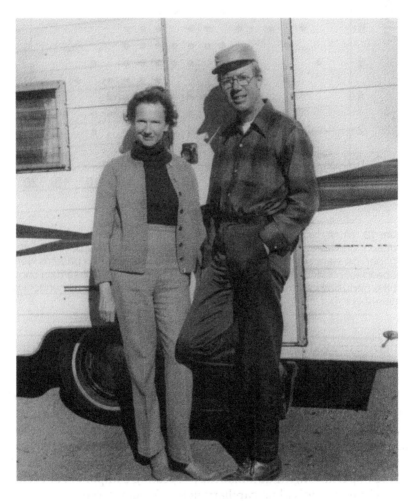

Figure 14. Estelle and Bob Grover ready for travel in 1974. Courtesy of R.F. Grover.

tion of the pulmonary arteries of patients who died of pulmonary hypertension or of the lungs from experimental animals. It was during the preceding summer that Bob and Estelle and Jack Reeves had studied the effect of high altitude on a number of species kept at 12,700 feet on Mt. Evans. The work led to 3 important papers that they published together. Between the experimental animals and the pre-pump days of cardiac surgery, there was no shortage of lungs to inject. Bob and I looked endlessly at the arterial branching patterns and wondered at the

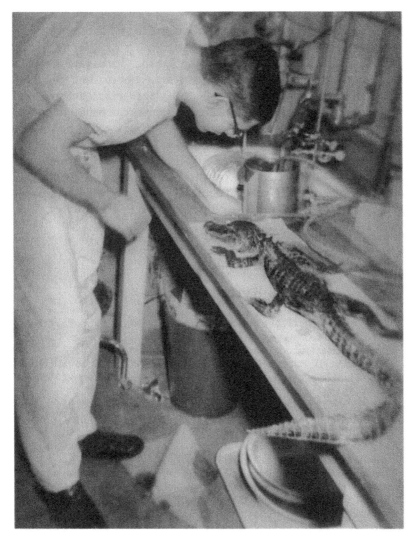

Figure 15. Wiltz Wagner with an experimental animal in 1960. Courtesy of R.F. Grover.

disappearance of the smallest vessels from the arteriograms as hypertension progressed.

That November, Bob invited me to his home for Thanksgiving dinner. There I first met Estelle, the fabulous cook, gardener, and Bob's constant companion during their research and many travels (Figure 14). After dinner, Bob and I sat on his couch and we sketched the anatomy of the heart and pulmonary circulation. This was the first of many times that we talked about the circulation. Our curiosity led to interesting experiments (Figure 15) and taught me that research, especially the kind that Bob and his colleagues did, was endless fun. Once I was in graduate school, Bob was my advisor. He and Estelle were always friendly and wonderfully supportive.

It was a real pleasure to watch Bob build the Cardiovascular Pulmonary Laboratory over the next 20 years, from not existing when he hired me, to a renowned laboratory where he was mentor to an amazing group of scientists; the impressive list of his trainees can be found on the Pulmonary Circulation Assembly website.[33] I am honored to be the Estelle Grover Lecturer and to publicly acknowledge the debt that so many of us owe to our scientific parents. Bob and Estelle Grover have produced an impressive scientific family consisting of many sons, daughters, grandchildren, and now great grandchildren who are themselves passing on the tradition of scientific excellence instilled by the Grovers.

Acknowledgments: Thanks are due to Drs. R.G. Presson, Jr., and T.M. Wagner for constructive criticism of the manuscript. Gary Schmitt provided excellent artwork.

References

1. Martin BA, Wright JT, Thommasen H, Hogg JC. Effect of pulmonary blood flow on the exchange between the circulating and marginating pool of polymorphonuclear leukocytes in dog lungs. *J Clin Invest* 1982;69:1277–1285.
2. Thommasen HV, Martin BA, Wiggs BR, et al. Effects of pulmonary blood flow on leukocyte uptake and release by dog lung. *J Appl Physiol* 1984;56: 966–974.
3. Hogg JC. Neutrophil kinetics and lung injury. *Physiol Rev* 1987;67:1249–1295.
4. Martin BA, Wiggs BR, Lee S, Hogg JC. Regional differences in neutrophil margination in dog lungs. *J Appl Physiol* 1987;63:1253–1261.
5. Doerschuk CM, Allard MF, Martin BA, et al. Marginated pool of neutrophils in rabbit lungs. *J Appl Physiol* 1987;63:1806–1815.
6. Doerschuk CM, Allard MF, Lee S, et al. Effect of epinephrine on neutrophil kinetics in rabbit lungs. *J Appl Physiol* 1988;65:401–407.
7. Hogg JC, McLean T, Martin BA, Wiggs BR. Erythrocyte transit and neutrophil concentration in the dog lung. *J Appl Physiol* 1988;65:1217–1225.
8. Clark ER, Clark EL. Observations on changes in blood vascular endothelium in living animals. *Am J Anat* 1935;57:385–438.
9. Lien DC, Wagner WW Jr, Capen RL, et al. Physiologic neutrophil seques-

tration in the canine pulmonary circulation: Visual evidence for localization in capillaries. *J Appl Physiol* 1987;62:1236–1243.

10. Lien DC, Worthen GS, Capen RL, et al. Neutrophil kinetics in the pulmonary microcirculation: Effects of pressure and flow in the dependent lung. *Am Rev Resp Dis* 1990;141:953–959.

11. Hanger CC, Wagner WW Jr, Janke SJ, et al. Computer simulation of neutrophil movement through the pulmonary capillary bed. *J Appl Physiol* 1993;74:1647–1652.

12. Von Euler US, Liljestrand G. Observations on the pulmonary arterial blood pressure in the cat. *Acta Physiol Scand* 1946;12:301–320.

13. Schmidt-Schöenbein GW, Shih YY, Chien S. Morphometry of human leukocytes. *Blood* 1980;56:866–875.

14. Weibel ER. Morphometrische analyse von zahl, volumen, und oberfläche der alveolen und kapillaren der menschlichen lunge. *Z Zellforsch Mikrosc Anat* 1962;57:648–666.

15. Gebb SA, Graham JA, Hanger CC, et al. Sites of leukocyte sequestration in the pulmonary microcirculation. *J Appl Physiol* 1995;79:493–497.

16. Wagner WW Jr, Filley GF. Microscopic observation of the lung in vivo. *Vasc Dis* 1965;2:229–241.

17. Wagner WW Jr. Pulmonary microcirculatory observations in vivo under physiologic conditions. *J Appl Physiol* 26375–377, 1969.

18. Wagner WW Jr, Barker DB, Filley GF. A photographic method for quantitating blood flow in the pulmonary microcirculation. *J Biol Photo Assn* 1967;35:95–108.

19. Wagner WW Jr, Latham LP, Gillespie MN, et al. Red cell transit times across pulmonary capillaries. *Science* 1982;218:379–380.

20. Wagner WW Jr, Latham LP, Hanson WL, et al. Vertical gradient of pulmonary capillary transit times. *J Appl Physiol* 1986;61:1270–1274.

21. Presson RG Jr, Hanger CC, Godbey PS, et al. The effect of increasing flow on the distribution of pulmonary capillary transit times. *J Appl Physiol* 1994;76:1701–1711.

22. Wagner PD. Diffusion and chemical reaction in pulmonary gas exchange. *Physiol Rev* 1977;57:257–312.

23. Presson RG Jr, Graham JA, Hanger CC, et al. Distribution of pulmonary capillary erythrocyte transit times. *J Appl Physiol* 1995;79:382–388.

24. Wagner WW Jr, Latham LP. Airway hypoxia causes pulmonary capillary recruitment in the dog. *J Appl Physiol* 1975;39:900–905.

25. Wagner WW Jr, Latham LP, Capen RL. Capillary recruitment during airway hypoxia: The role of pulmonary artery pressure. *J Appl Physiol* 1979; 47:383–387.

26. Hanson WL, Emhardt JD, Bartek JP, et al. The site of recruitment in the pulmonary microcirculation. *J Appl Physiol* 1989;66:2079–2083.

27. Jaryszak EM, Baumgartner WA, Peterson AJ, et al. Selected Contribution: Response of the pulmonary capillaries to sudden changes in flow. *J Appl Physiol* 2000;89:1233–1238.

28. Jaryszak EM, Baumgartner WA, Peterson AJ, et al. Video clip: Response of the pulmonary capillaries to sudden changes in flow. http://jap. physiology.org/cgi/content/full/89/3/1233.

29. Okada O, Presson RG Jr, Kirk KR, et al. Capillary perfusion patterns in single alveolar walls. *J Appl Physiol* 1992;72:1838–1844.

30. Okada O, Presson RG Jr, Godbey PS, et al. Temporal capillary perfusion patterns in single alveolar walls of intact dogs. *J Appl Physiol* 1994;76:380–386.

31. Presson RG Jr, Okada O, Godbey PS, et al. Stability of alveolar capillary opening pressures. *J Appl Physiol* 1994;77:1630–1637.
32. Wagner WW Jr, Todoran TM, Tanabe N, et al. Pulmonary capillary perfusion: Intra-alveolar fractal patterns and interalveolar independence. *J Appl Physiol* 1999;86:825–831.
33. Wagner WW Jr, Reeves JT. The Robert F. Grover Prize. In: Assembly Awards *http://www.thoracic.org/assemblies/pc/pc.html*.

Thrombosis

Thrombosis

Chapter 20

Coagulation and Fibrinolytic Factors in Pulmonary Hypertension

Carolyn H. Welsh, MD

Introduction

Clinical outcome data strongly suggest that thrombosis is important in the pathophysiology of pulmonary hypertension. Anticoagulant therapy is considered beneficial for primary pulmonary hypertension patients based on a retrospective study of 120 patients in which those receiving anticoagulation with warfarin lived longer.[1] In addition, the primary pulmonary hypertension registry patients who received warfarin therapy survived longer, even those patients without a vasodilator response; specifically, the 3-year survival increased from 31% to 62%.[2] There are fewer data to support a role for anticoagulation in persons with other types of pulmonary hypertension. In aminorex-induced pulmonary hypertension, anticoagulation improved survival from a mean of 6.1 years to 8.3 years,[3] suggesting that there is increased thrombosis in this type of pulmonary hypertension as well. How thrombosis participates in the natural history of pulmonary hypertension is not well delineated, but it may be mediated through bloodstream events, involving coagulation and fibrinolytic factors.

Acknowledgments: This work was supported in part by a Veterans Affairs Merit Review Grant award. Thanks to Laurie Graf, David Kressin for technical support and Kathy Hassell, MD, and Richard A. Marlar, PhD, for their help with the fibrinolytic and coagulation factor project.

From: Weir EK, Reeve HL, Reeves JT (eds). *Interactions of Blood and the Pulmonary Circulation*. Armonk, NY: Futura Publishing Company, Inc.; ©2002.

Overview: Circulating Coagulation and Fibrinolytic Factors

Circulating coagulation and fibrinolytic factors indirectly glimpse the pulmonary circulation. They are footprints of actual events at the endothelial cell surface and sample a secreted or released product. High circulating levels of an endothelial-associated clotting factor, such as thrombomodulin, tissue plasminogen activator (t-PA), or von Willebrand factor (vWF), may reflect either increased production, or alternatively increased degradation/loss of the factor from the endothelium. Low levels reflect decreased secretion, decreased production, or heightened metabolism. Alterations in these circulating levels may offer a picture of thrombotic properties of the endothelium. A confounding issue in the interpretation of circulating coagulation and fibrinolytic factors is that circulating factor levels reflect events in the systemic circulation as well as in pulmonary endothelium. There may be differences in factor levels, i.e., gradients, among venous, mixed venous, and arterial samples that can help determine which vascular bed may be affected to cause changes in plasma factor levels.[4] Nevertheless, venous sampling has determined characteristic findings in persons with pulmonary vascular disease. Despite this potential nonspecificity of plasma factor measurement, we believe that coagulation and fibrinolytic factors reflect pulmonary vascular events in pulmonary hypertension, and that plasma findings can be used to investigate the pulmonary endothelial environment.

The pulmonary circulation has unique features that may help explain changes in the procoagulant and anticoagulant profiles in the normal state and in the disease state. The pulmonary circulation is a high-flow, low-pressure circuit and normally experiences different (lower) levels of shear stress compared to the systemic arterial circulation. Endothelium in the pulmonary circulation is enriched in thrombomodulin, an endogenous anticoagulant, that may be particularly useful in clot prevention in an area of sluggish flow such as the pulmonary microvasculature. Second, the pulmonary microcirculation experiences higher oxygen tension than the systemic circulation. The pulmonary circulation has high levels of vasodilators, including nitric oxide and prostacyclin, with specificity for the lungs. These vasodilators have known antiplatelet aggregatory effects that may prevent local thrombosis under low flow conditions, although they have not had documented impact on plasma coagulation. Finally, the pulmonary circulation is unique in its interface with the airways, which may be a source of inflammation and thus promote procoagulant conditions. Perturbation of each of these 3 features, such as seen in pulmonary hypertension, high shear stress, hypoxemia, and inflammation, may alter local thrombotic conditions and coagulation factor release as discussed below.

Shear Stress

Shear stress experienced by the pulmonary circulation modulates vascular cell function and may affect thrombosis via changes in coagulation and fibrinolytic factors. Its major studied impact has been the enhancement of platelet aggregation under conditions of high flow and corresponding elevations of shear stress. At high levels of shear stress, platelet aggregation is vWF-dependent.[5] In human umbilical vein endothelial cells, acute exposure to moderate levels of shear stress over 24 hours leads to increased endothelial thrombomodulin expression.[6] Similar moderate to high shear stress levels (15–25 dynes/cm^2) for 24 hours have induced high t-PA secretion[7,8] with either no effect or an actual drop in plasminogen activator inhibitor-1 (PAI-1) release.[7] This may be an important local autoregulatory mechanism downregulating thrombosis since both t-PA and its product plasmin, the major fibrinolytic enzyme, inhibit shear-induced platelet aggregation. This offers a potential mechanism linking the complex platelet, coagulation, and fibrinolysis processes involved in thrombosis. The high levels of t-PA and plasmin under these high shear conditions appear to limit high shear stress-induced platelet aggregation[9] by causing proteolysis of the large functional vWF multimers essential for platelet aggregation.

Oxygen

The pulmonary circulation is exposed to varying oxygen concentrations, from low oxygen levels as blood enters the large pulmonary arteries to high saturations in the microcirculation and pulmonary veins. In the normal setting, the microcirculation sees a high oxygen tension, but this may change under pathological conditions. Oxidation with singlet oxygen inactivates clotting factors, including fibrinogen, V, VIII, X, and platelet aggregation in normal plasma in vitro[10] and may theoretically contribute to keeping the low flow pulmonary circulation free from microvascular clot formation. Hypoxia, a condition commonly associated with lung disease, can activate the procoagulant tissue factor pathway and reduce fibrinolyis in the endothelium.[11] Hypoxia is specifically associated with high levels of PAI-1, decreased t-PA, and subsequent fibrin accumulation.[12,13] Therefore, lowered oxygen exposure in pulmonary hypertension could contribute to the coagulation environment in the pulmonary circulation in ways that promote thrombosis.

Inflammation

Lung inflammation may cause endothelial vascular damage and initiate hypercoagulability. Cells exposed to inflammatory stimuli become procoagulant.[14-16] Apoptotic endothelial cells also become procoagulant with higher tissue factor, and lower endogenous anticoagulant levels of thrombomodulin, and tissue factor pathway inhibitor (TFPI).[17] Certainly the close proximity of the alveoli to the pulmonary circulation suggests that airway inflammation may contribute to hypercoagulability in humans with inflammatory lung disease. Clinical evidence to support this concept is present but sparse. Plasma coagulation factors have been measured in several populations with airway irritation. Air pollution increases serum viscosity, as measured in a large population.[18] Viscosity is largely a reflection of fibrinogen, with smaller contributions from alpha-2-macroglobulin and imunoglobulin M; and high fibrinogen levels are correlated with thrombosis, as discussed below. Therefore, the high viscosity may link airway inflammation and thrombosis. Cigarette smoke can also alter serum coagulation markers.[19] Specifically, heavy smokers have significantly reduced serum fibrinolytic activity as measured by a longer time to lysis compared to controls (males 286 ± 21 minutes in smokers compared to 236 ± 18 minutes in controls; females 315 ± 20 minutes compared to 193 ± 17 minutes).[19]

Although the mild pulmonary hypertension frequently seen in moderate to severe chronic obstructive lung disease (COPD) has been ascribed to hypoxic vasoconstriction, there may be an alternative pathogenetic explanation: that enhanced thrombosis potential leads to thromboembolic pulmonary hypertension. The data to support this hypothesis are through measures of circulating coagulation factors and from clinical observation. First, COPD exacerbations have been associated with hypercoagulability and venous thromboembolism. Using a global coagulation test, the modified recalcification time, acute bronchospasm was associated with heightened coagulation in 12 persons with COPD or asthma.[20] In 3 small series, COPD exacerbations were associated with an increased risk of venous thromboembolism.[21-23] Deep venous thrombosis by indium[111] platelet scanning was diagnosed in 45% (13/29) of serial COPD exacerbations reported by Winter.[21] In addition, Schonhofer reported that 21/196 (10.7%) patients with COPD exacerbations had a concomitant deep venous thrombosis, the majority of whom (18) were asymptomatic.[22] Third, autopsies in patients with end-stage lung disease and cor pulmonale who died of respiratory failure found that 14/19 had premortem venous thromboembolism.[23] These data suggest that COPD exacerbations are associated with a prothrombotic state and thrombosis.

Not only acute exacerbations but stable COPD as well may pose a prothrombotic risk. COPD patients in a small case control study had increased fibrinogen levels compared to age-matched controls (309 ± 10.3, n=63 vs. 256.3 ± 27, n=30, P=0.029), although there were no differences in C-reactive protein or factor VIII levels between groups (Welsh, unpublished data). Even stable COPD patients in another series had elevated levels of the prothrombin fragment F1.2, a marker of coagulation activation, in addition to high fibrinogen compared to controls.[24] In this study, both former and current smokers shared these procoagulant findings, making the procoagulant findings unlikely to be from a direct toxic effect of cigarette smoke.[24] In an ongoing study of risk factors for venous thromboembolism, COPD patients are disproportionately represented in the venous thromboembolism subject group compared to controls, 18% versus 6%, n=151 (Welsh, preliminary data), again potentially linking this lung disorder with venous thromboembolism. Finally, clinically unsuspected clots were identified as mobile central right pulmonary artery masses by transthoracic echocardiography in 12/25 COPD patients but in only 2/27 controls.[25]

These data link a hypercoagulable state with COPD clinical thrombosis, and thus provide an alternative hypothetical link of COPD to pulmonary hypertension. Inflammatory lung disease, such as COPD, may be a unique circumstance in which a hypercoagulable state induced by lung inflammation causes either pulmonary vascular clots or predisposes to systemic venous thromboembolism and perhaps associated pulmonary hypertension.

Are the Genetic Risk Factors for Venous Thromboembolism Important in the Development of Pulmonary Hypertension?

Genetic risk factors for venous thromboembolism have been associated with up to 30% of cases of venous thromboembolism. The 2 most common polymorphisms discovered to date are factor V_{Leiden} and the prothrombin 20,210 mutations. Other polymorphisms and plasma coagulation findings that are clinically demonstrated risk factors for venous thromboembolism include hyperhomocysteinemia, with or without the MTHFR 677 or MTHFR 1298 polymorphisms, high levels of lipoprotein (a) [Lp(a)], protein C deficiency, protein S deficiency, antithrombin III deficiency, elevated factor VIII levels, the angiotensin-converting enzyme D/D genotype, and a PAI-1 deletion mutation 4G/4G. Although these genetic polymorphisms increase risk for venous thromboembolism and theoretically should increase risk for pulmonary embolism, there is little to suggest that these are common findings in pulmonary hypertension per se. To date, the hereditary risks factors for venous thromboembolism are not more common in patients with primary pulmonary hypertension. In a series of pulmonary hypertension patients, 1/64 (1.5%) persons with primary pulmonary hypertension had factor V_{Leiden}, compared to 3 of 100 (3%) controls.[26] The thromboembolic pulmonary hypertension group had 3/46 (6.5%) with factor V_{Leiden}, again not significantly different from control incidence. In a group of patients with primary pulmonary hypertension (PPH), Elliott reported only 1 of 42 (2.4%) patients with factor V_{Leiden}, again showing no association of this common polymorphism with the pathogenesis of pulmonary hypertension.[27] Lipoprotein (a) [Lp(a)] has been measured, too. Lp(a) competes with plasminogen for binding to plasminogen receptors and thus acts to suppress fibrinolysis. In vitro, it regulates PAI-1.[28] Lp(a) concentrations in primary pulmonary hypertension were similar to controls, in contrast to chronic thromboembolic pulmonary hypertension where levels were elevated.[29] At the present time, the genetic polymorphisms for venous thromboembolism have been found as commonly for thromboembolic pulmonary hypertension as for venous thromboembolism itself, thus being detectable in a minority of cases. They are no more common in primary pulmonary hypertension than in a control population, and cannot be linked to its pathogenesis.

Autoimmune Aspects of Coagulation and Fibrinolytic Factors in Pulmonary Hypertension

Another potential link between thrombosis, coagulation factors, and pulmonary hypertension is the action of phospholipid-dependent antibodies including lupus anticoagulant, anticardiolipin antibodies, and other antiphospholipid (APL) antibodies to induce thrombosis. These antibodies are measured in plasma samples. Case reports and small case series describe the antiphospholipid syndrome as causal for 3 pulmonary vascular conditions: pulmonary hypertension, thrombosis with pulmonary embolism, and microthrombosis of the lung.[30] One notable patient with the anticardiolipin antibody had diffuse in situ thrombosis in the small pulmonary vessels of the lung at autopsy despite treatment with warfarin.[31] What is not clear is whether these antibodies, including the antibodies to components of the coagulation system or endothelium, reflect endothelial dysfunction or whether they actually initiate in situ thrombosis. Thus, the pathogenetic role as causal or simply as an epiphenomenon is uncertain.

The antiphospholipid antibodies on average may be more frequent in the pulmonary hypertensive population, especially for the pulmonary hypertensive patients with collagen vascular disease. In 38 patients with pulmonary hypertension, 11/37 (37%) patients with either primary pulmonary hypertension or pulmonary hypertension from lung or connective tissue disease had antiphospholipid antibodies (APL) antibodies, but none of 8 patients with postcapillary pulmonary hypertension and high wedge pressures from left ventricular dysfunction had APL antibodies.[32] Also, APL antibodies failed to correlate with the degree of pulmonary hypertension.[32] In a larger series, Wolf reported that 10% of primary pulmonary hypertension patients had APL antibodies (8/83) compared to 20% of patients with chronic thromboembolic pulmonary hypertension (25/116), some of the latter with much higher titers of antibodies.[26] No assay results are reported for any control subjects in this series. In a lupus clinic, 24 persons with pulmonary hypertension were identified and a large proportion, 68%, had circulating anticardiolipin antibodies or lupus anticoagulant.[33] In contrast, Isern failed to find frequent antiphospholipid antibodies in pulmonary hypertension, finding them in only 1.8% of 55 patients with primary or secondary pulmonary hypertension.[34] The assays used in this series may, however, have lacked appropriate sensitivity. Thus the association of these general autoantibodies to pulmonary hypertension appears weak.

Specific antibodies to coagulation and fibrinolytic factors have been reported as well.[35–37] These may be more germane in the development of a prothrombotic environment. Carson noted antithrombomodulin antibodies in 30% of persons with lupus anticoagulant and 10% of 200 patients with unexplained thrombosis.[35] Fritzler searched for the fibrin-bound anti-t-PA antibodies in serum from 128 patients with systemic sclerosis and found them in 25 (19%).[36] The patients with these t-PA antibodies were slightly more likely to have pulmonary hypertension (5/25, 20%).[36] Morse studied this same fibrin-bound t-PA antibody and noted its presence in 9.3% of 86 primary pulmonary hypertension patients but in only 2.5% (1/40) of patients with pulmonary hypertension from cardiac shunt.[37] Although these antibodies to coagulation or fibrinolytic factors may be more common for pulmonary hypertensive patients than are the general autoantibodies, their role in causing pulmonary hypertension is not clear. Their presence in only a minority of persons with pulmonary hypertension makes routine clinical use premature.

Specific Coagulation and Fibrinolytic Factors in Pulmonary Hypertension

Thrombomodulin

Endogenous anticoagulant properties of endothelium may be most useful in a low flow setting such as characterized by the pulmonary circulation. Four endogenous anticoagulant mechanisms have been localized to the vasculature including antithrombin III, thrombomodulin-activated protein C, tissue factor pathway inhibitor, and heparan sulfates, present on endothelium. The thrombomodulin-activated protein C is the best understood of these processes and may be uniquely important in the pulmonary circulation. Thrombomodulin is a glycoprotein receptor for thrombin located on endothelium. Its major anticoagulant mechanism is that, when binding thrombin to the endothelial cell, it activates protein C and inhibits further thrombin generation and clots by inactivating clotting factors Va and VIIIa (Figure 1).

Endothelium from vessels in body organs differs in its thrombotic profile and in particular in thrombomodulin content. The lung microvasculature appears to be enriched in thrombomodulin.[38,39] In the rabbit, lung thrombomodulin antigen levels are the highest of any organ[38] and there is a 5- to 12-fold increase in lung thrombomodulin compared to kidney concentrations in mice.[39] In the human lung, thrombomodulin is localized to capillary endothelium adjacent to alveoli, while vWF, another endothelial product, is localized to a somewhat different population of cells in slightly larger vessels and adjacent to connective tissue.[40] Although thrombomodulin is predominantly expressed in endothelium, after balloon-induced vessel injury it is also expressed by smooth muscle.[41] Thrombomodulin expression is altered by changes in flow. Moderate levels of shear stress (15 dynes/cm^2) induce a transient rise in thrombomodulin mRNA before a drop in levels by 9 hours. Thus, while thrombomodulin is concentrated in lung tissue, it may be more important in the microcirculation than in larger vessels,[40] and its expression is flow-regulated.[42]

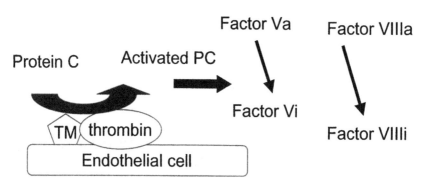

Figure 1. An important endogenous anticoagulation pathway. Thrombomodulin, an endothelial receptor for thrombin, binds thrombin and thereby activates protein C, which leads to inactivation of factors V and VIII. Thus, the prothrombotic molecule thrombin participates in endothelial-associated anticoagulation. TM = thrombomodulin; activated PC = activated protein C; Va = activated factor V; VIIIa = activated factor VIII; Vi = inactivated factor V; VIIIi = inactivated factor VIII.

Circulating thrombomodulin levels are in equilibrium with endothelial thrombomodulin, but are somewhat complex to interpret. Initial reports of circulating thrombomodulin in human disease described high levels in conditions such as acute respiratory distress syndrome, Wegener's granulomatosis, collagen vascular disease, and scleroderma.[43,44] Thrombomodulin levels are higher in congenital heart disease patients with pulmonary hypertension[44] compared to congenital heart disease patients without pulmonary hypertension and they rise after bypass procedures.[44] In contrast to acute illness, with a chronic state of low-grade injury such as might be seen in the pulmonary hypertensive state, thrombomodulin levels have been reported to be depressed.[45,46] In 2 case series where circulating thrombomodulin levels were measured in chronic primary and secondary pulmonary hypertension, they were lower than control values for the primary pulmonary hypertensive patients[45] or for both primary and secondary hypertension patients[46] (Table 1). This low thrombomodulin pattern is not a fixed finding, however, since levels can improve after therapy. Low thrombomodulin levels in plasma in chronic pulmonary thromboembolic hypertension increased after pulmonary endarterectomy.[47] Thus, circulating levels appear to have a complex relation to tissue levels, reflect pulmonary vascular events in persons without other vascular disease, and improve with treatment of pulmonary hypertension. There may be a biphasic pattern for plasma thrombomodulin with an acute increase and subsequent drop in circulating levels. Although most reports support a pulmonary vascular source of plasma thrombomodulin, it may be of systemic origin as well. In a large, 14,170-person case-cohort study, the Atherosclerosis Risk in Communities (ARIC) study, circulating thrombomodulin showed a strong inverse association with coronary artery disease, suggesting it is in equilibrium with systemic endothelial thrombomodulin as well.[48]

Table 1

Circulating Thrombomodulin Levels (ng/mL)

PPH	SPH	CHF/PHT	Control	Author
29±7* (12)	49±5 (25)		56±6 (14)	Welsh
29±3* (11)	22±2* (11)	85±17* (10)	44±2 (38)	Cacoub

PPH = primary pulmonary hypertension; SPH = secondary pulmonary hypertension; CHF/PHT = pulmonary hypertension from congestive heart failure.
* = significantly different from control; $P < 0.05$.

Tissue Factor Pathway Inhibitor (TFPI)

Tissue factor pathway inhibitor (TFPI) is a proteinase inhibitor that prevents tissue factor-induced blood coagulation. Tissue factor is an early initiating step in clot formation. TFPI is currently considered of lesser importance than antithrombin III or activated protein C as an endogenous anticoagulant. Circulating TFPI levels are low normal or deficient in pulmonary hypertension in 2 series.[45,49] Welsh reports somewhat lower levels in primary pulmonary hypertension than for secondary pulmonary hypertension or controls, although this is of borderline statistical significance[45] (115 ± 7 ng/mL, 157 ± 20 ng/mL, and 143 ± 22 ng/mL, respectively). Altman found that TFPI was diminished in pulmonary hypertension but only when right atrial pressure was 9 mm Hg or higher (47 ± 19 ng/mL). When right atrial pressure was less than 9 mm Hg, TFPI levels were comparable to control values (97 ± 32, 96 ± 62 ng/mL).[49] This may therefore be a second endogenous anticoagulant mechanism that is interrupted in pulmonary hypertension, predisposes to thrombosis, and can be monitored by blood draws.

Fibrinolysis

Fibrinolysis is the dissolution of a clot, which is an ongoing process important in vascular remodeling and wound healing, acting to keep vessels patent. Suppression of fibrinolytic activity leading to slowing of clot degradation has been reported on numerous occasions in pulmonary hypertension. Disturbances in fibrinolytic balance can include low free t-PA, and high levels of PAI-1, the primary t-PA inhibitor in blood, both leading to slowing of clot breakup (Figure 2). In addition, total t-PA may be elevated, reflecting both free and PAI-1-bound antigen. These 2 important fibrinolytic factors are both secreted by endothelium. Fibrinogen excess has been reported to lead to enhanced fibrin deposition, and lack of plasminogen, the substrate for plasminogen activator, could lead to sluggish clot lysis and be a risk for thrombosis as well (Figure 2).

Abnormalities leading to diminished fibrinolysis in pulmonary hypertension have been seen both in global measures of fibrinolysis such as euglobulin lysis time (ELT) as well as in the specific factors of fibrinolysis, t-PA, PAI-1 elevation (Figure 2), or a blunted venous occlusion response of t-PA. A primary pulmonary hypertension case report described low fibrinolytic activity as manifest by an elevated euglobulin lysis time and decreased plasminogen activation,[50] and a family with primary pulmonary hypertension showed elevated antiplasmin activity.[51]

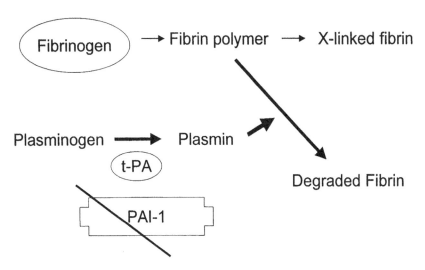

Figure 2. The process of fibrinolysis or dissolution of a clot. Thrombin cleaves fibrinogen to start fibrin deposition (not shown). Plasminogen is then activated to plasmin to initiate fibrinolysis. Plasmin degrades the fibrin polymers formed from fibrinogen and is activated by t-PA (tissue plasminogen activator), which is a rate-limiting step in fibrin degradation. PAI-1 is the important circulating inhibitor of t-PA.

Characteristic fibrinolytic factor findings include the following. Total t-PA levels, which include the antigen bound to the circulating inhibitor PAI-1 as well as free antigen, are variably high or normal in pulmonary hypertension.[45,49] and free t-PA levels are low to normal.[49] A higher rise of t-PA to a venous occlusion maneuver is seen in normal subjects, with a blunted response in pulmonary hypertensive patients, both in those with primary pulmonary hypertension and in those with thromboembolic pulmonary hypertension.[52,53] The findings of abnormal fibrinolysis are not fixed, but can respond to pulmonary hypertension therapy, such as reported by Boyer-Neumann, where prostacyclin decreases plasma levels of t-PA and PAI-1 in primary pulmonary hypertension.[54]

In addition to the low free t-PA, circulating PAI-1 levels are increased in persons with pulmonary hypertension.[45,49,55,56] PAI-1 regulates the fibrinolysis pathway and matrix turnover; it is the most important inhibitor of plasminogen activator in the blood. Hoeper showed PAI-1 was higher in arterial compared to mixed venous samples in primary pulmonary hypertensive patients, suggesting specific production in the pulmonary vascular bed.[55] High resting PAI-1 levels have been reported in thromboembolic pulmonary hypertension as well as in primary pulmonary hypertension.[52]

Newly described PAI-1 polymorphisms may shed light on predisposition to vascular disease, including pulmonary hypertension. These have not yet been investigated in pulmonary hypertension. A point deletion mutation in the promoter of plasminogen activator inhibitor type 1, the 4G allele, is associated with elevated PAI-1 levels.[57] Observational studies suggest that this 4G polymorphism is overrepresented in venous thromboembolism patients compared to healthy controls. The 4G/4G polymorphism interacts with the serum triglyceride levels; as triglyceride levels rise, PAI-1 levels are higher for 4G/4G than for 4G/5G or 5G/5G patients.[58] This may be a genetic predisposition to hypofibrinolysis comparable to the genetic variation seen in the endogenous anticoagulant system with factor V_{Leiden} leading to impaired activation of the protein C pathway. Genetic variations of this sort may be important in many circulatory disease processes, including pulmonary hypertension.

In addition to the fibrinolysis regulatory step of plasmin activation involving t-PA and PAI-1, other points in the fibrinolysis pathway may be altered in pulmonary hypertension (Figure 2). A single patient with a congenital plasminogen deficiency and pulmonary hypertension has been described. A 25-year-old with putative primary pulmonary hypertension had low levels of plasma plasminogen that the authors suggest was causal for the pulmonary hypertension.[59] Also, fibrinogen, which is the substrate for fibrin formation, is a marker of coronary artery risk for diabetes mellitus patients. Cleavage products of fibrinogen are mitogens for several cell types including endothelium as well as fibroblasts and smooth muscle cells and could be important in pulmonary hypertension.[60] Fibrinogen levels are elevated in pulmonary hypertension and are associated with the degree of pulmonary hypertension [45] ($p = 0.037, r = 0.3262$; see Table 4). Fibrinogen levels rise more after venous occlusion in pulmonary hypertensive patients than in controls[49] and are higher in those with pulmonary hypertension and a right atrial pressure of more than 9 mm Hg compared to those patients with a right atrial pressure less than 9.[49] Fibrinogen regulation, also, is under genetic control as well as environmental modification. Persons with the fibrinogen type AA show a higher fibrinogen rise to inflammation and a higher exercise response than do those with the GG alleles.[58] Both the PAI-1 4G/4G and fibrinogen AA polymorphisms have the potential to impact on pulmonary vascular responses and pulmonary hypertension and should be investigated further.

Fibrinolysis is correlated with systemic vascular disease including diabetes mellitus as well as pulmonary vascular disease. It may be that the findings of suppressed fibrinolysis, prolonged euglobin lysis time (ELT), and increased inhibitor PAI-1 are sequelae of endothelial injury or remodeling. Their presence in pulmonary hypertension may be nonspecific but is striking and consistent.

Coagulation Activation

Elevated markers of clot activation such as fibrinopeptide A have been reported in pulmonary hypertension,[52,56] but fibrinopeptide A is easy to trigger and therefore highly susceptible to artifactual elevation. Investigators have not consistently seen a rise with other coagulation activation assays to suggest continued clot or fibrinolysis activation, including fibrin degradation products, the prothrombin fragment F1.2, thrombin antithrombin complexes, or D-dimers.[45,49,55] Although there is no reproducible evidence for ongoing coagulation activation in pulmonary hypertension, the level of clot activation may be too subtle for the sensitivity of current tests.

Von Willebrand Factor

Alterations in vWF level, activity, and size have been investigated in numerous vascular diseases including pulmonary hypertension.[61,62] In pulmonary hypertension and atherosclerosis, elevations in the antigen level are considered a marker of endothelial dysfunction. vWF is a large multimeric glycoprotein synthesized by endothelium and megakaryocytes. It has several biological functions, including anchoring of platelet and endothelial cells to the matrix, and its action as an adhesive protein for platelets via both their GPIb and GPIIb-IIIa receptors.[61,62] In plasma, vWF carries factor VIII, and via this function as well as its platelet adhesive properties, it is an important participant in initiating thrombosis.

Several investigators have reported vWF abnormalities in pulmonary hypertension. These include increased levels of vWF antigen, loss of circulating high MW multimers and relative loss of vWF activity. First, several investigators have compared vWF levels in primary pulmonary hypertension to levels in other pulmonary hypertensive patients in small case series.[63–65] In those with congenital heart disorders or lung disease, vWF can be normal or elevated. High levels are also seen in cystic fibrosis patients with pulmonary hypertension.[63] In patients with pulmonary hypertension from congenital heart disease, levels are normal or modestly increased. In contrast, primary pulmonary hypertension patients show a more substantial vWF antigen elevation. There is a striking elevation of circulating vWF seen in primary pulmonary hypertension compared to other types of pulmonary hypertension for 6 of the 7 series reported (Table 2). Lopes found that circulating vWF antigen levels are more than double those in control subjects.[66] Welsh reports that vWF levels correlate with serum aspartate aminotransferase (SGOT) levels ($r=0.5209$, $P=0.0076$), supporting the hypothesis that this plasma coagulation marker may be associated with tissue injury.[45] One group of primary pulmonary hypertension patients had only a modest elevation of vWF antigen levels compared

Table 2

Von Willebrand Factor Antigen Levels (%)

Primary Pulmonary Hypertension	Control	Pulmonary Hypertension, Congenital Heart Disease	Secondary Pulmonary Hypertension	Author
239 (3)		138 ± 54 (25)	103 (3)	Rabinovitch, 1987
86 ± 25 (6)		102 ± 17 (12)	158 ± 24 (5)	Geggel, 1987
141 ± 13 (14)	104 ± 16 (15)		190 ± 19 (25)	Welsh, 1996
214 ± 91 (10)	91 ± 51		142 ± 74 (19)	Lopes, 1993, 1998
252 ± 58 (16)	97 ± 25 (16)			Hoeper, 1998
231 ± 89 (11)	87 ± 23 (20)	127 ± 68 (24)		Lopes, 2000

Numbers in parentheses are the number of subjects sampled.

to the other series in the literature[45] (Table 2). This was the only included series, to our knowledge, where some of the primary pulmonary hypertension patients received prostacyclin treatment at the time of blood draw. Thus, the blunted height of the vWF antigen peak compared to the other series may reflect a treatment effect of prostacyclin.

A second finding in pulmonary hypertension is that the vWF molecules may be abnormal in structure despite their presence in high levels. In primary pulmonary hypertension, there is loss of the high molecular weight multimers essential for platelet adhesiveness,[45,64,66] perhaps due to a sialic acid deficiency.[66] Third, measures of vWF activity level, ristocetin, are variably abnormal in pulmonary hypertension (Table 3), with a characteristic loss of activity for the degree of antigen elevation. When vWF activity/antigen levels are calculated, the majority of authors report

Table 3

Von Willebrand Factor Activity (%) Normal

Primary Pulmonary Hypertension	Control	Pulmonary Hypertension, Congenital Heart Disease	Secondary Pulmonary Hypertension	Author
91.7 (3)		98 ± 40 (21)	86 (2)	Rabinovich, 1987
197 ± 43 (6)		89 ± 11 (12)	153 ± 30 (5)	Geggel, 1987
128 ± 14 (14)	105 ± 10 (15)		143 ± 13 (26)	Welsh, 1996

Numbers in parentheses are the number of subjects sampled.

low ratios for persons with pulmonary hypertension. Lopes reports that activity decreases linearly with a drop in particle density.[66] The excessive amount of vWF antigens, therefore, may be poorly functional due to damaged endothelium or abnormal antigen degradation, possibly from shear stress in the pulmonary circulation.

Not only are antigen levels high, but high vWF may have prognostic value in pulmonary hypertension. Lopes showed that patients with primary pulmonary hypertension whose vWF antigen levels were greater than 245% predicted had poor short-term survival (n=40).[62] In congenital heart disease patients, levels were also correlated with survival, although average survival was longer for a given vWF value compared to the primary pulmonary hypertension patients. Lopes failed to find a correlation of vWF with survival for pulmonary hypertension from other causes, although the numbers are small. To see if treatment affects plasma markers, Friedman assessed vWF levels and activity in 64 primary pulmonary hypertension patients both before and during prostacyclin therapy.[67] vWF antigen levels decreased from 136 ± 89% to 56 ± 50%, while activity to antigen ratios rose from 0.8 to 1.2. Both of these trends suggest that prostacyclin treatment favorably impacted this marker of disease activity.[67] Thus, vWF appears to be higher in primary pulmonary hypertension than for other causes of pulmonary hypertension and is potentially a good marker for this type of pulmonary hypertension; it also provides prognostic information. Since these high antigen levels are seen in primary pulmonary hypertension out of proportion to their levels in other types of pulmonary hypertension of similar severity, they may ultimately correlate with the number or volume of the plexiform lesions characteristic of this disease rather than correlating with a generalized pulmonary endothelial dysfunction/injury. It is intriguing to think of the circulating vWF excess in this disease as a possible marker of the proliferative monoclonal endothelial cell expansion of endothelial cells[68] rather than reflective of the degree of "injury" from shear stress or other insult.[69]

Coagulation/Fibrinolytic Factor Profiles

After analysis of single factor test results, in our series of pulmonary hypertensive patients and controls, we asked whether there were patterns among the clotting and fibrinolytic factors in our series that described different types of endothelial dysfunction or severity of impairment.[45] First, we analyzed the degree of pulmonary artery pressure elevation for persons with either primary or secondary pulmonary hypertension versus the factor levels, to see if the degree of mean pulmonary artery pressure elevation correlated with more abnormal plasma coagulation or fibrinolytic factor levels (Table 4). The severity of pul-

Table 4

Pulmonary Artery Pressure Correlations with Coagulation and Fibrinolytic Factors

Coagulation Factor	Pearson's Correlation Coefficient (r)	Statistical Significance (p Value)
Fibrinolysis measurements		
Euglobulin lysis time (ELT)	0.6037	<0.0001
t-PA	0.2912	0.065
PAI-1	0.4245	0.0057
Fibrinogen	0.3262	0.037
Plasminogen	−0.1162	0.4694
Alpha-2-antiplasmin	−0.2614	0.8711
vWF antigen	0.2791	0.077
vWF activity (ristocetin)	0.1252	0.435
Thrombomodulin/protein C endogenous anticoagulation		
Thrombomodulin	−0.2798	0.076
Activated protein C	−0.3073	0.073
% Protein C activity	−0.2518	0.11
Protein S	−0.2394	0.13
TFPI	−0.0683	0.67
Antithrombin III	−0.1945	0.22
Markers of coagulation activation		
Thrombin-antithrombin Complexes	0.0908	0.57
Prothrombin fragment F 1.2	-0.0581	0.72

vWF = von Willebrand factor; t-PA = tissue plasminogen antigen; PAI-1 = plasminogen activator inhibitor-1; TFPI = tissue factor pathway inhibitor.

monary hypertension as measured by mean pulmonary artery pressure correlated with the euglobulin lysis time (Figure 3), elevated levels of PAI-1, and had a trend to higher t-PA levels ($P=0.065$). Second, the vWF antigen trended to higher levels with higher pulmonary artery pressure ($P=0.077$). Third, there was also a trend to lower circulating thrombomodulin with accompanying lower activated protein C activity ($P=0.051$ and 0.08, respectively). The parallel findings of diminished fibrinolysis, increased vWF antigen, and loss of the thrombomodulin/protein C pathway anticoagulant activity as pulmonary artery pressure was increasingly elevated support the concept of progressive endothelial dysfunction in the pulmonary hypertensive patient.

Next, we looked for patterns of low or high factors that tracked with each other and found 2 distinctive patterns. High vWF antigen levels correlated with high levels of thrombomodulin, high levels of t-PA, and preserved fibrinolytic function (low ELT) (Table 5). In contrast, the

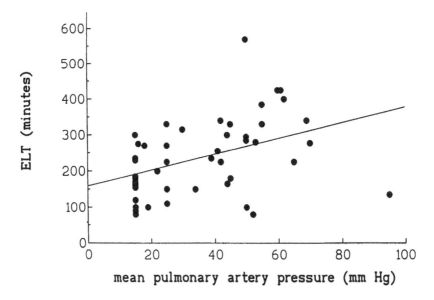

Figure 3. Prolonged fibrinolysis as measured with the global fibrinolyis test, euglobulin lysis time (ELT), correlates with the degree of pulmonary artery elevation (r=0.604, P<0.0001). Used with permission from *Chest*.[45]

Table 5

Coagulation/Fibrinolytic Factor Patterns: Correlation Between Procoagulant Markers of Endothelial Injury

	Pearson's Correlation Coefficient (r)	Statistical Significance (P value)
Increased ELT and:		
Decreased vWF activity	−0.54	<0.05
Decreased thrombomodulin	−0.58	<0.01
Increased PAI-1	0.59	<0.01
Increased alpha-2-antiplasmin	0.52	<0.05
Increased vWF antigen		
Increased thrombomodulin	0.43	<0.05
Increased t-PA	0.64	<0.001
Decreased ELT	-0.46	<0.05
For details of clotting tests used, see reference # 45		

ELT = euglobulin lysis time; vWF = von Willebrand factor; PAI-1 = plasminogen activator inhibitor-1; t-PA = tissue plasminogen activator.

higher euglobulin lysis times, which reflect diminished fibrinolysis, were associated with lower vWF, lower thrombomodulin, high PAI-1, and high levels of alpha-2-antiplasmin, another inhibitor of fibrinolysis. The first pattern, high vWF with preserved fibrinolytic function, may possibly represent acute endothelial damage or inflammation, while the second may implicate a more chronic damage pattern. Moreover, if high vWF denotes active inflammation or injury, the exceedingly high levels in primary pulmonary hypertension may parallel disease activity for which there are currently no good markers. The fibrinolytic findings are harder to understand but may be an adaptive or maladaptive response of endothelium involved with tissue growth or angiogenesis rather than reflecting the acute coagulation process. Prospective study to assess serial plasma samples in pulmonary hypertensive patients would be of great interest in addressing some of these speculations.

Conclusions and Perspectives

Low circulating thrombomodulin levels, low levels of tissue factor pathway inhibitor, prolonged fibrinolysis with increase in the PAI-1 inhibitor, and high vWF and fibrinogen are markers of intravascular injury or inflammation clearly reflective of pulmonary vascular events, although not always distinct from the systemic circulation. These are potentially easy to use as markers in the pulmonary circulation due to the large size of the vascular bed. They each have different biological roles with implications for severity of disease, stage of disease, or prognosis. In addition to viewing each marker in isolation, patterns of fibrinolytic and coagulation factors may be clinically useful in staging disease activity. Elevated vWF may be uniquely linked to primary pulmonary hypertension and its characteristic plexiform lesions, with high levels a hallmark of poor prognosis. Thrombomodulin depression may indicate a chronic process, while elevated fibrinogen may be associated with inflammation, COPD, or deep venous thrombosis. Serial coagulation measurements may be useful not only in prognostication for patients[62] but also in assessing the natural history of these perplexing disorders. As our understanding of thrombosis evolves, use of coagulation and fibrinolytic factors may play a more central role in clinical management of pulmonary hypertension as well, not only in monitoring response to therapy but in evaluation of new treatments.

References

1. Fuster V, Steele PM, Edwards WD, et al. Primary pulmonary hypertension: Natural history and the importance of thrombosis. *Circulation* 1984; 70:580–587.

2. Rich S, Kaufmann E, Levy PS. The effect of high doses of calcium-channel blockers on survival in primary pulmonary hypertension. *N Engl J Med* 1992;327:76–81.

3. Frank K, Gurtner HP, Kneual M, et al. Aminorex-induzierte, plexogene pulmonale arteriopathis: 25 jahre danach! *Z Kardiol* 1993;82:568–572.

4. Kalweit GA, Feindt P, Micek M, et al. Markers of activated hemostasis and fibrinolysis in patients with pulmonary malignancies: Comparison of plasma levels in central venous and pulmonary venous blood. *Thromb Res* 2000;97:105–111.

5. Alevriadou BR, Moake JL, Turner NA, et al. Real-time analysis of shear-dependent thrombus formation and its blockade by inhibitors of von Willebrand factor binding to platelets. *Blood* 1992;81:1263–1276.

6. Takada Y, Shinkai F, Kondo S, et al. Fluid shear stress increases the expression of thrombomodulin by cultured human endothelial cells. *Biochem Biophys Res Commun* 1994;205:1345–1352.

7. Diamond SL, Eskin SG, McIntire LV. Fluid flow stimulates tissue plasminogen activator secretion by cultured human endothelial cells. *Science* 1989;243:1483–1485.

8. Kawai Y, Matsumoto Y, Ikeda Y, et al. Effect of shear stress on hemostatic regulation in endothelium. *Rinsho Byori* 1994;42:1128–1136.

9. Kamat SG, Michelson AD, Benoit SE, et al. Fibrinolysis inhibits shear stress-induced platelet aggregation. *Circulation* 1995;92:1399–1407.

10. Stief TW, Kurz J, Doss MO, et al. Singlet oxygen inactivates fibrinogen, factor V, factor VIII, factor X, and platelet aggregation of human blood. *Thromb Res* 2000;97:473–480.

11. Yan S-F, Machkman N, Kisiel W, et al. Hypoxia/hypoxemia-induced activation of the procoagulant pathways and the pathogenesis of ischemia-associated thrombosis. *Arterioscler Thromb Vasc Biol* 1999;19:2029–2035.

12. Gertler JP, Perry L, L'Italien G, et al. Ambient oxygen tension modulates endothelial fibrinolysis. *J Vasc Surg* 1993;18:939–946.

13. Pinsky DJ, Liao H, Lawson CA, et al. Coordinated induction of plasminogen activator inhibitor-1 (PAI-1) and inhibition of plasminogen activator gene expression by hypoxia promotes pulmonary vascular fibrin deposition. *J Clin Invest* 1998;102:919–928.

14. Bevilacqua MP, Pober JS, Majeau GR, et al. Interleukin 1 induces biosynthesis and cell surface expression of procoagulant activity in human vascular endothelial cells. *J Exp Med* 1984;160:618–623.

15. Wakefield TW, Greenfield LJ, Rolfe MW, et al. Inflammatory and procoagulant mediator interactions in an experimental baboon model of venous thrombosis. *Thromb Haemost* 1993;69:164–172.

16. Nawroth PP, Handley DA, Esmon CT, et al. Interleukin 1 induces endothelial cell procoagulant while suppressing cell-surface anticoagulant activity. *Proc Natl Acad Sci USA* 1986;83:3460–3464.

17. Bombeli, T, Karsan A, Tait JF, et al. Apoptotic vascular endothelial cells become procoagulant. *Blood* 1997;89:2429–2442.

18. Peters A, Doring A, Wichmann HE, et al. Increased plasma viscosity during an air pollution episode: A link to mortality? *Lancet* 1997;349:1582–1587.

19. Billimoria JD, Pozner H, Metselaar B, et al. Effect of cigarette smoking on lipids, lipoproteins, blood coagulation, fibrinolysis and cellular components of human blood. *Atherosclerosis* 1975;21:61–76.

20. Pandit HB, Spillert CR, Shih RD. Determination of hypercoagulable state in acute bronchospasm. *J Am Osteopath Assoc* 1999;99:203–206.

21. Winter JH, Buckler PW, Bautista AP, et al. Frequency of venous thrombosis in patients with an exacerbation of chronic obstructive lung disease. *Thorax* 1983;38:605–608.
22. Schonhofer B, Kohler D. Prevalence of deep-vein thrombosis of the leg in patients with acute exacerbation of chronic obstructive pulmonary disease. *Respiration* 1998;65:173–177.
23. Calverley PMA, Howatson R, Flenley DC, et al. Clinicopathological correlations in cor pulmonale. *Thorax* 1992;47:494–498.
24. Alessandri C, Basili S, Violi F, et al. Hypercoagulability state in patients with chronic obstructive pulmonary disease. *Thromb Haemost* 1994;72:343–346.
25. Russo A, De Luca M, Vigna C, et al. Central pulmonary artery lesions in chronic obstructive pulmonary disease: A transesophageal echocardiography study. *Circulation* 1999;100:1808–1815.
26. Wolf M, Boyer-Neumann C, Parent F, et al. Thrombotic risk factors in pulmonary hypertension. *Eur Respir J* 2000;15:395–399.
27. Elliott CG, Leppert MF, Alexander GJ, et al. Factor V Leiden is not common in patients diagnosed with primary pulmonary hypertension. *Eur Respir J* 1998;12:1177–1180.
28. Etingin OR, Hajjar DP, Hajjar KA, et al. Lipoprotein (a) regulates plasminogen activator inhibitor-1 expression in endothelial cells: A potential mechanism in thrombogenesis. *J Biol Chem* 1991;266:2459–2465.
29. Ignatescu M, Kostner K, Zorn G, et al. Plasma Lp(a) levels are increased in patients with chronic thromboembolic pulmonary hypertension. *Thromb Haemost* 1998;80:231–232.
30. Asherson RA, Cervera R. Review: Antiphospholipid antibodies and the lung. *J Rheumatol* 1995;22:62–66.
31. Kerr JE, Poe R, Kramer Z. Antiphospholipid antibody syndrome presenting as a refractory noninflammatory pulmonary vasculopathy. *Chest* 1997; 112:1707–1710.
32. Karmochkine M, Cacoub P, Dorent R. High prevalence of antiphospholipid antibodies in precapillary pulmonary hypertension. *J Rheumatol* 1996;23:286–290.
33. Asherson RA, Higenbottam TW, Dinh Xuan AT, et al. Pulmonary hypertension in a lupus clinic: experience with twenty-four patients. *J Rheumatol* 1990;17:1292–1298.
34. Isern RA, Yaneva M, Weiner E, et al. Autoantibodies in patients with primary pulmonary hypertension: Association with anti-Ku. *Am J Med* 1992; 93:307–312.
35. Carson CW, Comp PC, Alireza RR, et al. Antibodies to thrombomodulin are found in patients with lupus anticoagulant and unexplained thrombosis. *J Rheumatol* 2000;27:384–390.
36. Fritzler MJ, Hart DA, Wilson D, et al. Antibodies to fibrin-bound tissue type plasminogen activator in systemic sclerosis. *J Rheumatol* 1995;22:1688–1693.
37. Morse JH, Barst RJ, Fotino M, et al. Primary pulmonary hypertension, tissue plasminogen activator antibodies, and HLA-DQ7. *Am J Resp Crit Care Med* 1997;155:274–278.
38. Debault LE, Esmon EL, Olson JR, et al. Distribution of the thrombomodulin antigen in the rabbit vasculature. *Lab Invest* 1986;54:172–178.
39. Ford VA, Stringer C, Kennel SJ, et al. Thrombomodulin is preferentially expressed in balb/c lung microvessels. *J Biol Chem* 1992;8:5446–5450.
40. Kawanani O, Jin E, Ghazizadeh, et al. Heterogeneous distribution of thrombomodulin and von Willebrand factor in endothelial cells in the human pulmonary microvessels. *J Nippon Med Sch* 2000;67:118–125.

41. Fink LM, Edit JF, Johnson K, et al. Thrombomodulin activity and localization. *Int J Dev Biol* 1993;37:221–226.
42. Malek AM, Jackman R, Rosenberg RD, et al. Endothelial expression of thrombomodulin is reversibly regulated by fluid shear stress. *Circ Res* 1994;74:852–860.
43. Stratton RJ, Pompon L, Coghlan JG, et al. Soluble thrombomodulin concentration is raised in scleroderma-associated pulmonary hypertension. *Ann Rheum Dis* 2000; 59:132–134.
44. Komai H, Haworth SG. Thrombomodulin and angiotension-converting enzyme activity during pediatric open heart operations. *Ann Thorac Surg* 1996;62:553–558.
45. Welsh CH, Hassell KL, Badesch, et al. Coagulation and fibrinolytic profiles in patients with severe pulmonary hypertension. *Chest* 1996;110:710–717.
46. Cacoub P, Karmochkine M, Dorent R, et al. Plasma levels of thrombomodulin in pulmonary hypertension. *Am J Med* 1996;101:160–164.
47. Sakamaki F, Kyotani S, Nagaya N, et al. Decreased plasma level of thrombomodulin in chronic pulmonary thromboembolism improved after pulmonary thromboendarterectomy. *Am J Resp Crit Care Med* 2000;161:634.
48. Salomaa V, Matei C, Aleksic N, et al. Soluble thrombomodulin as a predictor of incident coronary heart disease and symptomless carotid artery atherosclerosis in the Atherosclerosis Risk in Communities (ARIC) Study: A case-cohort study. *Lancet* 1999;353:1729–1734.
49. Altman R, Scazziota A, Rouvier J, et al. Coagulation and fibrinolytic parameters in patients with pulmonary hypertension. *Clin Cardiol* 1996;19:549–554.
50. Franz RC, Ziady F, Coetzee WJC, et al. A possible causal relationship between defective fibrinolysis and pulmonary hypertension. *S Afr Med J* 1979; 55:170–173.
51. Ingelsby TV, Singer JW, Gordon DS. Abnormal fibrinolysis in familial pulmonary hypertension. *Am J Med* 1973;55:5–14.
52. Olman MA, Marsh JJ, Lang IM, et al. Endogenous fibrinolytic system in chronic large-vessel thromboembolic pulmonary hypertension. *Circulation* 1992;86:1241–1248.
53. Huber K, Beckmann R, Frank H. Fibrinogen, t-PA and PAI-1 plasma levels in patients with pulmonary hypertension. *Am J Respir Crit Care Med* 1994;150:929–933.
54. Boyer-Neumann C, Brenot F, Wolf M, et al. Continuous infusion of prostacyclin decreases plasma levels of t-PA and PAI-1 in primary pulmonary hypertension. *Thromb Haemost* 1995;73:727–738.
55. Hoeper MMl, Sosada M, Fabel H. Plasma coagulation profiles in patients with severe primary pulmonary hypertension. *Eur Respir J* 1998;12:1446–1449.
56. Eisenberg PR, Lucore C, Kaufman K, et al. Fibrinopeptide A levels indicative of pulmonary vascular thrombosis in patients with primary pulmonary hypertension. *Circulation* 1990;82:841–847.
57. Sartori MT, Wiman B, Vettore S, et al. 4G/5G polymorphism of PAI-1 gene promoter and fibrinolytic capacity in patients with deep vein thrombosis. *Thromb Haemost* 1998;80:956–960.
58. Humphries SE, Panahloo A, Montgomery HE, et al. Gene-environment interaction in the determination of levels of haemostatic variables involved in thrombosis and fibrinolysis. *Thromb Haemost* 1997;78:457–461.
59. Okamura T, Tsuda Y, Murakawa M, et al. A patient with congenital plas-

minogen deficiency manifesting primary pulmonary hypertension. *Intern Med* 1993;32:332–335.

60. Herrick S, Blanc-Brude O, Gray A, et al. Fibrinogen. *Int J Biochem Cell Biol* 1999;31:741–746.

61. Ruggeri ZM. Structure and function of von Willebrand factor. *Thromb Haemost* 1999;82:576–584.

62. Lopes AAB, Maeda NY. Circulating von Willebrand factor antigen as a predictor of short-term prognosis in pulmonary hypertension. *Chest* 1998; 114:1276–1282.

63. Geggel RL, Carvalho ACA, Hoyer LW, et al. Von Willebrand factor abnormalities in primary pulmonary hypertension. *Am Rev Respir Dis* 1987; 135:294–299.

64. Rabinovitch M, Andrew M, Thom H, et al. Abnormal endothelial factor VIII associated with pulmonary hypertension and congenital heart defects. *Circulation* 1987;76:1043–1052.

65. Lopes AA, Maeda NY, Goncalves RC, et al. Endothelial cell dysfunction correlates differentially with survival in primary and secondary pulmonary hypertension. *Am Heart J* 2000;139:618–623.

66. Lopes AAB, Maeda NY. Abnormal degradation of von Willebrand factor main subunit in pulmonary hypertension. *Eur Respir J* 1995;8:530–536.

67. Friedman, Mears JG, Barst RJ. Continuous infusion of prostacyclin normalizes plasma markers of endothelial cell injury and platelet aggregation in primary pulmonary hypertension. *Circulation* 1997;96:2782–2784.

68. Voelkel NF, Cool C, Lee SD, et al. Primary pulmonary hypertension between inflammation and cancer. *Chest* 1998;114:225S–230S.

69. Chaouat A, Weitzenblum E, Higenbottam T. The role of thrombosis in severe pulmonary hypertension. *Eur Respir J* 1996;9:356–363.

Chapter 21

Molecular Approaches to Identify Mechanisms of Thrombus Stabilization in the Pulmonary Vasculature

Elisabeth Gharehbaghi-Schnell, PhD, and Irene M. Lang, MD

Chronic Thromboembolic Pulmonary Hypertension

Definition

Chronic thromboembolic pulmonary hypertension (CTEPH) is the result of single or recurrent pulmonary emboli arising from sites of venous thrombosis, thus leading to chronic obstruction of the central (main, lobar, and segmental) pulmonary arteries. These organized residua, over time, can lead to a reduction in pulmonary vascular conductance and compliance, and to an increased right ventricular workload, ultimately resulting in right ventricular failure. Each year approximately 600,000 people in the United States suffer a pulmonary embolic event. Of the 450,000 patients who survive, it is estimated that 0.1% fail to resolve their massive emboli appropriately and are candidates for the development of CTEPH.[1] Unfortunately, little information exists on the mechanisms responsible for the stabilization of thromboemboli in the pulmonary vasculature of these patients (e.g., elevated expression or lack of a specific protein). The natural history of pulmonary thromboemboli is to undergo

This research was supported in part by Austrian fellowship grants FWF P10559-MED, P13834-MED, Anton Dreher Stiftung, and Vermächtnis Josefine Hirtl zur Förderung der Medizinischen Forschung (to IML).

From: Weir EK, Reeve HL, Reeves JT (eds). *Interactions of Blood and the Pulmonary Circulation*. Armonk, NY: Futura Publishing Company, Inc.; ©2002.

total resolution, or resolution leaving minimal residua, with restoration of normal pulmonary hemodynamics. For reasons still unclear, thromboemboli in CTEPH patients fail to resolve and thus form endothelialized obstructions of the pulmonary vascular bed, including the major branches.

Pathophysiology

The pathophysiology of CTEPH remains unclear. Lack of disease recurrence after successful pulmonary thromboendarterectomy or lung transplantation, lack of risk factor sharing with deep vein thrombosis and acute pulmonary thromboembolism, and lack of clinically symptomatic episodes of pulmonary thromboembolism in the majority of patients has even suggested a nonthromboembolic origin of CTEPH.

Natural History

The majority of patients have a history of deep venous thrombosis (DVT) when carefully questioned. However, more than 60% of patients lack signs of past DVT at the time of diagnosis.[1] After an initial thromboembolic event that may or may not be symptomatic, the patients experience months to years of a "honeymoon period" without any clinical symptoms. Gradually, however, dyspnea on exertion develops. Clinical deterioration parallels the loss of right ventricular functional capacity. While right ventricular hypertrophy develops, additional changes in the pulmonary vascular bed develop and increase pulmonary vascular resistance (PVR). Histologically, CTEPH lesions are indistinguishable from pulmonary vascular lesions found in any other kind of pulmonary vascular hypertension.[2] It is suspected that the degree of "secondary" vascular changes determines the capability to normalize pulmonary pressures after successful pulmonary thromboendarterectomy. Right ventricular impairment is reversible with decrease of PVR.[3] While the initial major vessel red thrombi transform into whitish adherent masses of granulation tissue, high pulmonary vascular resistance and slow flow through multiple irregular vascular channels lined with dysfunctional endothelium cause further apposition of fresh red thrombus. Due to segmental underperfusion, alveolar dead space increases. Finally, right ventricular failure ensues. Hypoxemia becomes exaggerated by a combination of factors, including a decline in cardiac output with a fall in mixed venous oxygen saturation, worsening ventilation-perfusion relations, reopening of the foramen ovale, and development of small pulmonary arteriovenous fistulas in the lungs.

Animal Models of CTEPH

The difficulty of inducing CTEPH by repeated release of pre-formed clots from the inferior venae cavae of mongrel dogs[4] was resolved by a thorough biochemical dissection of factors contributing to increased vascular fibrinolytic activity in these animals.[5] It was found that high plasma levels of urokinase-type plasminogen activator (u-PA) activity are present in this species. Furthermore, u-PA is associated with canine platelets and mediates rapid clot lysis.

Coagulation and Fibrinolysis

No abnormalities of coagulation[1] and fibrinolysis[6] have been identified in patients with CTEPH. Recent data suggest that lupus anticoagulant, high levels of anticardiolipin, and anti-beta-2-glycoprotein-I antibodies are associated with chronic thromboembolic pulmonary hypertension.[7] Approximately 10% of CTEPH patients demonstrate lupus anticoagulant, and there exists an increased association with heparin-induced thrombocytopenia.[8] A recent study in a series of 20 CTEPH patients has demonstrated no increased prevalence of the factor V_{Leiden} mutation in CTEPH by using a PCR-based search for the R506G mutation.[9]

Molecular Dissection of the Vascular Remodeling Associated with Acute Pulmonary Thromboembolism[10]

Under the assumption that CTEPH thrombi result from the embolization of thrombi to the pulmonary vasculature, we designed experiments to understand the regulation of fibrinolytic genes in the first hours after a clinically submassive fatal pulmonary embolism. Because recent data suggest that the balance between plasminogen activators (PAs) and type 1 plasminogen activator inhibitor (PAI-1) plays a role in regulating cell migration within the extracellular matrix, we investigated the expression of these molecules by immunohistochemical and in situ hybridization analysis of pulmonary artery specimens from patients suffering from a fatal pulmonary embolism. The data were compared with the expression of these molecules both in patients' noninvolved pulmonary arteries and in organ donor pulmonary arteries. Regions of initial organization and vascular remodeling were identified by a modified trichrome stain and by the presence of proliferating cell nuclear antigen (PCNA), a cell marker of proliferation. Staining for tissue-type PA antigen was low to undetectable in endothelial cells directly in contact with the fibrin-platelet thromboembolus and in areas in which the endothelial cell lining was replaced by cell growth into the thrombus. Urokinase-like PA (u-PA) expression was detected in mononuclear cells within the thrombus in the initial phase of thromboembolism and within cells migrating into the thrombus during the later stages of organization. PAI-1 expression was elevated in the monolayer of endothelial cells underlying the fresh platelet-fibrin thromboembolus and in a PCNA-positive cell population present between the pulmonary arterial intima and the thromboembolus that represents early organization. Increased expression of PAI-1 may play a role in inhibiting proteolysis and fostering the localization of the acute fibrin-platelet thrombus to the vascular wall, which is followed by the upregulation of u-PA in migrating cells during the reorganization process.

Serial Analysis of Differential Gene Expression in Pulmonary Thromboemboli and Pulmonary Arteries of Patients with CTEPH

Introduction

Recent research has focused on local gene expression within pulmonary arterial thromboemboli and pulmonary arteries from CTEPH patients. By a candidate gene approach utilizing in situ techniques, increased expression of plasminogen activator inhibitor type 1 (PAI-1) was found in small thrombus neovessels, thus potentially promoting small vessel thrombosis and thrombus growth from within.[11] On the other hand, elevated PAI-1 gene expression was also identified at a specific stage in the natural course of organization of acute pulmonary thromboemboli.[10] This thorough investigation of the patterns of gene expression during the vascular remodeling associated with organization of acute pulmonary thromboemboli has shed new light on the events leading to restoration of normal pulmonary blood flow after venous thromboembolism. One hypothesis emerging from these studies is that, by a mechanism yet to be defined, deep venous thrombi undergo extensive organization in the vascular compartment of the deep femoral and pelvic veins. When such thrombi are embolized, even well-functioning machineries of fibrinolysis and thrombolysis do not suffice to remove these organized materials and lead to CTEPH. In other studies, the expression of a potent inhibitor of factor IXa and factor XIa (i.e., protease nexin-2/amyloid beta-protein precursor, A beta PP) in the organized vascular occlusions harvested from patients with this disease was demonstrated.[12] Clot vessel hemorrhage is a feature of CTEPH thrombus histology and it is speculated to be a powerful stimulator for angiogenesis.

Expression of Angiogenic Growth Factors Within Chronic Nonresolving Pulmonary Thromboemboli: Defining Basic Mechanisms Involved in the Remodeling of Atherosclerotic Tissues and Chronic Pulmonary Thromboemboli

Chronic nonresolving pulmonary thromboemboli represent poorly understood vascular obstructions that arise from thromboemboli, but are thought to expand in situ by various mechanisms, e.g., in situ thrombosis, angiogenesis, and smooth muscle proliferation. To test the hypothesis that mechanisms of vascular remodeling and compensatory vessel enlargement of systemic arteries underlie the chronic expansion of nonresolving pulmonary thromboemboli, a gene expression analysis approach was taken. Although a clear distinction between predominantly proliferative and regressive lesions could be made in coronary artery lesions, growth patterns varied within a single chronic thromboembolus.

First, areas were identified in which the majority of cells were undergoing apoptosis by morphology and positive immunoreactivity with a TUNEL stain. In addition, areas with numerous PCNA-positive cells were found, colocalizing with neovessels and stellate smooth muscle cells that were morphologically similar to neointimal smooth muscle cells of coronary plaques. Second, candidate angiogenic growth factors were analyzed by immunohistochemistry. Intense immunoreactivity for bFGF and platelet-derived endothelial cell growth factor was detected. Vast extracellular deposits of a protein cross-reacting with monospecific antibodies directed against transforming growth factor (TGF)-β1–3 protein were identified. Because lipoprotein(a) can interfere with the co-localization of plasmin activity and, hence, the activation of TGF-β, we extended our analysis of growth factors to include this molecule. Extracellular deposits of lipoprotein(a) were present around the vascular lumen in thromboembolic specimens. In contrast, vascular endothelial cell growth factor that was readily identified in placenta was immunologically confined to few cells within the thromboemboli. In situ hybridization analysis compared signals in a proliferating tumor (e.g., mammary carcinoma) with signals in cells within chronic thromboemboli. Basic fibroblast growth factor was detected only in endothelial cells, while TGF-β and PD-ECGF expression was localized in smooth muscle cells. Distinct groups of cells were found expressing vascular endothelial cell growth factor (VEGF).

The data indicate that organization of nonresolving pulmonary thromboemboli is regulated by a diverse set of growth factors predominantly expressed by vascular smooth muscle cells. Based on these data, we wished to obtain a quantitative measure of the level of expressed genes. Under the assumption that differences in gene expression between pulmonary artery and pulmonary thromboemboli might provide a clue to mechanisms of thrombus persistence, a classic differential display approach was chosen.[13]

Differential Gene Expression in Chronic Pulmonary Thromboemboli and Pulmonary Arteries

After differential display and confirmation of clones by reverse Northern analysis, 67 different clones were identified. From these, 9 were unknown and 58 were molecules found in the database. As expected, most of the clones had been isolated in their 3-untranslated region. Among the genes in the database were a number of genes involved in lipid metabolism, e.g., lipoprotein lipase (LPL), LDL-C, a brefeldin A-sensitive peripheral Golgi protein required for normal Golgi function, apoER2,[14] and LRP-6,[15] a recently discovered novel member of the LDL lipoprotein receptor proteins.

Conclusion

After pursuing candidate gene research over the past few years and investigating detailed gene expression patterns within chronic pulmonary vascular occlusions, we recently chose a differential display expression cloning strategy to elucidate the mechanisms underlying the failure to resolve pulmonary thromboemboli. While familial cases of primary pulmonary hypertension have permitted the search for a single gene that has been recently identified as bone morphogenic protein receptor II (BMPRII), a member of the transforming growth factor beta receptor superfamily,[16] CTEPH does not demonstrate a heritable trait. Therefore, gene expression studies at the tissue level are justified. Messenger RNA display of hundreds of genes, comparing pulmonary arteries and pulmonary arterial thromboemboli of CTEPH patients, has demonstrated a remarkable loss of genetic repertoire in chronic clots in comparison with the expression profile of the parent pulmonary artery. This observation is in contrast to the observation of very focal neoangiogenesis, macrophage accumulation, and calcification within distinct areas of chronic thromboemboli. Our data suggest that the genes expressed at these sites are also expressed at some lower level in the pulmonary artery and do not appear as differentially regulated genes.

Furthermore, it was observed that CTEPH thromboemboli are remarkably devoid of fat. If found, fat accumulates in foci. In line with this finding, several genes involved in lipid metabolism were differentially regulated. Dysregulation of lipid metabolism is a key mechanism underlying atherosclerosis. Because atherosclerosis is associated with vascular remodeling, an adaptive process that is aimed at the preservation of a patent lumen,[17] a shutdown of this process may result in progressive occlusion. We have not systematically investigated plasma lipids and lipoproteins in CTEPH patients. The only existing data that relate to lipoprotein metabolism and CTEPH report elevated levels of Lp(a) in patient plasmas.[18]

In conclusion, while elevated local expression of PAI-1 may promote ongoing thrombosis within chronic thrombi, and local expression of beta-APP may cause hemorrhage, thus igniting abnormal angiogenesis, the pathogenesis of CTEPH remains to be determined. Whether differential downregulation of lipid-regulating genes and altered lipid metabolism in chronic thrombi is associated with a key pathogenic mechanism underlying failure to lyse and subsequent progressive vascular occlusion is the subject of further studies.

We would like to acknowledge the contributions of Shahrzad Rezaie-Majd, MD, Manuela Mühlbauer, BA, Diana Bonderman, MD, Johannes Jakowitsch, PhD, Martin Czerny, MD, Bruno Podesser, MD, Gerald Maurer, MD, Raymond Schleef, PhD, Richard Channick, MD, William Auger, MD, Peter Fedullo, MD, Lewis Rubin, MD, and Stuart Jamieson, MD.

References

1. Moser KM, Auger WR, Fedullo PF. Chronic major-vessel thromboembolic pulmonary hypertension. *Circulation* 1990;81:1735–1743.
2. Moser KM, Bloor CM. Pulmonary vascular lesions occurring in patients with chronic major vessel thromboembolic pulmonary hypertension. *Chest* 1993;103:685–692.
3. Dittrich HC, Chow LC, Nicod PH. Early improvement in left ventricular diastolic function after relief of chronic right ventricular pressure overload. *Circulation* 1989;80:823–830.
4. Marsh JJ, Konopka RG, Lang IM, et al. Suppression of thrombolysis in a canine model of pulmonary embolism. *Circulation* 1994;90:3091–3097.
5. Lang IM, Marsh JJ, Konopka RG, et al. Factors contributing to increased vascular fibrinolytic activity in mongrel dogs. *Circulation* 1993;87:1990–2000.
6. Olman MA, Marsh JJ, Lang IM, et al. Endogenous fibrinolytic system in chronic large-vessel thromboembolic pulmonary hypertension. *Circulation* 1992;86:1241–1248.
7. Martinuzzo ME, Pombo G, Forastiero RR, et al. Lupus anticoagulant, high levels of anticardiolipin, and anti-beta-2-glycoprotein-I antibodies are associated with chronic thromboembolic pulmonary hypertension. *J Rheumatol* 1998;25:1313–1319.
8. Auger WR, Permpikul P, Moser KM. Lupus anticoagulant, heparin use, and thrombocytopenia in patients with chronic thromboembolic pulmonary hypertension: A preliminary report. *Am J Med* 1995;99:392–396.
9. Lang IM, Klepetko W, Pabinger I. No increased prevalence of the factor V Leiden mutation in chronic major vessel thromboembolic pulmonary hypertension (CTEPH) [letter]. *Thromb Haemost* 1996;76:476–477.

10. Lang IM, Moser KM, Schleef RR. Elevated expression of urokinase-like plasminogen activator and plasminogen activator inhibitor type 1 during the vascular remodeling associated with pulmonary thromboembolism. *Arterioscler Thromb Vasc Biol* 1998;18:808–815.

11. Lang IM, Marsh JJ, Olman MA, et al. Expression of type 1 plasminogen activator inhibitor in chronic pulmonary thromboemboli. *Circulation* 1994; 89:2715–2721.

12. Lang IM, Moser KM, Schleef RR. Expression of Kunitz protease inhibitor-containing forms of amyloid beta-protein precursor within vascular thrombi. *Circulation* 1996;94:2728–2734.

13. Liang P, Averboukh L, Keyomarsi K, et al. Differential display and cloning of messenger RNAs from human breast cancer versus mammary epithelial cells. *Cancer Res* 1992;52:6966–6968.

14. Kim DH, Iijima H, Goto K, et al. Human apolipoprotein E receptor 2: A novel lipoprotein receptor of the low density lipoprotein receptor family predominantly expressed in brain. *J Biol Chem* 1996;271:8373–8380.

15. Brown SD, Twells RCJ, Hey PJ, et al. Isolation and characterization of LRP6, a novel member of the low density lipoprotein receptor gene family. *Biochem Biophys Res Com* 1998;248:879–888.

16. Deng Z, Morse J, Slager SL, et al. Familial primary pulmonary hypertension (gene PPH1) is caused by mutations in the bone morphogenic protein receptor-II gene. *Am J Hum Genet* 2000;67:737–744.

17. Glagov S, Weisenberg E, Zarins CK, et al. Compensatory enlargement of human atherosclerotic coronary arteries. *N Engl J Med* 1987;316:1371–1375.

18. Ignatescu M, Kostner K, Zorn G, et al. Plasma Lp(a) levels are increased in patients with chronic thromboembolic pulmonary hypertension. *Thromb Haemost* 1998;80:231–232.

Chapter 22

Hypoxia-Induced Activation of Early Growth Response (Egr)-1:

A Novel Pathway Mediating the Vascular Response to Oxygen Deprivation

Shi Fang Yan, MD, David J. Pinsky, MD, and David M. Stern, MD

Introduction

The cellular response to oxygen deprivation occurs on multiple levels, including rapid changes in ion flux and generation of eicosanoids,[1] and a reprogramming of biosynthetic activities.[2] Differential cloning strategies have revealed the identity of many oxygen-regulated proteins (ORPs) and have shown them to facilitate the cellular response to environmental challenge. For example, an oxygen-regulated protein with a molecular mass of 150 kDa (termed ORP150) is a member of the heat shock protein 70 (HSP70) family; it is an inducible chaperone present in the endoplasmic reticulum and enhances cell viability in response to oxygen deprivation.[3,4] As might be expected, some ORPs overlap with proteins induced in cells as the result of other stresses, such as glucose deprivation.[5] Thus, ORP80 (an ORP with a molecular mass of 80 kDa) has proven to be identical to a protein induced by glucose depletion (termed glucose-regulated protein 80 or GRP80).[6]

The most significant step enhancing our understanding of mechanisms underlying the pattern of protein induction in cells subjected to oxygen deprivation was the discovery of a DNA motif in the erythro-

This work was supported by grants from the USPHS and the Surgical Research Fund of Columbia University.

From: Weir EK, Reeve HL, Reeves JT (eds). *Interactions of Blood and the Pulmonary Circulation*. Armonk, NY: Futura Publishing Company, Inc.; ©2002.

poietin promoter termed the "hypoxia-response element" (HRE), and the characterization of hypoxia-inducible factor-1 (HIF-1), which binds to the HRE.[7,8] For example, one of the best-known adaptive responses to hypoxia is the increase in red cell mass marshaled to enhance the oxygen carrying capacity of the blood. Thus, attention was initially focused on the erythropoietin gene as a model system for hypoxia-induced gene expression. The pioneering studies of Dr. Gregg Semenza led to the identification of HIF-1, a key transcription factor that regulates the expression of multiple genes in which HREs have been found.[9,10] Aside from erythropoietin, this includes the angiogenic agent vascular endothelial growth factor (VEGF),[11,12] multiple glycolytic enzymes,[13,14] and the noninsulin-dependent glucose transporter (GLUT1),[15] as well as multiple other genes. In each case, the adaptive benefit of these genes is evident; VEGF promotes increased vascularity at sites of insufficient oxygen delivery, and elevated levels of GLUT1 and glycolytic enzymes facilitate glucose uptake and utilization by anaerobic pathways, respectively. Several recent reviews of HIF-1 provide more information on the biology of this transcription factor and its mechanism of regulating expression of target genes.[9,10,16]

However, there is another facet of the vascular response to hypoxia that is well known clinically, but does not seem, at the outset, to exert a protective effect. Increased deposition of fibrin in hypoxic vasculature has been noted for over 20 years, and a theory was suggested some time ago proposing that venous thrombi begin on the parietal aspect of the venous valve pocket because oxygen tension is lowest at this point in response to limb stasis.[17,18] These observations led us to develop a model of hypoxia-induced fibrin deposition and to determine mechanisms underlying activation of coagulation. Our studies have led to the recognition of an HIF-1-dependent pathway promoting expression of the procoagulant regulator tissue factor, as well as other genes, and have elucidated a new facet of the cellular response to oxygen deprivation.

Hypoxia-Mediated Induction of Tissue Factor

Mice subjected to normobaric hypoxia (oxygen tension of 6%) demonstrated vascular fibrin deposition within several hours, as determined by immunoblotting and immunohistochemistry with an antibody specific for fibrin (this antibody was reactive with gamma-gamma chain crosslinks).[19,20] Fibrin deposition in this setting appeared to result from induction of tissue factor, the procoagulant cofactor that initiates coagulation in vivo. Tissue factor, undetectable in the inner vessel wall and mononuclear phagocytes (MPs) under homeostatic conditions, was induced in response to hypoxia, especially in vascular smooth muscle cells and MPs.[19,21] That tissue factor was the trigger for fibrin formation was shown by inhibition of the latter in hypoxic animals treated with blocking anti-tissue factor IgG.[19] The thrombin inhibitor, hirudin, also suppressed vascular fibrin deposition in hypoxic animals,[19] indicating that tissue factor-mediated initiation of coagulation was followed by thrombin formation, leading to fibrin formation.

In order to analyze mechanisms underlying tissue factor expression, we first sought to determine if transcriptional regulation was operative. Levels of tissue factor mRNA were increased in hypoxic lung, and studies in mononuclear phagocytes and HeLa cells showed that oxygen deprivation (pO_2 ≈13 torr) caused a similar increase in tissue factor transcripts.[21] Nuclear run-on analysis in cultured cells showed an approximate 10-fold increase in the rate of transcription of tissue factor under hypoxia, indicating a central role for transcriptional control in the upregulation of this gene under oxygen deprivation. Analysis of the tissue factor promoter did not show the presence of HIF-1 DNA binding motifs, suggesting that a mechanism distinct from HIF-1-HRE interaction might be operative. Transfection studies with a series of tissue factor promoter-luciferase reporter constructs focused our attention on a portion of the promoter containing a trio of overlapping DNA binding motifs for Sp1 and early growth response (Egr) (this has been termed the serum response region of the promoter).[22] Complementary electrophoretic mobility shift assays (EMSA) and transient transfection studies showed that interaction of Egr-1 with the Egr DNA binding motif in the tissue factor gene promoter was responsible for hypoxia induction of the tissue factor.[21] Egr-1 is a member of a family of zinc finger transcription factors that was first identified by its characteristic rapid induction following exposure of cells to growth stimulants.[23,24] Further studies focused on its possible role in development. For example, in vitro studies suggested that Egr-1 might be critical for differentiation of hematopoietic cells along the monocyte lineage.[25,26] However, with the development of Egr-1 null mice,[27,28] our perspective on Egr-1 has required considerable revision. Since these mice display a virtually normal phenotype in the absence of stress, attention has focused on the response of Egr-1 null mice to physiological (fertility)[28] and pathophysiological (hypoxia, experimental nephrotic syndrome, etc.)[21,29] challenges.

Using Egr-1 null mice, we examined their capacity to express tissue factor and display vascular fibrin deposition in response to oxygen deprivation (≈6% oxygen).[21] While wild-type controls showed induction of tissue factor mRNA and antigen under hypoxia, this response was severely blunted in the Egr-1 null mice that showed a minimal increase in tissue factor. Consistent with these data, fibrin deposition was observed in the vasculature of hypoxic wild-type mice, but not in Egr-1 null mice. These data focused our attention on Egr-1 expression under hypoxic conditions. Lung from wild-type animals exposed to a range of oxygen concentrations showed rapid induction of Egr-1 transcripts by 30 minutes.[30] At this time, maximal induction of Egr-1 mRNA (approximately 18-fold) occurred at 6% oxygen, and fell off in a dose-dependent manner up to 10% oxygen (it reached the normoxic baseline by 12% oxygen) (Figure 1 A, B). In contrast to these results with Egr-1, another transcription factor that also binds to GC-rich DNA motifs, Sp1, was not induced by hypoxia (Figure 1 C, D), nor was β-actin (Figure 1 E, F). Thus, Egr-1 induction occurred rapidly, specifically, and at levels of oxygen tension where host response mechanisms for adaptation to hypoxia are clearly operative. At an oxygen concentration of 10%, time course experiments were performed to track expression of Egr-1 transcripts in the lung.[30] Induction of Egr-1 occurred in a biphasic manner (Figure 2 A, B); a rapid increase (≈5-fold) occurred within 30 minutes and steadily decayed over the next 8 hours. Then, at 24 and 48 hours, Egr-1 expression appeared to increase again. In contrast to these results with Egr-1, levels of Sp1 (Figure 2 C, D) and β-actin (Figure 2 E, F) transcripts were unchanged over this time period at 10% oxygen. At the 48-hour time point, induction of Egr-1 remained dependent on oxygen concentration from 6% to 10% oxygen, and levels of Egr-1 transcripts/antigen were paralleled by comparable induction of tissue factor. Although further experiments will be required to fully map out the time course for Egr-1 expression in response to hypoxia beyond 48 hours, these data demonstrate that the rapid expression of Egr-1 shortly after oxygen deprivation is followed by a second phase at later times. In each case, Egr-1 induction is sensitive to the concentration of oxygen over a range of 6–10%.

As levels of Egr-1 in hypoxic lung were closely coupled to increased Egr-1 DNA binding activity in nuclear extracts (and Egr-1 was virtually undetectable in normoxic lung), it appeared that expression of Egr-1 was the limiting factor for induction of tissue factor. Since Egr-1 expression was especially evident in vascular smooth muscle cells and MPs, it was logical to turn to cultured MPs to assess underlying mechanisms.[31] Hypoxia caused an increase in the rate of transcription of Egr-1, indicating control at the transcriptional level. Analysis of the Egr-1 promoter did not, again, show evidence of HREs of the type that interacts with HIF-1. Consistent with these data, studies with a line of mutant hepatoma cells with nonfunctional HIF-1β/ARNT (thereby preventing assembly of active HIF-1, a heterodimer of HIF-1α/β)[32] showed identical expression of Egr-1 transcripts and induction of Egr-1 DNA binding activity in response to hypoxia, as was observed in wild-type hepatoma cells (with functional HIF-1).[31] These observations were consistent with the concept that induction of Egr-1 under hypoxic conditions reflected a novel pathway not previously described.

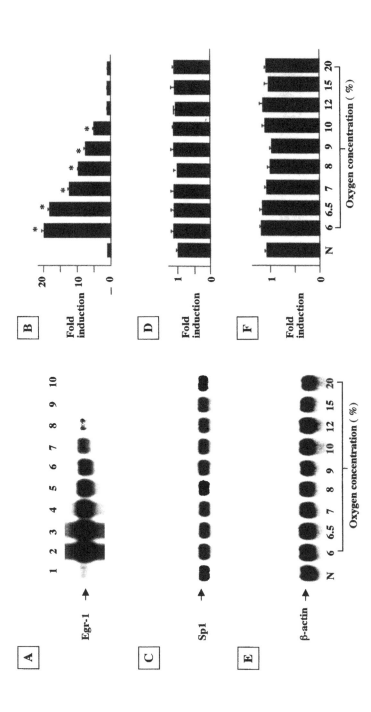

Figure 1. Expression of Egr-1 (A, B), Sp1 (C, D) and β-actin (E, F) transcripts in lungs from mice exposed to the indicated concentration of oxygen for 30 minutes. Panels A, C, and E show Northern blots (20 μg of total RNA added per lane) and panels B, D, and F show densitometric analysis of 3–5 experiments similar to those shown in A, C, and E. * indicates *P*<0.001. Adapted and used with permission from reference 30.

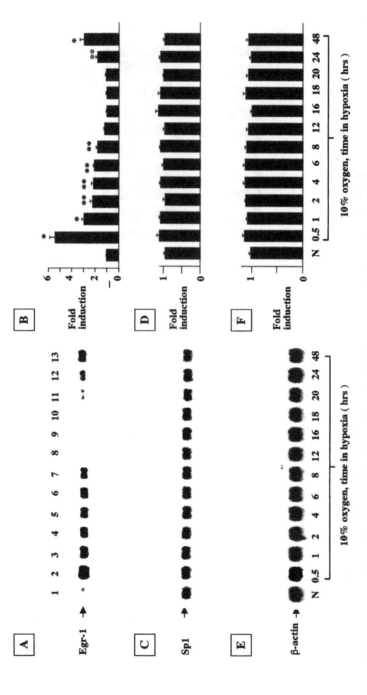

Figure 2. Expression of Egr-1 (A, B), Sp1 (C, D), and β-actin (E, F) transcripts in lungs from mice exposed to an atmosphere with 10% oxygen for the indicated times, up to 48 hours. Panels A, C, and E show Northern blots (20 μg of total RNA added per lane) and panels B, D, and F show densitometric analysis of 3–5 experiments similar to those shown in A, C, and E. * indicates $P < 0.001$ and ** indicates $P < 0.05$. Adapted and used with permission from reference 30.

Intracellular Signaling Events Leading to EGR-1 Activation Under Oxygen Deprivation

Transient transfection studies with Egr-1 promoter-luciferase reporter constructs using a line of mononuclear phagocytes indicated that the serum response elements (SRE) in the Egr-1 promoter were essential for hypoxia induction.[31] Specifically, a particular configuration of the SRE, namely one in which the SRE was flanked by 2 ets binding sites (EBS) resulting in the following trio, EBS-SRE-SBE, appeared to confer hypoxia inducibility. These observations suggested that an ets factor, probably Elk-1, in complex with serum response factor (SRF) was likely to be responsible for the increase in Egr-1 expression observed with oxygen deprivation.[31] This led us to predict a series of events, involving protein kinase C, raf, MEK, and mitogen-activated protein kinases (erk 1/2), that would ultimately lead to phosphorylation/activation of Elk-1. Experiments were performed to confirm the involvement of each part of the pathway. In terms of protein kinase C (PKC), our attention was focused on the βII isoform. While overexpression of constitutively active forms of PKC alpha, beta, and delta all induced expression of Egr-1, only expression of a plasmid-encoding dominant-negative PKC-βII had an inhibitory effect. Thus, once PKC isoforms are activated (by whatever mechanism), similar downstream targets may be recruited, but hypoxia exerts its specific effect at the level of selective activation of the βII isoform of PKC. Further support for the role of PKC-βII was obtained from translocation studies, demonstrating that hypoxia caused this isoform to become membrane-associated, and from autophosphorylation experiments.[31] However, the most compelling data implicating PKC-β was obtained using PKC-β null mice (since PKC-βI and βII are products of the same gene, they are both deleted in the PKC-β null mice).[33] When these mice were subjected to hypoxia (6% oxygen), they did not display vascular fibrin formation or tissue factor expression. Furthermore, hypoxia caused only a small increase in Egr-1 transcripts/antigen, compared with robust increases for each of these in wild-type controls subjected to oxygen deprivation.

Studies in PKC-β null mice shed further light on mechanisms linking activation of PKC-β to phosphorylation of Elk-1 and transcription of Egr-1. Activated PKC-βII phosphorylates raf, thereby activating this kinase. A role for raf activation in the pathway leading to Egr-1 transcription was shown by the inhibitory effect of transfecting a cultured macrophage line with an expression of plasmid-encoding dominant-negative raf.[33] Similar experiments were performed with respect to activation of mitogen-activated kinase erk 1/2. These studies established that MEK1/2 activated erk 1/2, and that these events were in the pathway that led to phosphorylation of Elk-1.

Hypothesis

These studies have established a novel pathway through which hypoxia triggers activation of PKC-βII and Egr-1, allowing them to recruit their cellular targets as part of the response to oxygen deprivation. Thus, the PKC-βII/Egr-1 pathway is likely to have profound effects on the expression of a range of genes. Aside from the setting of acute hypoxia and fibrin deposition, what type of pathophysiological settings might this pathway be involved in?

A logical extension of this work would be to determine if chronic hypoxia utilizes the PKC-βII/Egr-1 pathway for vascular remodeling. Pulmonary hypertension is associated with enhanced production of extracellular matrix components, including tenascin C.[34-36] Murine tenascin C has been shown to have functional Egr-1 sites in the promoter.[37] Matrix metalloproteinases are also involved in the vascular hypertrophy accompanying pulmonary hypertension.[34,36] Membrane type 1 metalloproteinase (MT1-MMP) has also been shown to have functional Egr-1 sites in the promoter.[38] Future studies will be required to see if these associations result in cause-effect relationships with Egr-1 and pulmonary vascular remodeling in chronic hypoxia.

With respect to Egr-1, this work contributes to an emerging paradigm in which rapid activation of this transcription factor is part of a vascular stress response.[39,40] Following mechanical injury to the vessel wall[40] or angioplasty,[41] rapid activation of Egr-1 has been observed. Administration of a DNA enzyme that cleaved Egr-1 mRNA prevented restenosis in a rat model of vascular damage. Egr-1 might also be relevant in more chronic settings, such as atherosclerosis and emphysema. A recent report has documented increased Egr-1 expression in cellular elements in the expanded intima of atherosclerotic plaques.[42] Furthermore, high levels of Egr-1 were also observed in emphysematous lung removed at the time of lung reduction surgery.[43] In the latter case, Egr-1 expression was observed in a wide range of cells, including vascular and bronchial smooth muscle, alveolar macrophages, and lung epithelium. The important future challenge in this area is to determine if the association of Egr-1 with a particular disorder contributes to the pathogenesis of organ dysfunction. In this context, Egr-1 null mice are particularly useful. For example, multiple previous studies have demonstrated an association of Egr-1 with ischemic episodes in the kidney and heart.[44-46] In preliminary studies, we have been able to confirm these results in a model of lung ischemia, and, using Egr-1 null mice, to identify cytokine/chemokine genes regulated by Egr-1 and to show a protective effect in the absence of Egr-1.[47]

Taken together, our results have led to the elucidation of an HIF-1-independent pathway that highlights a quite different aspect of the adaptive response to oxygen deprivation. Future studies will be required to determine beneficial/detrimental effects of the PKC-βII/Egr-1 pathway in hypoxia. However, it is possible that the activation of procoagulant mechanisms in hypoxemic lung is a primordial response in which ischemic tissue is walled off from normal tissue.

References

1. Michiels C, Arnould T, Knott I, et al. Stimulation of prostaglandin synthesis by human endothelial cells exposed to hypoxia. *Am J Physiol* 93;264: C866-C874.
2. Heacock C, Sutherland R. Induction characteristics of oxygen regulated proteins. *Int J Radiat Oncol Biol Phys* 1986;12:1287–1290.
3. Kuwabara K, Matsumoto M, Ikeda J, et al. Purification and characterization of a novel stress protein, the 150 kDa oxygen regulated protein (ORP150), from cultured rat astrocytes and its expression in ischemic gerbil brain. *J Biol Chem* 1996;271:5025–5032.
4. Ozawa K, Kuwabara K, Tamatani M, et al. ORP150 suppresses hypoxia-induced apoptotic cell death. *J Biol Chem* 1999;274:6397–6404.
5. Lee A. Mammalian stress responses: Induction of the glucose-regulated protein family. *Curr Opin Biol* 1992;4:267–273.
6. Roll D, Murphy B, Laderoute K, et al. Oxygen regulated 80 kDa protein and glucose regulated 78 kDa protein are identical. *Molec Cell Biochem* 1991;103:141- 148.
7. Bunn H, Poyton R. Oxygen sensing and molecular adaptation to hypoxia. *Physiol Revs* 1996;76:839–885.
8. Semenza G, Roth P, Fang H-M, Wang G. Transcriptional regulation of genes encoding glycolytic enzyme by HIF-1. *J Biol Chem* 1994;269:23757–23763.
9. Semenza G. Regulation of mammalian oxygen homeostasis by HIF-1. *Annu Rev Cell Dev Biol* 1999;15:551–578.
10. Semenza G. Perspectives on oxygen sensing. *Cell* 1999;98:281–284.
11. Shweiki D, Itin A, Soffer D, Keshet E. VEGF induced by hypoxia may mediate hypoxia-initiated angiogenesis. *Nature* 1992;359:843–845.
12. Forsythe J, Jiang B, Iyer N, et al. Activation of VEGF gene transcription by HIF- 1. *Molec Cell Biol* 1996;16:4604–4613.
13. Semenza G, Jiang B-H, Leung S, et al. Hypoxia response elements in the aldolase A, enolase 1, and lactate dehydrogenase A gene promoters contain essential binding sites for HIF-1. *J Biol Chem* 1996;271:32529–32537.
14. Firth J, Ebert B, Pugh C, Ratcliffe P. Oxygen regulated elements in the phosphoglycerate kinase-1 and lactate dehydrogenase A genes: Similarities with the erythropoietin 3' enhancer. *Proc Natl Acad Sci USA* 1994;91:6496–6500.
15. Ebert B, Firth J, Ratcliffe P. Hypoxia and mitochondrial inhibitors regulate expression of GLUT 1 via distinct cis-acting sequences. *J Biol Chem* 1995; 270:29083–29089.
16. Zhu H, Bunn HF. Oxygen sensing and signaling: Impact on the regulation of physiologically important genes. *Respir Physiol* 1999;115:239–247.
17. Hamer J, Malone P, Silver I. The pO_2 in venous valve pockets: Its possible bearing on thrombogenesis. *Br J Surg* 1981;68:166–170.
18. Malone P. The sequestration and margination of platelets and leukocytes in veins during conditions of hypokinetic and anemic hypoxia: Potential

significance in clinical postoperative venous thrombosis. *J Pathol* 1978;125: 119–129.

19. Lawson C, Yan S-D, Yan S-F, et al. Monocytes and tissue factor promote thrombosis in a murine model of oxygen deprivation. *J Clin Invest* 1997;99: 1729–1738.

20. Lahiri B, Koehn J, Canfield R, et al. Development of an immunoassay for the COOH-terminal region of the gamma chains of human fibrin. *Thromb Res* 1981;23:103–112.

21. Yan S-F, Zou Y-S, Gao Y, et al. Tissue factor transcription driven by Egr-1 is a critical mechanism of murine pulmonary fibrin deposition in hypoxia. *Proc Natl Acad Sci USA* 1998;95:8298–8303.

22. Cui M-Z, Parry G, Oeth P, et al. Transcriptional regulation of the tissue factor gene in human epithelial cells is mediated by Sp1 and Egr-1. *J Biol Chem* 1996;271:2731–2739.

23. Milbrandt J. A nerve growth factor induced gene encodes a possible transcriptional regulatory factor. *Science* 1988;238:797–799.

24. Gashler A, Sukhatme V. Egr-1: Prototype of a zinc finger family of transcription factors. *Prog Nucl Acids Res Molec Biol* 1995;50:191–224.

25. Krishnaraju K, Nguyen H, Liebermann D, Hoffman B. The zinc finger transcription factor Egr-1 potentiates macrophage differentiation of hematopoietic cells. *Molec Cell Biol* 1995;15:5499–5507.

26. Nguyen H, Hoffman-Liebermann B, Liebermann D. The zinc finger transcription factor Egr-1 is essential for and restricts differentiation along the macrophage cell lineage. *Cell* 1993;72:197–209.

27. Lee SL, Wang Y, Milbrandt J. Unimpaired macrophage differentiation and activation in mice lacking the zinc finger transcription factor NGFI-1 (Egr-1). *Molec Cell Biol* 1996;16:4566–4572.

28. Lee S, Sadovsky Y, Swirnoff A, et al. Luteinizing hormone deficiency and female infertility in mice lacking the transcription factor NGFI-A (Egr-1). *Science* 1996;273:1219–1221.

29. Svaren J, Sevetson B, Apel E, et al. NAB2, a corepressor of NGFI-A (Egr-1), and Krox20, is induced by proliferative and differentiative stimuli. *Molec Cell Biol* 1996;16:3545–3553.

30. Yan S-F, Lu J, Zou Y-S, et al. Pulmonary expression of early growth response- 1: Biphasic time course and effect of oxygen concentration. *J Appl Physiol* 2000;88:2303–2309.

31. Yan S-D, Lu J, Zou Y-S, et al. Hypoxia-associated induction of early growth response-1 gene expression. *J Biol Chem* 1999;274:15030–15040.

32. Wood SM, Gleadle J, Pugh C, et al. The role of ARNT in hypoxic induction of gene expression. *J Biol Chem* 1996;271:15117–15123.

33. Leitges M, Schmedt C, Guinamard R, et al. Immunodeficiency in protein kinase C- beta-deficient mice. *Science* 1996;273:788–791.

34. Jones P, Cowan K, Rabinovitch M. Tenascin-C, proliferation and subendothelial accumulation of fibronectin in progressive pulmonary vascular disease. *Am J Pathol* 1997;150:1349–1360.

35. Cowan K, Jones P, Rabinovitch M. Elastase and matrix metalloproteinase inhibitors induce regression, and tenascin-C antisense prevents progression, of vascular disease. *J Clin Invest* 2000;105:21–34.

36. Rabinovitch M. Diseases of the pulmonary vasculature. In Topol E (ed): *Comprehensive Cardiovascular Medicine.* Philadelphia, PA: Lippincott-Raven Publishers; 1998:3001–3029.

37. Copertino D, Edelman G, Jones F. Multiple promoter elements differen-

tially regulate the expression of the mouse tenascin gene. *Proc Natl Acad Sci USA* 1997;94:1846–1851.

38. Haas T, Stitelman D, Davis S, et al. Egr-1 mediates extracellular matrix-driven transcription of membrane type 1 matrix metalloproteinase in endothelium. *J Biol Chem* 1999;274:22679–22685.

39. Khachigian L, Collins T. Inducible expression of Egr-1-dependent genes: A paradigm of transcriptional activation in vascular endothelium. *Circ Res* 1997;81:457–461.

40. Khachigian L, Lindner V, Williams A, Collins T. Egr-1-induced endothelial gene expression: A common theme in vascular injury. *Science* 1996;271:1427–1431.

41. Santiago F, Lowe H, Kavurma M, et al. New DNA enzyme targeting Egr-1 mRNA inhibits vascular smooth muscle proliferation and regrowth after injury. *Nat Med* 1999;5:1264–1269.

42. McCaffrey T, Fu C, Du B, et al. High-level expression of Egr-1, and Egr-1-inducible genes, in mouse and human atherosclerosis. *J Clin Invest* 2000;105:653–662.

43. Zhang W, Yan S-D, Zhu A, et al. Expression of EGR-1 in late-stage emphysema. *Am J Pathol* 2000;157:1311–1320.

44. Brand T, Sharma H, Fleischmann K, et al. Proto-oncogene expression in porcine myocardium subjected to ischemia and reperfusion. *Circ Res* 1992;71:1351–1360.

45. Ouellette A, Malt R, Sukhatme V, Bonventre J. Expression of two "immediate early" genes, Egr-1 and c-fos, in response to renal ischemia and during compensatory renal hypertrophy in mice. *J Clin Invest* 1990;85:766–771.

46. Safirstein R, Price P, Saggi S, Harris R. Changes in gene expression after temporary renal ischemia. *Kidney Intl* 1990;37:1515–1521.

47. Yan S-F, Fujita T, Okada K, et al. Early growth response-1 is a master switch in the pathogenesis of ischemic stress. *Circulation*. In press.

Chapter 23

Long-Term Sequelae Following Pulmonary Thromboendarterectomy

William R. Auger, MD

Introduction

Pulmonary hypertension secondary to chronic thromboembolic involvement of the pulmonary vascular bed can lead to profound disability characterized by a progressive decline in functional capacity and exertional dyspnea. Although appreciated as a sequela of pulmonary embolic disease in the 1950s by Hollister and Cull,[1] the antemortem diagnosis of this disease was rare, and few, if any, therapeutic alternatives existed. The first planned surgical treatment for chronic pulmonary embolism was reported by Hurwitt et al.,[2] and although unsuccessful, they laid the foundation for the pursuit of a surgical remedy for this debilitating disorder. In 1961, the first successful pulmonary thromboendarterectomy (PTE) was performed.[3] With advances in diagnostic capabilities, surgical techniques, and postoperative management over the last 4 decades, what was once considered a uniformly fatal form of pulmonary hypertension can now be effectively treated. Following PTE surgery, it is possible for afflicted patients not only to experience restoration of normal pulmonary hemodynamics but also long-term survival, functional status, and quality of life can be substantially improved.

Perioperative Mortality and Long-Term Survival

Early reports of the surgical treatment for chronic thromboembolic pulmonary hypertension (CTEPH) suggested that while removal of

From: Weir EK, Reeve HL, Reeves JT (eds). *Interactions of Blood and the Pulmonary Circulation*. Armonk, NY: Futura Publishing Company, Inc.; ©2002.

chronic thromboembolic material from the proximal pulmonary vascular bed was surgically feasible and frequently successful in restoring favorable pulmonary hemodynamics, the mortal risk of the procedure was extremely high. Chitwood and colleagues,[4] in a review of the world's experience in 85 patients having undergone PTE surgery between 1960 and 1983, reported a combined mortality rate of 22%. At one center included in their review, perioperative mortality was as high as 40%. However, despite these discouraging figures, progress in the surgical approach to these patients was sustained primarily because medical therapies were ineffective, the potential for substantial improvement in hemodynamic and functional status with surgery was well documented, and survival in untreated patients was extremely poor. In patients with documented thromboembolic disease who presented with pulmonary hypertension, Riedel and colleagues demonstrated a relationship between survival and the degree of pulmonary hypertension at initial evaluation.[5] Patients with a mean pulmonary artery pressure between 31 and 40 mm Hg experienced a 50% survival rate over a 10-year follow-up period. At an initial mean pulmonary artery pressure of 41–50 mm Hg, survival rates declined to 20% over 10 years, and to 5% if the mean pulmonary artery pressure was greater than 50 mm Hg. Furthermore, the 2-year survival rate in this latter group was only 20% (Figure 1). These data are in sharp contrast to the

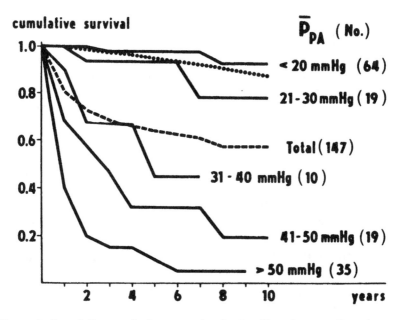

Figure 1. Cumulative survival curves of patients with pulmonary thromboembolism according to initial mean PA pressures. Reprinted with permission from Reidel M, et al.[5]

survival rate of patients following PTE surgery (Figure 2). In a long-term outcome study conducted by Archibald et al.,[6] 532 post-PTE patients exhibited a 75% probability of survival beyond 6 years. Although the majority of post-hospital deaths in this group were not related to pulmonary vascular disorders, persistent pulmonary hypertension or recurrent pulmonary emboli occurred in 22 of the 51 patients who died.

Since 1990, several centers from around the world have reported a growing experience with the surgical approach to patients with CTEPH. Mortality figures, however, continue to vary considerably among centers (Table 1).[7,8,16,17] Although speculative, it is reasonable to suggest that patient selection, as well as the surgical and postoperative management experience of the center, impact mortality figures. In the 30-year history of performing PTE surgeries at the University of California, San Diego, there has been a trend toward lower perioperative mortality rates.[18] Between 1970 and 1983, the 17 patients undergoing PTE surgery at UCSD had a 17.6% in-hospital mortality rate. From January 1984 to November 1989, the mortality rate of 171 operated patients was 15.2%. With the current care providers in the PTE program, between the end of 1989 and 1992, 7.2% of 207 operated patients died; since 1993, in 875 patients, the mortality rate has declined to 6.6%.

Factors affecting perioperative mortality have not been completely

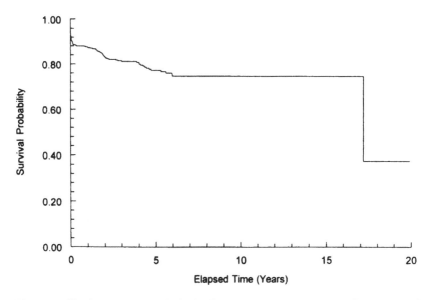

Figure 2. Kaplan-Meier survival plot in post-PTE patients; time from date of surgery until time of death or last follow-up. Reprinted with permission from Archibald CJ, et al.[6]

Table 1

PTE Surgery: Perioperative Mortality Rates, 1990–2000

	No. of Patients	Mortality %
Jault et al.,[7] France, 1990	33	20
Daily/Moser,[8] San Diego CA, 1990	149	11.4
Jamieson/Moser,[9] San Diego CA, 1993	150	8.7
Simmoneau et al.,[10] France 1995	11	18
Hartz et al.,[11] Chicago IL, 1996	34	23
Mayer et al.,[12] Germany, 1996	119	24
Mayer et al.,[13] Germany, 1997	32	9.3
Nakajima et al.,[14] Japan, 1997	30	13.3
Gilbert et al.,[15] Baltimore, MD, 1998	17	23.5
Miller et al.,[16] Philadelphia, PA, 1998	25	24
UCSD (unpublished data), 1999	1181	8.4
Cerveri et al.,[17] Pavia, Italy, 2000	34	8.8

defined. Moser and colleagues[19] listed several factors which appeared to impact the chance of survival postoperatively: New York Heart Association functional class IV status preoperatively, age older than 70 years, marked obesity, the presence of significant comorbid diseases, the severity of the preoperative pulmonary vascular resistance, the presence of right ventricular failure, as manifested by high right atrial pressures, and "perhaps" the duration of pulmonary hypertension. More recently, Hartz et al.[11] found that a preoperative pulmonary vascular resistance greater than 1100 dynes/s/cm^{-5} and mean pulmonary artery pressure greater than 50 mm Hg predicted a higher likelihood of operative mortality. Gilbert et al.[15] reported an increased operative risk for obese patients. A prolonged cardiopulmonary bypass time and failure to achieve at least a 50% reduction in pulmonary vascular resistance following PTE surgery was found by Daily and colleagues to predict in-hospital death.[20]

Given the complexities of the surgical procedure and postoperative care, the attributable causes of death following PTE surgery vary considerably. Cardiac arrest, cerebrovascular accidents, myocardial injury, uncontrollable postoperative mediastinal bleeding, sepsis syndrome, and multiorgan failure are listed in several reports.[11,21,22] However, persistent pulmonary hypertension postendarterectomy with resulting right ventricular failure and acute reperfusion lung injury represent the major causes of death after this operation. With the UCSD experience, between January 1984 and November 1995, one or both of these devastating clinical problems postoperatively accounted for 54.2% of the reported deaths in 651 patients.[18]

Pulmonary Hemodynamic Outcome Following PTE

For the majority of patients undergoing a pulmonary thromboendarterectomy, the surgical removal of the chronic thromboembolic residua from the proximal pulmonary vascular bed results in a significant decline in mean pulmonary arterial pressure, accompanied by an augmentation in cardiac output. As blood flow is restored to previously occluded lung regions, the decline in right ventricular afterload generally occurs immediately following the endarterectomy, the surgeon often noting an improvement in right ventricular contractility and a reduction in heart size even prior to chest closure. This immediate hemodynamic response has been reported by several groups.[9,11,13,14,23] Representative data available from UCSD is presented in Table 2.[24]

The sustainment of the hemodynamic result over the years following surgery has been similarly gratifying. Follow-up right heart catheterization was obtained 6 to 24 months after PTE surgery in 47 of the first 150 operated patients at UCSD.[23] The results are presented in Table 3. Mayer and colleagues[12] documented equally impressive results in 65 post-PTE patients reassessed 13–48 months (mean 27 months) after surgery. Mean pulmonary artery pressure at follow-up was significantly reduced when compared to pre- and postoperative values (preoperative 49 ± 19 mm Hg, postoperative 31 ± 8 mm Hg, follow-up 23 ± 10 mm Hg). Although not statistically significant compared with immediate postoperative values (cardiac index 2.6 ± 0.5 L/min/m²), the follow-up cardiac index in this group (2.9 ± 0.5 L/min/m²) achieved significance over preoperative (2.0 ± 0.7 L/min/m²) values. And finally, mean pulmonary vascular resistance was significantly reduced (198 ± 72 dynes/sec/cm⁻⁵) compared

---

Table 2

Preoperative and Postoperative Pulmonary
Hemodynamics in 457 Patients Undergoing
PTE Surgery at UCSD Between 1994 to 1997

	Preoperative	Postoperative
PA mean pressure (mm Hg)	47.9 ± 13.1	28.1 ± 9.6*
PA systolic pressure (mm Hg)	79.3 ± 21.4	46.2 ± 16.2*
Cardiac output (L/min)	3.92 ± 1.30	5.66 ± 1.51*
PVR (dynes/sec/cm⁻⁵)	877 ± 452	267 ± 192*

PA = pulmonary artery; PVR = pulmonary vascular resistance.
*$P<.0001$.

Reprinted with permission from Archibald CJ, Auger WR, Fedullo PF. Outcome after pulmonary thromboendarterectomy. *Semin Thorac Cardiovasc Surg* 1999;11(2):164–171.

Table 3

Pulmonary Hemodynamics Obtained in 47 Patients,
6 to 24 Months After PTE Surgery

	Preoperative	Postoperative	Follow-Up
PA mean pressure (mm Hg)	48 ± 12	27 ± 8*	24 ± 10
PA systolic pressure (mm Hg)	80 ± 21	44 ± 15*	39 ± 17**
Cardiac output (L/min)	3.7 ± 1.2	6.0 ± 1.1*	4.8 ± 1.0***
PVR (dynes/sec/cm⁻⁵)	971 ± 551	232 ± 111*	282 ± 251

PA = pulmonary artery; PVR = pulmonary vascular resistance.
*$P<$.001 vs. preoperative value.
**$P<$.0015 vs. postoperative value.
***$P<$.0001 vs. postoperative value.
Reprinted with permission from Moser KM, Auger WR, Fedullo PF, et al. Chronic thromboembolic pulmonary hypertension: Clinical picture and surgical treatment. *Eur Respir J* 1992;5:334–342.

with preoperative (1015 ± 454 dynes/sec/cm⁻⁵) and immediate postoperative (322 ± 154 dynes/sec/cm⁻⁵) values. Included in this group were 3 patients exhibiting a modest increase in pulmonary vascular resistance between postoperative and follow-up measurements.

Although it was once thought that prolonged exposure to high pulmonary artery pressures would cause irreversible damage to the right ventricle, several clinical studies of CTEPH patients have refuted these concerns. Obtaining right ventricular endomyocardial biopsies at the time of surgery, Bradley and colleagues[25] demonstrated normal myocardium (5%), myocyte hypertrophy only (80%), and mild focal fibrosis in addition to hypertrophy (12.5%) in 40 PTE patients biopsied. The mean duration of cardiopulmonary symptoms in this group of patients was 4.8 ± 5.2 years, consistent with the presence of longstanding pulmonary hypertension. This study showed that despite this duration of significant right ventricular afterload, clinically important right ventricular fibrosis or end-stage unrecoverable heart disease was not observed. Further evidence for resiliency of the right ventricle following adequate reduction in right ventricular afterload with a successful endarterectomy is found in echocardiographic studies of right heart geometric changes following surgery. Performing 2-dimensional echocardiography 8 ± 8 days before and 6 ± 4 days after PTE surgery in 30 patients, Dittrich and colleagues[26] reported a significant decrease in end-diastolic right ventricular size postoperatively, accompanied by a more normal position of the interventricular septum, a moderate increase in left ventricular end-diastolic size, a reduction in right atrial size, and reduction in the dimension of the inferior vena cava (Figure 3). Menzel et al.[27] re-

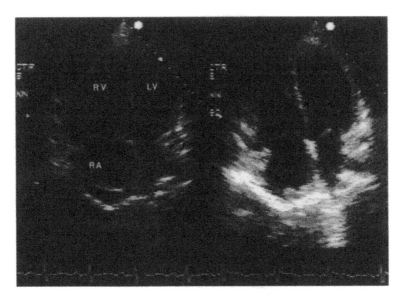

Figure 3. Apical 4-chamber echocardiograms in CTEPH patients before (left) and 7 days after (right) PTE surgery. Preoperative pulmonary vascular resistance (PVR) was 1080 dynes/sec/cm^{-5}; postoperative PVR was 226 dynes/sec/cm^{-5}. Substantial reduction in right heart chamber size is noted. Reprinted with permission from Dittrich HC, et al.[26]

ported similar findings in 14 PTE patients 18 ± 12 days following surgery. Further improvement in right heart dimensions at long-term follow-up has been documented by Mayer et al.[12] At a mean follow-up period of 27 months, end-diastolic right ventricular area (cm^2) decreased from 33.8 ± 8.5 preoperatively to 26.1 ± 5.8 immediately postoperatively and to 21.5 ± 5.1 at follow-up. The corresponding values for end-systolic right ventricular area (cm^2) were 29.9 ± 7.4 preoperatively, 23.2 ± 5.9 postoperatively, and 14.7 ± 4.3 at follow-up. This was accompanied by normal interventricular septal position in 52 of 65 patients studied. This study is a testimony to the lasting improvement in right heart function and the reversal of right ventricular hypertrophy following long-term reduction in right ventricular afterload.

Although the improvement in pulmonary hemodynamics following endarterectomy can be readily understood, the vascular changes occurring after surgery are more difficult to explain. Postoperative perfusion lung scans commonly show what has been termed "pulmonary vascular steal," i.e., a redistribution of blood flow away from the previously perfused segments into the newly endarterectomized lung regions. Olman et al.[28] have suggested that this may be secondary to a development of varied vascular resistances in the pulmonary vessels following endarterectomy . . . a "low resistance" area in the endarterectomized

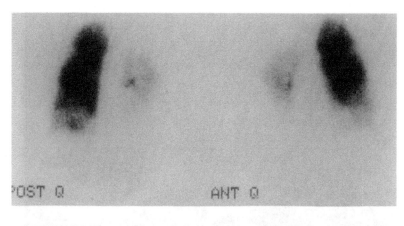

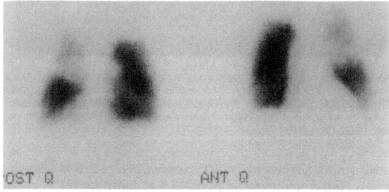

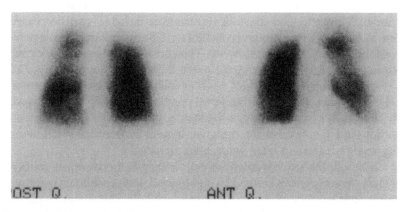

Figure 4A. Upper panel: Preoperative perfusion lung scan showing lobar/segmental defects, (L) lung, and segmental defects (R) lower lobe. Middle panel: Postoperative lung scan demonstrating redistribution of blood flow from previously perfused lung regions into newly endarterectomized lung segments. Lower panel: Follow-up scan 5 months postendarterectomy showing improvement in perfusion to "vascular steal" regions. Reprinted with permission from Archibald CJ, et al.[24]

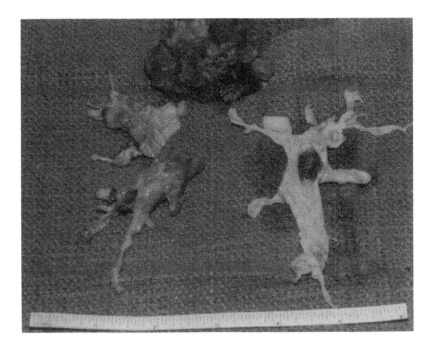

Figure 4B. Chronic thromboembolic material removed at surgery in patient whose lung scans are depicted in Figure 4A.

lung region and a "high resistance" area in the lung region that was not involved with chronic thromboembolic residua. This may be a reasonable postulate since Moser and Bloor[29] have described the development of small vessel changes, indistinguishable from those seen in primary pulmonary hypertension, in the nonoccluded vascular bed of CTEPH patients. However, a disturbance in vasomotor tone post-PTE cannot be discounted as an alternative explanation. Furthermore, in a long-term follow-up study, Moser and colleagues[30] show that this redistribution in pulmonary perfusion improves in most patients (Figure 4 A, B). It was suggested that "remodeling" of the small vessel changes may account for this improvement, which is manifested as a more homogeneous perfusion pattern by lung scan over time.

Functional Status and Quality of Life Following Surgery

Although several groups experienced in the care of patients with CTEPH have demonstrated sustained improvement in pulmonary hemodynamics after PTE surgery,[10,12,23] limited information is available on the long-term effects of this operation on functional status and quality of life. In a group of 9 patients, Rich and colleagues[31] measured quality of life at a mean of 14.3 months following PTE surgery. They demonstrated that fewer cardiopulmonary symptoms and improved functional status was experienced by these individuals as compared to patients with end-stage cardiac disease. Other investigators have reported postoperative improvement in New York Heart Association (NYHA) functional class, which appears to be maintained over time in the majority of patients[12,23,32] (Table 4).

In a large cross-sectional study, Archibald and coworkers[6] examined the functional status and quality of life in a cohort of 308 patients having undergone PTE surgery between 1970 and 1994. Three self-administered questionnaires were distributed by mail: (1) a PTE Follow-up Questionnaire addressing NYHA class status, prevalence of cardiopulmonary symptoms, walking distance, stair climbing ability, work status, and health care utilization; (2) the UCSD Shortness of Breath Questionnaire,[33] which rates severity of dyspnea during 23 activities of daily living; and (3) the Rand 36-Item Health Survey (SF-36),[34] which assesses information related to quality-of-life issues (physical function, role limitations due to physical function, emotional well-being, role limitations due to emotional problems, bodily pain, social function, energy/fatigue, and general health). The respondents consisted of 181 men and 127 women, with a mean age of 56.2 years at the time of survey, and an average of 3.3 years (median 2.3 years, range 1–16 years) following PTE surgery.

The majority of patients, or 93% of the 306 respondents, identified themselves as NYHA Class I or II functional status. Furthermore, most patients (63% of 303 answering the survey) reported no dyspnea walking on a level surface, or they only sometimes (25% of those surveyed)

Table 4

NYHA Functional Status of 65 Long-Term Survivors Following PTE Surgery

Class	Preoperative	Follow-Up*
IV	24	0
III	38	3
II	3	16
I	0	46

*13 to 48 months preoperatively (mean, 27 months).

Adapted and reprinted with permission from Mayer E, Dohm M, Hoke U, et al. Mid-term results of pulmonary thromboendarterectomy for chronic thromboembolic pulmonary hypertension. *Ann Thorac Surg* 1996;61:1788–1792.

experienced shortness of breath with this activity. In response to the PTE Follow-up Questionnaire, when asked to rate their shortness of breath since surgery, 73.2% of patients reported their dyspnea to be "much improved," 22.9% were "improved," 2.6% "about the same," and <1% were "worse." Consistent with these responses, the majority of patients noted considerable walking and stair climbing capabilities: 56 of 306 patients claimed they could walk "indefinitely," with a median distance of 10 city blocks (5,280 feet) reported by the remaining 250 patients; only 8 patients reported an ability to ambulate 60 feet or less.

The PTE Follow-up Questionnaire also addressed the issue of supplemental oxygen use postoperatively. Of the 275 respondents, 89.6% were no longer using oxygen supplementation, with the mean duration of oxygen use post-PTE of 7.1 weeks (range 1–64 weeks). This improvement in oxygenation status postoperatively has also been demonstrated by other groups[35,36] and is felt to reflect resolution of the post-sternotomy restrictive impairment and postoperative ventilation-perfusion maldistribution.

One of the most notable results of this cross-sectional study was evaluation of employment status after surgery. One hundred thirty-three patients, or 43.3% of the surveyed group, returned to work after their PTE. Although 51 of these individuals were employed prior to the operation, 82 patients were able to resume gainful employment. Furthermore, 35 patients (11.4%) were able to perform volunteer work, and 100 patients (32.6%) reported the renewed ability to do housework. Unfortunately, 63 patients, or 20.5% of the respondents, were disabled prior to surgery and remained disabled.

The assessment of quality-of-life issues with the Rand Survey was similarly encouraging as to the potential benefits of a thromboendarterectomy. The patients' impression of their overall health status postoperatively revealed that 53 of 298 respondents felt that they were in "excellent health," 92 patients (31%) reported "very good health," 102 (34%) reported "good health," 39 (13%) felt their health status was "fair," and 7 (2%) reported "poor health." In comparing each of the 8 health concepts with normals and a cohort of pre-PTE patients,[37] the post-PTE patient groups scored higher in every category relative to the preoperative patients. When compared to normal mean scores, the post-PTE patients scored significantly lower in 4 of the categories (physical function, role limits due to physical function, general health, and emotional well-being), with similar scores in social function and role limits due to emotional problems. Of note were the higher scores recorded for post-PTE patients for energy/fatigue and the reports of less bodily pain.

Archibald and coworkers also attempted to address health care utilization following surgery.[6] Patients were asked about the number of hospitalizations and emergency visits since their PTE that could be attributed to residual CTEPH postoperatively or to the treatment of the patients' CTEPH (such as complications of anticoagulation). These investigators demonstrated that for the patients surveyed, 83.4% (256 patients) reported no disease-related hospitalizations, with the number of hospitalizations for the time since surgery (range 1–16 years) averaging only 0.13 ± 0.48 per year (range 0–6.17, 78 hospitalizations for 51 patients). Similarly, the number of disease-related, emergency-related visits for the time since surgery averaged 0.07 ± 0.23 visits per year (range 0–2.49, 44 visits for 17 patients). An extension of these observations comes in a prospective study conducted by the same investigators. In a group of 56 PTE patients operated at UCSD, the number of disease-related hospitalizations (1.86 vs. 0.93 per year), days hospitalized (14.1 vs. 6.89 per year), and emergency visits (1.26 vs. 0.26 per year) significantly decreased in the first year postoperatively compared to preoperative utilization of health resources.[37] This beneficial effect of PTE surgery was sustained in a similar cohort of 25 patients over a 4-year postoperative period.[32]

Future Challenges

The majority of CTEPH patients who undergo a pulmonary thromboendarterectomy experience a remarkable reversal of fate. With a postsurgical decrement in pulmonary arterial pressures and improvement in right heart function, a patient's sense of well-being, functional status, and quality of life can be restored. However, this outcome is not seen in every CTEPH patient. An estimated 10–15% of operated patients are left with a degree of pulmonary hypertension that continues to functionally limit them. One may speculate that the incidence of persistent pulmonary hypertension postoperatively may be reduced if improved diagnostic capabilities or historical clues could differentiate patients with primarily large vessel chronic thromboembolic disease from those with extensive small vessel arteriopathy. More effort is required to recognize CTEPH earlier in its course and, as a result, potentially limit the extent of the secondary small vessel changes that appears to occur in the unobstructed vascular bed. This may be the most effective strategy in decreasing the incidence of persistent pulmonary hypertension postendarterectomy and, as a consequence, may decrease the mortality and morbidity associated with this problem. For these same reasons, further investigative efforts need to be directed toward understanding the pathophysiology of reperfusion lung injury with the intent of developing effective therapeutic strategies for preventing and treating this devastating condition. For those patients with persistent pulmonary hypertension following PTE surgery, the optimal therapeutic approach is yet to be defined. Long-term pulmonary vasodilator therapy, such as continuous intravenous prostacyclin, remains an option but requires careful and controlled investigation. And although recurrence of CTEPH is seen in approximately 1% of operated patients,[38] those at risk, prevention strategies, and results of reoperation require ongoing analysis. And finally, well-designed, prospective outcome research in this patient population remains critical in understanding the "natural history" of this disease following surgery. Only with this approach will the long-term benefits of this unique operation be best defined.

References

1. Hollister LE, Cull VL. The syndrome of chronic thrombosis of the major pulmonary arteries. *Am J Med* 1956;21:312–320.
2. Hurwitt ES, Schein CJ, Rifkin J, et al. A surgical approach to the problem of chronic pulmonary artery obstruction due to thrombosis or stenosis. *Ann Surg* 1958;177:157–165.
3. Snyder WA, Kent DC, Baisch BF. Successful endarterectomy of chronically occluded pulmonary artery: Clinical report and physiologic studies. *J Thorac Cardiovasc Surg* 1963;45:482–489.
4. Chitwood WR, Sabiston DC, Wechsler AS. Surgical treatment of chronic unresolved pulmonary embolism. *Clin Chest Med* 1984;5:507–536.
5. Riedel M, Stanek V, Widimsky J, et al. Long-term follow-up of patients with pulmonary thromboembolism: Late prognosis and evaluation of hemodynamic and respiratory data. *Chest* 1982;81:151–158.
6. Archibald CJ, Auger WR, Fedullo PF, et al. Long-term outcome after pulmonary thromboendarterectomy. *Am J Respir Care Med* 1999;160:523–528.
7. Jault F, Cabrol C, Gandjbakhch I, et al. Results of thromboendarterectomy of chronic pulmonary embolism. *Arch Mal Coeur Vaiss* 1990;83:205–208.
8. Daily PO, Dembitsky WP, Iversen S, et al. Current early results of pulmonary thromboendarterectomy for chronic pulmonary embolism. *Eur J Cardiothorac Surg* 1990;4:117–123.
9. Jamieson SW, Auger WR, Fedullo PF, et al. Experience and results with 150 pulmonary thromboendarterectomy operations over a 29-month period. *J Thorac Cardiovasc Surg* 1993;106:116–127.
10. Simonneau G, Azarian R, Brenot F, et al. Surgical management of unresolved pulmonary embolism: A personal series of 72 patients. *Chest* 1995; 107:52S–55S.
11. Hartz RS, Byrne JG, Levitski S, et al. Predictors of mortality in pulmonary thromboendarterectomy. *Ann Thorac Surg* 1996;62:1255–1259.
12. Mayer E, Dahm M, Hake U, et al. Mid-term results of pulmonary thromboendarterectomy for chronic thromboembolic pulmonary hypertension. *Ann Thorac Surg* 1996;61:1788–1792.
13. Mayer E, Kramm T, Dahm M, et al. Early results of pulmonary thromboendarterectomy in chronic thromboembolic pulmonary hypertension. *Z Kardiol* 1997;86:920–927.
14. Nakajima H, Masuda M, Mogi K. The surgical treatment for chronic pulmonary thromboembolism: Our experience and current review of the literature. *Ann Thorac Cardiovasc Surg* 1997;3(1):15–21.
15. Gilbert TB, Gaine SP, Rubin LJ, et al. Short-term outcome and predictors

of adverse events following pulmonary thromboendarterectomy. *World J Surg* 1998;22:1029–1032.

16. Miller WT Jr, Osiason AW, Langlotz CP, et al. Reperfusion edema after thromboendarterectomy: Radiographic patterns of disease. *J Thorac Imaging* 1998;13:178–183.

17. Cerveri I, Corsico A, Fulgoni P, et al. Monitoring of cardiopulmonary function in patients after thromboendarterectomy for chronic thromboembolic pulmonary hypertension. (CTPH). *Am J Resp Crit Care Med* 2000; 161(3):A637.

18. Auger WR, Fedullo PF, Moser KM, et al. In-hospital mortality has decreased for patients undergoing pulmonary thromboendarterectomy. *Am J Resp Crit Care Med* 1996;153:A92 (abstract).

19. Moser KM, Auger WR, Fedullo PF. Chronic major vessel thromboembolic pulmonary hypertension. *Circulation* 1990;81:1735–1743.

20. Daily PO, Dembitsky WP, Iverson S, et al. Risk factors for pulmonary thromboendarterectomy. *J Thorac Cardiovasc Surg* 1990;99:670–680.

21. Moser KM, Daily PO, Peterson KL, et al. Thromboendarterectomy for chronic, major vessel thromboembolic pulmonary hypertension: Immediate and long-term results in 42 patients. *Ann Intern Med* 1987;107:560–565.

22. Fedullo PF, Auger WR, Channick RN, et al. Chronic thromboembolic pulmonary hypertension. *Clin Chest Med* 1995;16:353–374.

23. Moser KM, Auger WR, Fedullo PF, et al. Chronic thromboembolic pulmonary hypertension: Clinical picture and surgical treatment. *Eur Respir J* 1992;5:334–342.

24. Archibald CJ, Auger WR, Fedullo PF. Outcome after pulmonary thromboendarterectomy. *Sem Thorac Cardiovasc Surg* 1999;11(2):164–171.

25. Bradley SP, Auger WR, Moser KM, et al. Right ventricular pathology in chronic pulmonary hypertension. *Am J Card* 1996;78:584–587.

26. Dittrich HC, Nicod PH, Chow LC, et al. Early changes of right heart geometry after pulmonary thromboendarterectomy. *J Am Coll Cardiol* 1988;11: 937–943.

27. Menzel T, Wagner S, Mohr-Kahaly S, et al. Reversibility of changes in left and right ventricular geometry and hemodynamics in pulmonary hypertension: Echocardiographic characteristics before and after pulmonary thromboendarterectomy. *Z Kardiol* 1997;86(11):928–935.

28. Olman MA, Auger WR, Fedullo PF, et al. Pulmonary vascular steal in chronic thromboembolic pulmonary hypertension. *Chest* 1990;98:1430–1434.

29. Moser KM, Bloor CM. Pulmonary vascular lesions occurring in patients with chronic major vessel thromboembolic pulmonary hypertension. *Chest* 1993;103:685–692.

30. Moser KM, Metersky ML, Auger WR, et al. Resolution of vascular steal after pulmonary thromboendarterectomy. *Chest* 1993;104:1441–1444.

31. Rich M, Riegel B, Goeka I, et al. Quality of life after thromboendarterectomy. Presented at the Sixth Annual Conference, Nursing Research: Making It Part of Your Practice. San Diego, CA, February 21, 1992.

32. Archibald CJ, Auger WR, Fedullo PF, et al. Prospective four-year follow-up after pulmonary thromboendarterectomy: Functional status and health care utilization. *Am J Resp Crit Care Med* 1999;159:A456

33. Eakin EG, Prewitt LM, Ries AL, et al. Validation of the UCSD Shortness of Breath Questionnaire. *J Cardiopulm Rehab* 1998;113:619–624.

34. Ware JE Jr, Sherbourne CD. A 36-item short-form health survey (SF-36): Results from the Medical Outcomes Study. *Med Care* 1992;30:467–472.

35. Tanabe N, Okada O, Nakagawa Y, et al. The efficacy of pulmonary thromboendarterectomy on long-term gas exchange. *Eur Respir J* 1997;10:2066–2072.
36. Kapitan KS, Clausen JL, Moser KM. Gas exchange in chronic thromboembolism after pulmonary thromboendarterectomy. *Chest* 1990;98:14–19.
37. Archibald CJ, Auger WR, Fedullo PF, et al. Prospective analysis of functional status and quality of life after pulmonary thromboendarterectomy. *Am J Resp Crit Care Med* 1998;157:A587.
38. Mo M, Kapalanski DP, Mitruka SM, et al. Reoperative pulmonary thromboendarterectomy. *Ann Thorac Surg* 1999;68:1770–1777.

Index

Printed and bound by CPI Group (UK) Ltd, Croydon, CR0 4YY

16/04/2025

14658822-0004